AF614755

METHODS IN MOLECULAR BIOLOGY™

Series Editor
John M. Walker
School of Life Sciences
University of Hertfordshire
Hatfield, Hertfordshire, AL10 9AB, UK

For other titles published in this series, go to
www.springer.com/series/7651

Photodynamic Therapy

Methods and Protocols

Edited by

Charles J. Gomer

University of Southern California and Children's Hospital Los Angeles, Los Angeles, CA, USA

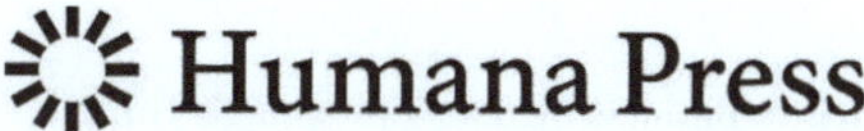

Editor
Charles J. Gomer
University of Southern California
Keck School of Medicine
Children's Hospital
Los Angeles
4650 Sunset Blvd.
Los Angeles CA 90027
USA
cgomer@chla.usc.edu

ISSN 1064-3745 e-ISSN 1940-6029
ISBN 978-1-60761-696-2 e-ISBN 978-1-60761-697-9
DOI 10.1007/978-1-60761-697-9
Springer New York Dordrecht Heidelberg London

Library of Congress Control Number: 2010921916

Printed on acid-free paper

Humana Press is part of Springer Science+Business Media (www.springer.com)

Preface

Biological interactions of visible light with photosensitizers have been studied for over a century while controlled clinical applications of light and photosensitizers to treat solid tumors (photodynamic therapy) have been evolving since the mid-1970s. There are hundreds of excellent publications describing basic, preclinical, and clinical applications of PDT for both malignant and non-malignant disorders. However, I believe this book provides the first comprehensive description of methods and protocols specifically related to relevant mechanistic, dosimetric, preclinical, and clinical procedures used in current PDT research.

Thinking "outside the box" is a cliché that seems to garner too much play these days in areas of biomedical science. However, back in the early 1970s, Tom Dougherty, working at Roswell Park, exhibited true out-of-the-box scientific thinking along with a naive determination that successfully brought a totally new therapeutic procedure to the clinic. Tom provides a very interesting and enjoyable history in the introductory chapter of the book on exactly how PDT got its start in his laboratory at Roswell Park. As Tom's first graduate student, I was fortunate to be working in his laboratory during that exciting time period.

During those early days of PDT-directed research, it was assumed that when cells were exposed to a photosensitizer, porphyrin derivatives being among the most often used, and visible light, that photochemically generated reactive oxygen species killed these cells by simply damaging cell membranes and/or vital subcellular structures. This certainly plays a role in PDT-mediated cell kill, but as is clearly observed and described in this book, numerous signal transduction and cell death pathways are also involved. The in vivo situation is even more complex. A growing number of studies are demonstrating that immunological, tumor microenvironmental, and vascular responses are all contributing to PDT treatment outcomes. Photophysical methods to monitor treatment responses are now providing real-time analysis of PDT doses and PDT efficacy. Finally, effective clinical trials remain the primary long-term objective of all PDT research. A variety of PDT applications for both malignant and non-malignant diseases and disorders are now showing promise. The goal of this book is to provide the reader with current and useful protocols that can be used to evaluate mechanisms and applications of PDT. Leading PDT scientists and clinicians have contributed to this book by providing chapters with clear roadmaps, methodologies, and suggestions that should prove beneficial to new investigators just starting out in PDT research as well as seasoned investigators changing the direction of their research.

I would like to thank all of the contributors of this book for their efforts, enthusiasm, and patience. I also want to thank John Walker, Series Editor, for his consistent encouragement and assistance.

Charles J. Gomer

Contents

Contributors

PATRIZIA AGOSTINIS • *Department of Molecular and Cell Biology, Catholic University of Leuven, Leuven, Belgium*

OMAR ALQAWI • *Department of Pathology and Molecular Medicine, McMaster University, Hamilton, ON, Canada*

KRISTIAN BERG • *Department of Radiation Biology, Institute for Cancer Research, The Norwegian Radium Hospital, Montebello, Oslo, Norway*

MERRILL A. BIEL • *Virginia Piper Cancer Institute, Minneapolis, MN; Department of Otolaryngology, Surgery and Family Practice, University of Minnesota, Minneapolis, MN, USA*

ANETTE BONSTED • *Department of Radiation Biology, Institute for Cancer Research, The Norwegian Radium Hospital, Montebello, Oslo, Norway*

SÉBASTIEN BONTEMS • *Laboratory of Virology and Immunology, GIGA-R, B34 +2, CHU, Liege, Belgium*

THERESA M. BUSCH • *Department of Radiation Oncology, School of Medicine, University of Pennsylvania, Philadelphia, PA, USA*

YIHUI CHEN • *PDT Center, Cell Stress Biology, Roswell Park Cancer Institute, Buffalo, NY; Department of Nuclear Chemistry, SUNY, Buffalo, NY, USA*

ISABELLE COUPIENNE • *Laboratory of Virology and Immunology, GIGA-R, B34 +2, CHU, Liege, Belgium*

TIANHONG DAI • *Wellman Center for Photomedicine, Massachusetts General Hospital, Boston, MA; Department of Dermatology, Harvard Medical School, Boston, MA, USA*

SCOTT C. DAVIS • *Thayer School of Engineering, Dartmouth College, Hanover, NH, USA*

MICHAEL DEWAELE • *Department of Molecular and Cell Biology, Catholic University of Leuven, Leuven, Belgium*

THOMAS J. DOUGHERTY • *Roswell Park Cancer Institute, Buffalo, NY, USA*

MYRNA ESPIRITU • *Department of Pathology and Molecular Medicine, McMaster University, Hamilton, ON, Canada*

ANGELA FERRARIO • *The Saban Research Institute, Children's Hospital Los Angeles, University of Southern California, Los Angeles, CA, USA*

SUMMER L. GIBBS-STRAUSS • *Thayer School of Engineering, Dartmouth College, Hanover, NH, USA*

CHARLES J. GOMER • *Departments of Pediatrics and Radiation Oncology, Keck School of Medicine, The Saban Research Institute, Children's Hospital Los Angeles, University of Southern California, Los Angeles, CA, USA*

MICHAEL R. HAMBLIN • *Wellman Center for Photomedicine, Massachusetts General Hospital, Boston, MA; Department of Dermatology, Harvard Medical School, Boston, MA; Harvard-MIT Division of Health Sciences and Technology, Cambridge, MA, USA*

ANDERS HØGSET • *PCI Biotech AS, Oslo, Norway*

LIYI HUANG • *Wellman Center for Photomedicine, Massachusetts General Hospital, Boston, MA; Department of Dermatology, Harvard Medical School, Boston, MA, USA; Department of Infectious Diseases, First Affiliated College & Hospital, Guangxi Medical University, Nanning, China*

NADINE S. JAMES • *PDT Center, Cell Stress Biology, Roswell Park Cancer Institute, Buffalo, NY, USA*

PETRAS JUZENAS • *Department of Radiation Biology, Institute for Cancer Research, The Norwegian Radium Hospital, Montebello, Oslo, Norway*

ASTA JUZENIENE • *Department of Radiation Biology, Institute for Cancer Research, The Norwegian Radium Hospital, Montebello, Oslo, Norway*

DAVID KESSEL • *Wayne State University School of Medicine, Detroit, MI, USA*

MLADEN KORBELIK • *B.C. Cancer Agency, Vancouver, BC, Canada*

HERWIG KOSTRON • *Department of Neurosurgery, Medical University of Innsbruck, Innsbruck, Austria*

MARIAN LUNA • *The Saban Research Institute, Children's Hospital Los Angeles, University of Southern California, Los Angeles, CA, USA*

WIM MARTINET • *Division of Pharmacology, University of Antwerp, Antwerp, Belgium*

EMMA MAZUREK • *Juravinski Cancer Centre and McMaster University, Hamilton, ON, Canada*

JOSEPH MISSERT • *PDT Center, Cell Stress Biology, Roswell Park Cancer Institute, Buffalo, NY, USA*

JOHAN MOAN • *Department of Radiation Biology, Institute for Cancer Research, The Norwegian Radium Hospital, Montebello, Oslo, Norway; Institute of Physics, University of Oslo, Oslo, Norway*

NANCY L. OLEINICK • *Case Western Reserve University, Cleveland, OH, USA*

RAVINDRA K. PANDEY • *PDT Center, Cell Stress Biology, Roswell Park Cancer Institute, Buffalo, NY, USA*

MICHAEL S. PATTERSON • *Juravinski Cancer Centre and McMaster University, Hamilton, ON, Canada*

JACQUES PIETTE • *Laboratory of Virology and Immunology, GIGA-R, B34 +2, CHU, Liege, Belgium*

BRIAN W. POGUE • *Thayer School of Engineering, Dartmouth College, Hanover, NH, USA*

LINA PRASMICKAITE • *Department of Radiation Biology, Institute for Cancer Research, The Norwegian Radium Hospital, Montebello, Oslo, Norway*

MUNAWAR SAJJAD • *PDT Center, Cell Stress Biology, Roswell Park Cancer Institute, Buffalo, NY; Department of Nuclear Chemistry, SUNY, Buffalo, NY, USA*

KIMBERLEY S. SAMKOE • *Thayer School of Engineering, Dartmouth College, Hanover, NH, USA*

PÅL K. SELBO • *Department of Radiation Biology, Institute for Cancer Research, The Norwegian Radium Hospital, Montebello, Oslo, Norway*

GURMIT SINGH • *Department of Pathology and Molecular Medicine, Juravinski Cancer Centre, McMaster University, Hamilton, ON, Canada*

MARIE-THERESE R. STRAND • *Department of Radiation Biology, Institute for Cancer Research, The Norwegian Radium Hospital, Montebello, Oslo, Norway*

TOM VERFAILLIE • *Department of Molecular and Cell Biology, Catholic University of Leuven, Leuven, Belgium*

ERNST WAGNER • *Pharmaceutical Biology-Biotechnology, Department of Pharmacy, Ludwig-Maximilians-Universitaet, Munich, Germany*

ANETTE WEYERGANG • *Department of Radiation Biology, Institute for Cancer Research, The Norwegian Radium Hospital, Montebello, Oslo, Norway*

SAM WONG • *The Saban Research Institute, Children's Hospital Los Angeles, University of Southern California, Los Angeles, CA, USA*

Chapter 1

Introduction

Thomas J. Dougherty

Abstract

In this book you will find chapters describing the most up-to-date information concerning the important clinical applications and methodology of photodynamic therapy. This introduction will provide some background on general mechanisms, cellular targets, and note a few significant new findings relevant to photodynamic action in clinical practice. A short description of the development of photodynamic therapy at Roswell Park Cancer Institute is included.

Key words: Photodynamic therapy, PDT development, newer advances, Roswell Park Cancer Institute.

1. Photodynamic Therapy (PDT) Treatment

Delivery of treatment by PDT is straightforward. Inject a photosensitizer systemically or apply it topically, wait a period of time for distribution and then direct the proper wavelength of light onto the area to be treated for a time sufficient to destroy the cancer (preferably selectively). While it takes some time to properly define these various parameters (especially the selectivity), it is mainly a matter of trial and error. A reviewer of an early grant application of mine pointed out that PDT could not possibly kill all the tumors directly. He was right of course since the resulting tumor destruction, initiated by formation of singlet oxygen (**Fig. 1.1**) is quite complex, involving not only direct cell kill by necrosis and apoptosis but also indirect effects including induction of immunological effects and importantly, initiation of tumor anoxia resulting from destruction of the tumor vasculature. There

C.J. Gomer (ed.), *Photodynamic Therapy*, Methods in Molecular Biology 635,
DOI 10.1007/978-1-60761-697-9_1,

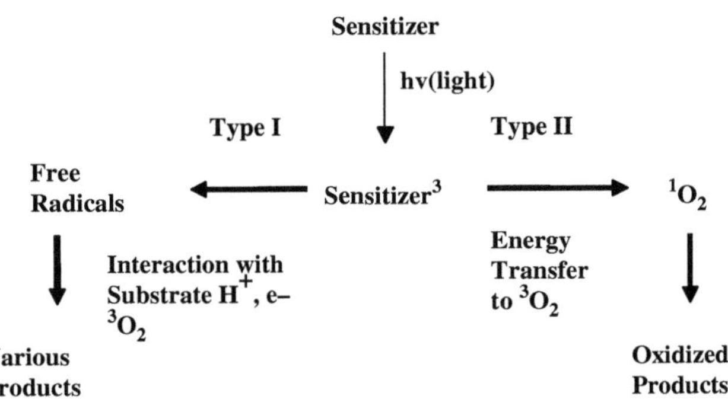

Fig. 1.1. Mechanism of formation of singlet oxygen via the Type II pathway. The competing Type I-free radical pathway is of little importance in PDT; however, free radicals likely form secondarily to the singlet oxygen oxidation of PDT cellular targets shown in **Fig.1.2**. Superscripts refer to electronic states.

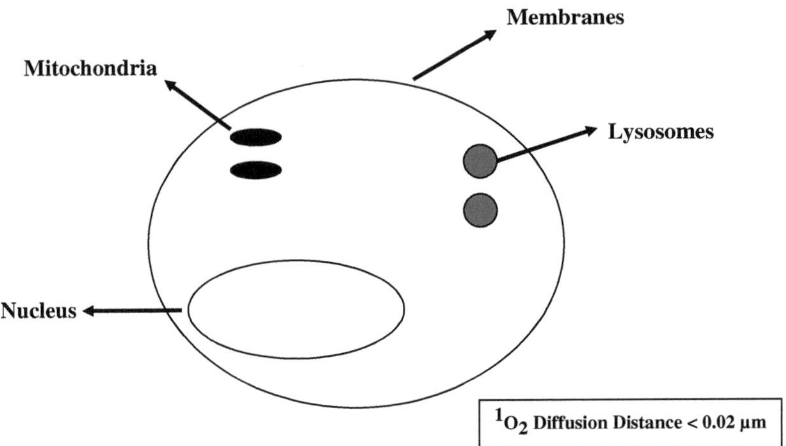

Fig. 1.2. Some intracellular damage sites oxidized by singlet oxygen and/or secondary-free radical species during PDT. The short diffusion distance of singlet oxygen limits damages mainly to the sites of photosensitizer localization.

are also numerous target sites within the cell itself depending on the particular photosensitizer used (**Fig. 1.2**). Many articles and reviews as well as chapters in this book will describe these mechanisms and their clinical applications in detail.

2. PDT Development at Roswell Park Cancer Institute (RPCI)

Since many readers will know little of the history of PDT, at least as it occurred at Roswell Park Cancer Institute (RPCI), I am including some of this here.

PDT at RPCI (originally known as Roswell Park Memorial Institute after its founder, Roswell Park, MD) came about beginning in 1972 as a result of several serendipitous events described below.

After receiving my PhD in physical-organic chemistry from The Ohio State University in 1960, I spent several years at the DuPont Company near Buffalo, NY, where I learned photochemistry from a consultant at DuPont, George Hammond, then Head of the Department of Chemistry at California Institute of Technology, and considered the "father of photochemistry." We had become friends and when I told him that I had decided that industry was not for me and that I wanted to work at RPCI he offered to write a letter of recommendation for me which got me in the door as a postdoctoral student. I started at RPCI in 1970 and spent most of the first year in the library learning as much as I could about cancer, in particular how I could use my knowledge of chemistry and photochemistry in cancer treatment. I found a possibility in the problem of resistance of hypoxic cancers to radiation therapy. I began by attempting to make drugs that would produce oxygen when irradiated by x-rays.

Having no background in cancer biological techniques I looked around for people at RPCI who would be willing to help me. One of these was the Institute Director, George Moore, who in addition to administering the Institute also carried on a busy operating schedule and a active research laboratory. While learning cell culture techniques in his laboratory one of the techs warned me that the chemical I was using to test cell viability by fluorescence would kill all the cells if left in the light (fluorescein diacetate which is converted enzymatically to fluorescent fluorescein only by viable cells). This sure sounded like photochemistry to me so of course I tried it by putting the culture in the sunlight. Sure enough it killed all the cells! I decided to change my research direction to trying to use photochemical means to kill cancer cells. Back to the library! I learned that this process (dyes plus light to destroy cells) dated back to the late nineteenth century in Germany where Paramecium were shown to be killed when exposed to an acridine dye and light. However, nothing was known about how it worked (the term *photodynamic* came along later). I could not find any instance where it had been used in humans (My search at that time was the old fashioned way, library searches by hand (before the Internet!). Later I did find some information in the older literature). I began my experiments by testing fluorescein which worked in the cell culture experiments. I injected it into a mouse that had an experimental mammary tumor and exposed the tumor to fluorescein's longest absorption band in the green, produced from a filtered Xenon lamp. While the tumor growth slowed a little, it was not very significant. I realized that the problem was twofold; the fluorescein did not stay in the tumor long enough (a few minutes) and the green light was not penetrating deep enough into the tumor. Since it was clear that only red light would go deeper into the tumor, I further searched the literature and found that the Mayo Clinic had been using the fluorescence property of a red light-absorbing porphyrin (referred to as hematoporphyrin derivative, Hpd, structure unknown) in humans to detect tumors. I managed to make some Hpd and injected it into a tumor-bearing mouse and exposed the tumor to the red light (the parameters were a complete guess).The tumors did not just slow down, they disappeared! *Wow* – this looked good!

I applied for a research grant to the NCI which was rejected out of hand by the Radiation Study Section with the comment: “It’s an elegant idea but impractical to treat cancer since light does not penetrate tissue.” I reapplied including a photo from the literature showing red light penetrating all the way through a human breast (they were trying to find tumors this way) and also suggested that the grant be reviewed by a different Study Section. It went to the Medicine Study Section and was funded! (Subsequent grants went back in the Radiation Study Section since they thought this was their area of expertise. It took quite a while until this was in fact the case.) After we worked out how to make Hpd reproducibly and had out carried many more animal experiments studying all the variables of treatment, I approached some of the clinical staff to see if any would be interested in trying this in cancer patients. Most thought I was crazy except for Dr. Arnold Mittleman, an internationally well-known surgeon here and a very unique individual who was always open to new approaches to cancer treatment. Of course we needed FDA approval to do this. The problem was that neither I nor anyone else here knew the first thing about how to obtain this approval. Bench to patient research (now commonly known as “Translational Research”) was not a common practice at this time. So we learned how by talking to the people at the FDA who were quite helpful in guiding us through the process and we eventually received permission (IND) to treat patients. Dr. Mittleman carried out the first ever clinical trial of PDT in patients with any solid cancer exposed to the outside of the patient (we did not have lasers then) and who had expended all other options. We found that PDT killed cancers in humans just like it did in mice, although it took some time to find the correct parameters, since the mouse data could not be directly translated to humans, no surprise. As an aside, this being my first exposure to cancer patients I was surprised by their willingness to try an experimental treatment which they well knew would not help them but might help someone else. These are truly amazing people!

Eventually we isolated an “active” fraction from Hpd, known to be a very complex mixture of porphyrin oligomers with both ester and ether linkages. A major advantage of this isolation and preliminary structure identification was that it allowed us to obtain patents on this material (Photofrin) which is critical to be able to license the rights to a company capable of carrying out the final step in the FDA approval process (very expensive and complex multi-center, randomized Phase III clinical trials) leading to commercialization and availability to all cancer patients. We had carried out numerous Phase I clinical studies at Roswell (mainly toxicology studies although considerable efficacy data were also collected) as had several other institutions to whom we had supplied Photofrin. After several, often frustrating attempts at licensing which are not worth going into here, we finally succeeded in licensing Photofrin to a large pharmaceutical company with the expertise to complete the approval process and to market PDT. The first health agency approval came in Canada in 1993 for treatment of obstructive esophageal cancer and bladder cancers. This was followed in 1995 in the United States, Japan, and Europe with subsequent approvals in these countries for obstructive lung cancer, early-stage lung cancer, and high-grade dysplasia in Barrett's esophagus.

3. Significant Newer Advances in PDT

3.1. Scientific

3.1.1. The Recognition of Immunological Effects in PDT

The work of Golllnick and that of Korbelick, described in this book, has clearly demonstrated the importance of immunological induction by PDT in contributing to complete eradication of various tumors in animals. While these effects are more difficult to identify in humans they are very likely operative in at least some cancers treated by PDT.

3.1.2. Low Dose Rate Treatment Conditions

This effect has clinical relevance (see below) and has been explored in our laboratory by Barbara Henderson and her group who have shown that at a set drug dose, the area of tumor necrosis is greater at low-light dose rates of 7–20 mw (whole tumor) compared to higher dose rates of 50–100 mw. This is at least partly a result of oxygen depletion at high-treatment doses rates.

3.2. Clinical

3.2.1. Clinical Efficacy of Low Dose Rates

Some of the more recent exciting clinical work is being carried out by Light Sciences Oncology (see their web site). It has long been their intension to apply PDT to larger tumors than those generally treated. They have in fact accomplished this with the combination of their photosensitizer, LS11, a chlorine-type molecule formerly known as Npe6, and a special implantable "fiber" consisting of multiple light-emitting diodes (LEDs). The light is delivered at low dose rates over several hours to deliver the prescribed light dose. Treatment for metastatic colon cancer to the liver and primary hepatomas is in advanced Phase III clinical trials outside the United States. These studies when approved will bring PDT to a large number of patients formerly considered to be ineligible for PDT.

3.2.2. The Application of PDT to Treatment of Early-Stage Head and Neck Cancers

The work of Biel, described in this book, and which has been ongoing for several years using Photofin-PDT has not led to FDA approval since it has not been followed up by the current producer of Photofrin. This is unfortunate since his results are certainly impressive and have been recently confirmed at RPCI by Rigual et al. It should be noted, however, that Foscan-PDT is approved in Europe for this indication (but has not been allowed by the United States). Each of these photosensitizers noted suffer from side effects of cutaneous photosensitivity and the latter by lack of selectivity. This may be alleviated by using photosensitizers without these drawbacks as noted below.

3.2.3. New Photosensitizing Agents

Our group has evaluated a very large number of new photosensitizing agents developed by Pandey et al. among which is a series of pyropheophorbide ethers which have been subjected to an extensive QSAR study. The optimal drug was the hexyl ether (HPPH) which has been studied in several Phase I/II and Phase II studies including cancers of the skin, lung, esophagus, and currently head and neck. A total of more than 120 patients have been included in these studies which has demonstrated (1) no systemic toxicity, (2) no long-term cutaneous photosensitivity, and (3) efficacy which appears to be similar to that of Photofrin. Our preliminary results in head and neck cancer are similar to those reported by Biel and by us using Photofrin. HPPH currently is licensed in China and shortly will be licensed elsewhere outside the United States.

Photodynamic therapy is still alive after 37 years and there is every indication that it will be around for a long time to come.

Chapter 2

Death and Survival Signals in Photodynamic Therapy

Michael Dewaele, Tom Verfaillie, Wim Martinet, and Patrizia Agostinis

Abstract

Photodynamic therapy (PDT) is an anticancer modality utilizing the generation of singlet oxygen and other reactive oxygen species through visible light irradiation of a photosensitive dye accumulated in the cancerous tissue. Upon exposure of cancer cells to the photodynamic stress, multiple signaling cascades are concomitantly activated and depending on the subcellular location of the generated ROS and the intensity of the oxidative damage, they dictate whether cells will cope with the stress and survive or succumb and die. Different methodologies have been developed to allow the discrimination of cell death subroutines at the morphological, ultrastructural, and biochemical levels and to scrutinize signaling cascades in response to PDT. Here we describe a selection of useful techniques to characterize apoptosis and autophagy and to monitor the activation status of the MAPK- and Akt-mTOR pathways after PDT.

Key words: PDT, hypericin, signal transduction, protein kinases, apoptosis, autophagy, Odyssey.

1. Introduction

The present classification of cell death modalities, which includes apoptosis, autophagic cell death, and necrosis, is largely based on their distinguishable morphologies and biochemical hallmarks (1).

Apoptosis, or type 1 cell death, is regarded as the most widespread mode of cell death and is a major in vitro and in vivo response to PDT (2–4). Apoptosis is characterized by cell shrinkage, chromatin condensation and DNA fragmentation, membrane blebbing, activation of caspases, and, in vivo, phagocytosis by neighboring cells. In contrast, necrosis, also known as type 3 cell death, is characterized by cellular swelling, rapid loss

C.J. Gomer (ed.), *Photodynamic Therapy*, Methods in Molecular Biology 635,
DOI 10.1007/978-1-60761-697-9_2, © Springer Science+Business Media, LLC 2010

of plasma membrane integrity, and the absence of caspase signaling. This type of cell death occurs typically in response to excessive photodynamic injury to cellular components. During the last decades a number of techniques to discriminate apoptosis from necrosis have been extensively developed. These include measurements of DNA fragmentation, mitochondrial membrane permeabilization and release of mitochondrial intermembrane proteins in the cytosol, activation of caspases, and ultrastructural analysis of cell death morphologies by transmission electron microscopy. More recently, we and others have shown that PDT can activate autophagy which can result in an autophagic cell death, or type 2 cell death, which is morphologically defined (especially by transmission electron microscopy) as a type of cell death accompanied by large-scale autophagic vacuolization of the cytoplasm in the absence of chromatin condensation (4). Autophagy, literally "self-eating" in Greek, takes place at constitutively low levels in all eukaryotic cells as a main survival mechanism to maintain vital functions during nutrient-limiting conditions and to rid cells from aberrant or unnecessary organelles, toxic metabolites, or intracellular pathogens (5). Autophagy stimulation is observed under conditions of chronic metabolic stress, such as those found in the tumor microenvironment, as well as following acute damage to vital cellular components, as observed following a variety of anticancer treatments (6). The hallmark of autophagy is the formation of double-membraned vacuoles, called autophagosomes, that sequester cytoplasmic components as well as organelles, which eventually fuse with lysosomes to become a single-membraned autolysosome, where the cargo is degraded by lysosomal hydrolases. The detection and quantification of the autophagosomes present in the cells, the evaluation of the autophagic flux, and the activation status of signaling pathways regulating autophagy, such as the Akt-mTOR and the mitogen-activated protein kinases (MAPKs), are frequently used methods to analyze the stimulation of this catabolic process after cellular stress.

Because of the relevance of these signaling pathways in the regulation of the cell's fate, we describe here a selection of techniques used to monitor and characterize apoptotic cell death and autophagy and MAPK- and Akt-driven pathways in cell lines exposed to PDT.

2. Materials

2.1. Photosensitization and Cell Culture Media

1. Hypericin is synthesized from emodin anthraquinone according to Falk et al. (7), dissolved in dimethyl sulfoxide (DMSO) to attain 1,000X working stocks, and stored in dark conditions at −18°C.

2. Cell culture medium is prepared as follows: 500 ml DMEM (Dulbecco's Modified Eagle's Medium) supplemented with 100 units/ml penicillin, 100 μg/ml streptomycin, 2 mM L-glutamine (all from Gibco, Invitrogen, Carlsbad, CA, USA), and 10% (v/v) FBS (fetal bovine serum; HyClone, Thermo Fisher Scientific, Waltham, MA). This medium will be referred to as "serum-containing DMEM" in the protocols. After preparation store at 4°C.

2.2. Preparation of Protein Lysates

1. HEPES lysis buffer: 25 mM 4-(2-hydroxyethyl)-1-piperazine ethane sulfonic acid (HEPES) pH 7.5, 0.3 M NaCl, 1.5 mM $MgCl_2$, 20 mM β-glycerol-phosphate, 2 mM ethylenediaminetetraacetic acid (EDTA), 2 mM ethylene glycol tetraacetic acid (EGTA), 1 mM dithiothreitol (DTT), 1% (v/v) Triton X-100, 10% (v/v) glycerol, 10 μg/μl leupeptin, 5 μg/μl aprotinin, 1 mM phenyl methane sulphonyl fluoride (PMSF), 1 mM Na_3VO_4, and 50 mM NaF. Store aliquots at –18°C.

2.3. Gel Electrophoresis and Western Blotting

1. Determination of protein concentration: BCA™ protein assay kit (Pierce, Rockford, IL, USA).
2. 6X Loading buffer: 0.35 M Tris–HCl pH 6.8, 10% (w/v) SDS, 36% (v/v) glycerol, and 0.01% (w/v) bromophenol blue. Store aliquots at –20°C. For the aliquot in use, add 5% (v/v) β-mercaptoethanol.
3. TBS-T (Tris-buffered saline with Tween): 25 mM Tris–HCl pH 7.4, 150 mM NaCl, and 0.1% Tween. Store at RT.
4. Blocking buffer: 5% non-fat milk powder (Nestlé Belgilux NV, Brussels, Belgium) in TBS±T.
5. Secondary HRP-labeled antibody for ECL: Horse anti-mouse and goat anti-rabbit (Cell Signaling Technology, Danvers, MA, USA) diluted 1:2,000 in blocking buffer.
6. Secondary IR-labeled antibody for Odyssey: Alexa Fluor® 680 goat anti-rabbit IgG "highly cross-adsorbed" (Invitrogen, Carlsbad, CA, USA) diluted 1:5,000 in blocking buffer; DyLight 800 conjugated goat anti-mouse IgG (H+L) (Thermo Fisher Scientific, Rockford, IL, USA) diluted 1:5,000 in blocking buffer.

2.4. Assessment of Apoptosis in PDT-Treated Cells

2.4.1. Determination of Caspase Activity

1. Rabbit anti-caspase 3 (recognizing the proform and processed active forms) and mouse anti-poly(ADP-ribose) polymerase (PARP) recognizing the full protein and the caspase-cleaved PARP fragment (BIOMOL International LP, Plymouth Meeting, PA, USA).

2. Assay buffer: 100 mM HEPES pH 7.4, 10% (w/v) sucrose, 1% (v/v) Triton X-100, 2.5 mM EDTA, 5 mM DTT, 1 mM PMSF, 2 μg/ml pepstatin, and 2 μg/ml leupeptin. Store at 4°C.
3. Fluorescent substrates (7-amino-4-methylcoumarin (AMC)) and inhibitors (fluoromethyl ketone (FMK)) for the different caspases (Bachem GmbH, Weil am Rhein, Germany).

2.4.2. Determination of DNA Fragmentation by Sytox Green Staining

1. DNA extraction buffer: 0.2 M Na_2HPO_4 and 0.1 M nitric acid brought to pH 7.8 with NaOH.
2. DNA staining solution: 1 μM Sytox green (Invitrogen, Carlsbad, CA, USA) in PBS and 0.2 mg/ml DNase-free RNase.

2.4.3. Assessment of Mitochondrial Outer and Inner Membrane Permeabilization

1. Digitonin buffer: 0.01% (w/v) digitonin (Sigma-Aldrich, St. Louis, MO, USA) (stock solution: 1% in methanol, store at RT) and 1 mM EDTA diluted in PBS.
2. Stabilization buffer: 20 mM HEPES pH 7.5, 250 mM sucrose, 10 mM KCl, 1.5 mM $MgCl_2$, 1 mM EDTA, 1 mM EGTA, 1 mM DTT, 10 μg/ml leupeptin, 1 mM PMSF, and 10 μg/ml aprotinin.
3. Streptolysin O (Sigma-Aldrich, St. Louis, MO, USA).
4. Mouse anti-actin antibody (The Developmental Studies Hybridoma Bank, University of Iowa, Iowa City, IA, USA), mouse anti-cytochrome oxidase subunit IV antibody (Molecular Probes, Invitrogen, Carlsbad, CA, USA), and mouse anti-cytochrome *c* antibody (BD Biosciences, Franklin Lakes, NJ, USA).
5. DiOC6(3) (3,3′-dihexyl oxacarbocyanine iodide; Molecular Probes, Invitrogen, Carlsbad, CA, USA).

2.5. Transmission Electron Microscopy (TEM) for the Study of Cell Death

1. 0.033 M veronal acetate buffer: This buffer is prepared as follows. First, a veronal acetate stock solution is prepared by dissolving 9.71 g sodium acetate trihydrate and 14.71 g sodium 5,5-diethylbarbiturate in 500 ml ultrapure water. The veronal acetate stock solution can be stored for several weeks at 4°C. Subsequently, 6 g saccharose is dissolved in a small volume of water. After addition of 20 ml veronal acetate stock, the pH is adjusted to 7.2–7.4 using acetic acid. The solution is made up to 100 ml with ultrapure water, yielding 6% saccharose in 0.05 M veronal acetate buffer. Finally, two volumes of the latter buffer, 0.5 volume of 6% OsO_4, and 0.5 volume of water are mixed to obtain 0.033 M of veronal acetate buffer-containing 4% saccharose.
2. Reynolds solution: First, slightly heat (and stir) 17.6% sodium citrate. Slowly add 13.3% lead nitrate and leave

for 30 min at room temperature. Adjust to pH 10.5 with sodium hydroxide Titrisol. This stock solution can be stored at room temperature for several weeks. Prior to use, adjust to pH 12.4 with sodium hydroxide Titrisol. This pH is critical as pH > 12.45 will lead to precipitation whereas pH < 12.35 will give poor staining.

2.6. Monitoring Autophagy

1. Mouse anti-LC3 antibody (NanoTools, Antikörpertechnik GmbH & Co, Teningen, Germany).
2. pBABE-GFP-LC3 vector (Dr. J. Debnath, Dept. Cell Biology, Harvard Medical School, Boston, MA, USA).
3. Bafilomycin A1 (Sigma-Aldrich, St. Louis, MO, USA) is dissolved in DMSO to attain a 1,000X stock solution of 100 μM.

2.7. Monitoring MAPK and Akt-mTOR Signaling Cascades

1. Stripping buffer: 62.5 mM Tris–HCl pH 6.7, 2% (w/v) sodium dodecyl sulfate (SDS), and 100 mM β-mercaptoethanol (BME).
2. Mouse anti-p38 MAPK antibody; rabbit anti-phospho-p38 (Thr180/Tyr182) antibody; rabbit anti-Akt antibody; mouse anti-phospho-Akt (Ser473) antibody; rabbit anti-p70S6 antibody; mouse anti-phospho-p70S6 (Thr389) antibody; mouse anti-S6 ribosomal protein antibody; and rabbit anti-phospho-S6 ribosomal protein (Ser235/236) antibody (Cell Signaling Technology, Danvers, MA, USA) diluted 1:1,000 in blocking buffer; rabbit anti-JNK1 antibody was prepared as described in (8); rabbit anti-phospho-JNK 1 and 2 (Thr183/Tyr185) antibody (BioSource^{TM}, Invitrogen, Camarillo, CA, USA) diluted 1:1,000 in blocking buffer.

3. Methods

Here we describe a compendium of different techniques that are used to assess morphological and biochemical hallmarks of apoptosis, autophagy, and regulation of MAPK and Akt-mTOR signaling pathways after cell photosensitization (PDT). At the beginning of the different subchapters we will provide background, step-by-step protocols, and applications and discuss some alternative techniques which can be applied. Since the variety of photosensitizers used in PDT cannot be completely covered, we will focus on the photodynamic effects evoked by light activation of the naturally occurring photosensitizer hypericin, which upon cellular uptake has been shown to localize predominantly to the ER compartment (9, 10).

3.1. Photosensitization (PDT)

1. Seed cells to attain a confluency of 75–80% at the time of irradiation. After attachment, incubate the cells with fresh serum-containing DMEM supplemented with 1X hypericin solution. The concentration of hypericin and the duration of incubation are determined and optimized for every cell line. Usually a range between 0.05 and 1 μM hypericin is used in most experiments.
2. Incubate the plates protected from light exposure at 37°C.
3. If pharmacological compounds (e.g., inhibitors) are used, add 1 h prior to irradiation (*see* **Note 1**).
4. Collect the medium in Falcon tubes and cover the cells in pre-warmed PBS for the duration of the irradiation period.
5. Place the cell culture plates on a plastic diffuser sheet above a set of seven L18W30 fluorescent lamps (Osram). The fluence rate of the lamps is 4.5 mW/cm^2 as measured with an IL 1,400 radiometer (International Light, Newburyport, MA). The fluence or light dose (J/cm^2) is calculated by multiplying the fluence rate with the time of irradiation. Usually a light dose between 1.9 and 2.7 J/cm^2 is used.
6. Replace PBS with the original medium and put the plates back in the incubator at 37°C protected from light until further analysis.

3.2. Preparation of Protein Lysates

1. At the required time points, remove the plates from the incubator and put them on ice. Collect the medium in Falcon tubes. Wash the cells once with 5 ml pre-chilled PBS.
2. Scrape off the cells from the plate in 5 ml pre-chilled PBS on ice and collect the suspension in a new Falcon tube. Centrifuge both suspensions (floating cells and attached cells) at 500×*g* for 5 min.
3. Aspirate the supernatants and resuspend the pellets combined in HEPES lysis buffer in a total volume adapted to the size of the pellet (50–100 μl). Transfer the samples to pre-chilled eppendorfs.
4. Perform lysis on ice for 15 min followed by centrifugation at 16,000×*g* for 15 min at 4°C to pellet cell debris, nuclei, and membranous components. Remove the supernatant carefully (without disturbing the pellet) and transfer it to new pre-chilled eppendorfs. Immediately store at –20°C.

3.3. Gel Electrophoresis and Western Blotting

1. Determine protein concentration and prepare samples to obtain equal protein loading (e.g., 20–40 μg, *see* **Note 2**). Add 1:6 volume of 6X loading buffer to the samples. Spin down and boil the samples for 5 min in a heating block at 100°C.
2. Load samples on a precast Criterion™ XT gel and separate samples by SDS-PAGE (Criterion™ Cell; Bio-Rad

Laboratories, Hercules, CA, USA). 4–12% Bis–Tris gels are chosen to allow good separation of proteins ranging between 100 and 10 kDa. To separate higher MW proteins in the range of 75–250 kDa, 3–8% Tris-Acetate gels are used. Stop gel electrophoresis just before the bromophenol blue-stained front runs off the gel.

3. Enclose the gel in a blotting cassette (Criterion™ Blotter; Bio-Rad Laboratories, Hercules, CA, USA) and transfer proteins to a Protran 2-μm pored nitrocellulose paper (Perkin-Elmer, Boston, MA, USA).
4. Block the membrane for 1 h in a 5% non-fat milk powder solution: For chemiluminescent detection (ECL) the milk powder is dissolved in TBS-Tween. For infrared (IR) fluorescence detection with the Odyssey near-IR detection (LiCor Biosciences, Lincoln, NE, USA) system, the milk powder is dissolved in TBS without Tween (*see* **Note 3**).
5. Incubate the membrane with the appropriate primary antibody diluted in blocking buffer, ON at 4°C with gentle shaking.
6. Wash the membrane three times for 10 min in an excess amount of TBS-Tween.
7. Incubate the membrane with a secondary antibody in blocking buffer for 2 h at 4°C with gentle shaking: For ECL – 1:2,000 dilution of the HRP-labeled secondary antibody (ab), for Odyssey – 1:5,000 dilution of the IR-labeled secondary ab, and incubate and wash the membranes in dark conditions.
8. Wash the membrane three times for 10 min in an excess amount of TBS-Tween.
9. For ECL: Cover the membrane with the ECL reagent mixture (ECL Western blotting substrate, Pierce, Rockford, IL, USA) for 1 min and place it between two transparent plastic sheets. Wipe out excess amounts of reagents and expose the membrane to a light-sensitive film Cronex5 medical X-ray film (AGFA-Gevaert, Mortsel, Belgium) in a light-safe cassette. The duration of the exposure of the membrane to the light-sensitive film varies, depending on the primary antibody used. For Odyssey: the membranes are scanned on the Odyssey InfraRed Imager.

3.4. Assessment of Apoptosis in PDT-Treated cells

In this section we will detail protocols to detect and quantify apoptotic cell death, based on the determination of DNA fragmentation, assays of mitochondrial outer and inner membrane permeabilization and release of mitochondrial intermembrane proteins and caspase activity following hypericin–PDT. Additionally we detail a protocol for the discrimination of cell death morphology by TEM analysis.

3.4.1. Determination of Caspase Activity

At the biochemical level apoptosis entails the activation of caspases, a highly conserved family of cysteine-dependent aspartate-specific proteases. All caspases share an active-site cysteine residue and the specific requirement for a four-amino acid recognition motif that terminates in aspartic acid for cleavage. Caspases are synthesized as proenzymes or zymogens, consisting of a prodomain of variable length, followed by p20 and p10 subunits containing residues critical for the recognition of the substrate and the catalytic activity. Caspases are activated in response to an apoptotic signal by proximity-induced dimerization at a multimeric protein complex (initiator caspases), which is followed by autocatalytic processing, or by limited proteolysis by an upstream caspase (effector caspases) (11). In both cases the end result is the separation of the prodomain from the p20 and p10 subunits generating an active heterotetramer. Proteolytic activation of caspases can be detected by the appearance of the p20 and p10 fragments and the concomitant decrease in the inactive zymogen by Western blotting. It is generally accepted that once activated, the effector caspases are responsible for most of the stereotypic morphological and biochemical changes observed during apoptosis by cleaving a restricted subset of vital substrates like the nuclear protein poly(ADP-ribose)polymerase (PARP). Activation of caspases does not occur during necrotic or autophagic cell death. Thus, detection of caspase activity during the cell death process and its sensitivity to inhibition by inhibitors of caspases can be used to discriminate between apoptosis (caspase-mediated) and other cell death modalities. Measurement of caspase activity requires the use of synthetic substrates for caspases. These substrates are usually tetrapeptides with aspartate at the position P1, within the primary structure "XXXD," conjugated with a fluorogenic AMC (7-amino-4-methylcoumarin) or AFC (7-amino-4-trifluoromethylcoumarin) group. Hydrolysis of the substrate by active caspase results in the release of free AMC or AFC groups which are fluorescent and can be measured in a fluorometer.

3.4.1.1. Determination of Caspase Processing and Substrate Proteolysis by Western Blotting

Western blot procedures are performed according to the protocols detailed in **Section 3.3**. The caspase 3 and PARP antibodies are both diluted 1:5,000 in blocking buffer. A representation of caspase 3 processing and PARP cleavage after hypericin–PDT treatment is displayed in **Fig. 2.1**.

3.4.1.2. Caspase Activity Assay

1. Lysates for this caspase activity assay are made according to protocol in **Section 3.2** with a specific lysis buffer detailed as the "assay buffer" in **Section 2.4.1**. In this assay buffer, the proteasome inhibitor cocktail is modified not to compromise caspase activity.

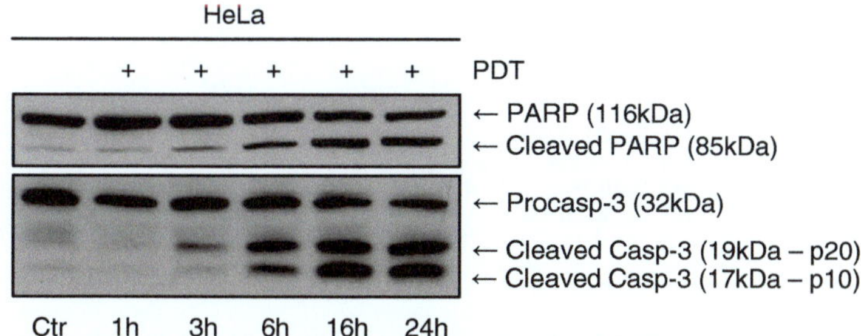

Fig. 2.1. PDT-induced caspase-3 activation and substrate cleavage. At the indicated time points after irradiation (controls are incubated with hypericin but not irradiated) total protein lysates were made and processed for Western blotting according to protocols in **Sections 3.3** and **3.4.1**. Chemiluminescent detection reveals the increased accumulation of the active p10 and p20 fragments of caspase-3, which parallels the proteolytic processing of its downstream substrate PARP.

2. On a 96-well plate, incubate lysates containing 50 μg of proteins with 50 μM of the fluorescent substrate Ac-DEVD-AMC (for caspase 3 and 7) in a total volume of 250 μl assay buffer at 37°C for 30 min (*see* **Note 4**). A condition carrying only assay buffer with the fluorescent substrate is used as a negative control.
3. Measure kinetics of DEVD-AMC cleavage for 40 min with a 2 min interval between the readings, with fluorospectrometer pre-warmed to 37°C. For AMC the excitation is at 360 nm and the emission is measured at 460 nm.
4. Normalize the raw data by subtracting the value of the negative control from the raw data per time point. Plot the normalized data vs time. The best fitting curve is calculated and the slope of the curve can be used to calculate the amount of fluorescence produced per minute.

3.4.2. Determination of DNA Fragmentation by Sytox Green Staining

DNA fragmentation is a hallmark of apoptosis. Activation of various apoptotic nucleases during cell death results in the formation of high molecular weight (>50 kbp) and nucleosome-sized (200 bp) DNA fragments. Based on this apoptotic parameter, different techniques, which include separation of DNA ladders by agarose gel electrophoresis, fluorescence imaging of nuclear fragmentation with 4′,6-diamidino-2-phenylindole dihydrochloride (DAPI), Hoechst, or propidium iodide (PI), and terminal deoxynucleotidyl transferase-mediated dUTP nick end labeling (TUNEL), have been developed (*see* **Note 6**). A particularly useful technique is the determination of the cell's "hypoploid" or sub-G1 DNA content by flow cytometry. This technique provides information on the distribution of the cell population within the major phases of the cell cycle, while estimating the frequency

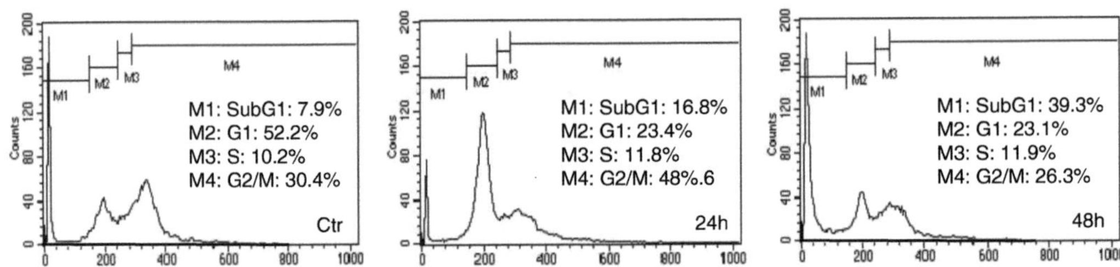

Fig. 2.2. PDT-induced DNA fragmentation in HeLa cells. At 24 and 48 h after hypericin–PDT treatment, the cells were harvested and stained with Sytox Green according to protocol in **Section 3.4.2** and compared with control cells (hyp-incubated but not irradiated). DNA fragmentation in the population of cells increases over time (indicated by the SubG1 fraction) as a late event in the degradation phase of apoptosis.

of apoptotic cells with a hypoploid DNA amount. Typically, a healthy population of nonsynchronized cells will exhibit a biphasic peak of $2n$ (G1) and $4n$ (G2) cells. Upon apoptosis induction a fraction of cells showing a lower DNA fluorescent pattern, as the result of DNA fragmentation, appears as a "sub-G1 peak." For hypericin–PDT, we use Sytox Green, a green fluorescent DNA dye, as detailed below (**Fig. 2.2**).

1. After irradiation of the cells on 10-cm culture dishes, collect the medium in a Falcon tube and wash the cells once with 5 ml PBS pre-warmed at 37°C.
2. Trypsinize cells with 1 ml of pre-warmed (37°C) trypsin solution. Since the integrity of the cells has to be maintained to the highest possible extent this procedure is preferred over scraping the cells of the plate.
3. Stop trypsinization by adding 1 ml serum-containing DMEM and collect the cells in the Falcon tube.
4. Centrifuge the cells for 5 min at 100×*g*. Aspirate the supernatant and resuspend the pellet in 300 μl PBS and transfer it into eppendorfs.
5. Add 1.5 ml of ice-cold 70% ethanol (EtOH) and allow fixation overnight (ON) at –20°C.
6. Centrifuge the cells for 10 min at 2,500×*g* and aspirate the EtOH carefully. Wash once with 1.5 ml PBS and centrifuge for 10 min at 2,500×*g*.
7. Aspirate the supernatant and resuspend the pellet in 0.5 ml PBS. Add 1 ml DNA extraction buffer. Incubate 5 min at room temperature (RT).
8. Centrifuge for 10 min at 2,500×*g* and aspirate off the supernatant. Resuspend the pellet in 0.5 ml DNA staining solution (*see* **Note 7**). Incubate for 30 min at RT.
9. Perform flow cytometric analysis.

3.4.3. Assessment of Mitochondrial Outer and Inner Membrane Permeabilization

Detection of outer membrane (OM) permeabilization relies mainly on the analysis of the subcellular redistribution of proteins that are usually retained within the intermembrane space (IMS) (i.e., the space formed between the inner and outer membrane of the mitochondria) by the OM, following PDT. This is usually performed by immunoblot detection of such proteins, which include primarily cytochrome *c*, but can also be extended to other proapoptotic molecules trapped in the IMS, such as AIF, EndoG, Smac/DIABLO, and Omi/HtrA2 (12), upon isolation of different subcellular fractions (e.g., cytosol and mitochondria). Usually this approach requires that a mild detergent permeabilizing the plasma membrane while leaving intact the mitochondrial membrane, such as digitonin, is used to avoid that IMS proteins' leak out during organelle and subcellular preparation. Since IMS proteins are released with variable kinetics, depending on the type of photosensitizer and the cells used (4), it is advisable to perform kinetic studies and monitor the subcellular localization of several IMS proteins rather than of a single one. Assessment of IM permeability, which often occurs during cell death, relies on the use of IM-permeant lipophilic cations that accumulate in the mitochondrial matrix. Since under normal circumstances, the $\Delta\psi_m$ ranges from 120 to 180 mV (the intramitochondrial side being electronegative), these lipophilic cations concentrate in the mitochondrial matrix driven by the $\Delta\psi_m$ following the Nernst equation. These fluorochromes include, but are not limited to, rhodamine 123 (Rh 123), tetramethyl rhodamine ethyl and methyl esters (TMRE and TMRM, respectively), chloromethyl-*X*-rosamine (CMXRos, also known as MitoTracker Red), 5,5′,6,6′-tetrachloro-1,1′,3,3′-tetraethylbenzimidazolcarbocyanine iodide (JC-1), and 3,3′-dihexyloxacarbocyanine iodide (DiOC6(3)). The choice of the fluorochrome is dictated by their spectral properties, since this analysis is performed in living cells loaded with the fluorescent dye. For hypericin, which has a maximal absorption spectrum at 595 nm, we load the cells with the carbocyanine DiOC6(3) (max. abs. 484 nm) followed by quantification of the cell population with high (untreated) or low DiOC6(3) staining (PDT treated) by flow cytometric analysis (**Fig. 2.3**).

Additionally, two-color immunofluorescence staining (*see* **Section 3.4.3.3**) can be employed to visualize the co-localization of IMS proteins, such as cytochrome *c* or AIF, with specific mitochondrial markers (e.g., cytochrome *c* oxidase subunit IV) or using organelle-specific fluorescent markers (e.g., MitoTracker® Red CMXRos). Often nuclear counterstaining and/or the use of antibodies specific for active caspases are used to provide supplementary information about the apoptotic cascade induced by PDT.

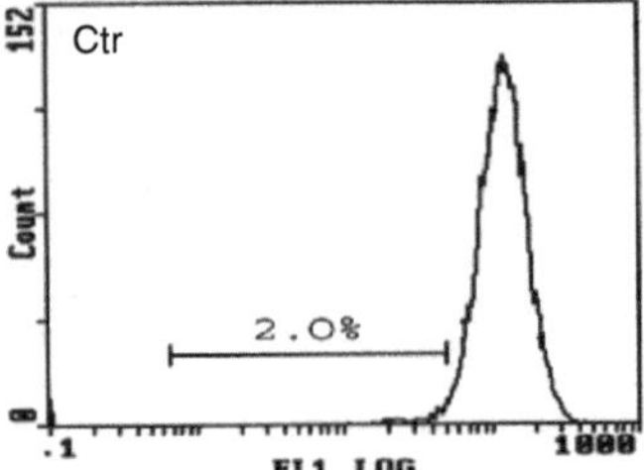

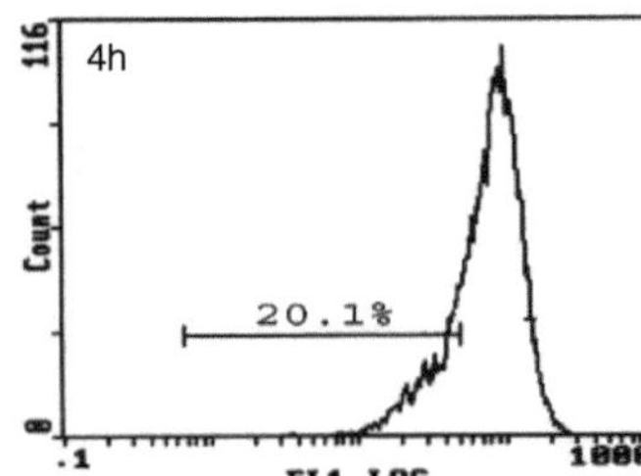

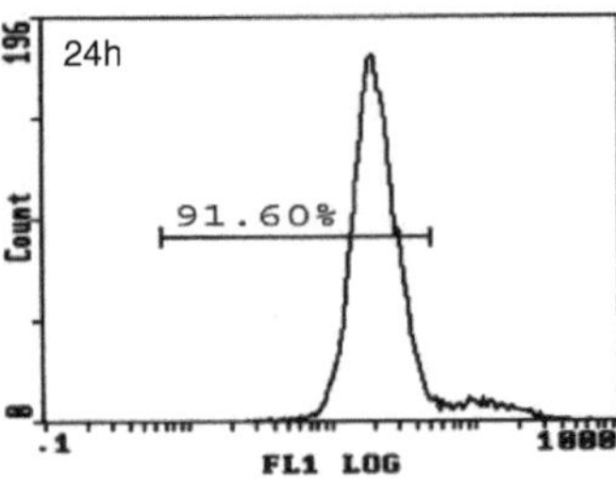

Fig. 2.3. PDT-induced mitochondrial membrane depolarization in HeLa cells. At 4 and 24 h after hypericin–PDT treatment, the cells were harvested and stained with DiOC6(3) according to protocol in **Section 3.4.3** and compared with the control cells (hyp-incubated but not irradiated). The gate indicates the increasing fraction of cells with depolarized mitochondria over time. The mitochondrial depolarization is an early event in the induction of apoptosis and clearly precedes the DNA fragmentation depicted in Fig. 2.2.

3.4.3.1. Subcellular Fractionation with Digitonin

1. At the required time points after PDT, remove the plates from the incubator and place them on ice. Collect the medium in a Falcon tube and spin down detached cells at 100×*g*. Meanwhile, wash the cells in the culture plates once with 5 ml ice-cold PBS, aspirate the PBS, and add 5 ml fresh ice-cold PBS.
2. Resuspend cell pellet in ice-cold PBS. Scrape off the cells from the plate in the PBS on ice and collect the suspension in the Falcon with resuspended cell solution (in this way both attached and floating cells are collected). Centrifuge the suspension mildly at 100×*g* for 5 min to avoid physical rupture of the membranes and organelles.
3. Aspirate the supernatant and resuspend the pellet shortly in 150 μl of digitonin buffer. Collect the suspension in pre-chilled eppendorfs and immediately centrifuge for 20 min at 16,000×*g* at 4°C. Only a short incubation in the soft detergent digitonin will break the plasma membrane without compromising the integrity of the organelle membranes. A fast transfer of the resuspended pellet to the eppendorfs and the subsequent centrifugation are therefore essential steps in this experimental approach (*see* **Note 8**).
4. Transfer the supernatant (supernatant A), without disturbing the pellet (pellet A) to a pre-chilled eppendorf. Supernatant A contains all soluble proteins, including the released mitochondrial intermembrane proteins. Pellet A contains the intact cells, the intact organelles, and the plasma membrane.
5. Resuspend the pellet A in 150 μl of HEPES lysis buffer and incubate on ice for 15 min. Centrifuge the lysates at 16,000×*g* for 15 min at 4°C.
6. Transfer the supernatant (supernatant B) without disturbing the pellet (pellet B) to a new pre-chilled eppendorf. This

supernatant contains proteins recovered from the organelle fraction and plasma membrane.

7. Measure protein concentration of supernatant A and B and perform Western blotting for cytochrome *c*, using a 1:1,000 dilution of the anti-cytochrome *c* antibody.
8. Check the purity of the soluble and mitochondrial fractions by the specific immunodetection of cytoplasmic, like actin (anti-actin antibody is diluted 1:50,000) or mitochondrial proteins, like cytochrome oxidase subunit IV (anti-cytochrome *c* oxidase subunit IV is diluted 1:1,000), in the respective subcellular fractions.

3.4.3.2. DiOC6(3) Staining for Mitochondrial Inner Membrane Depolarization

1. After treatment, wash the cells once with 5 ml of pre-heated PBS at 37°C and trypsinize them with 1 ml pre-warmed trypsin solution for 5 min.
2. Stop trypsinization by adding 1 ml serum-containing DMEM and collect the cells in a Falcon tube.
3. Centrifuge the cells (100×*g* for 5 min) and resuspend the pellet carefully in serum-containing DMEM with 40 nM of DiOC6(3) (*see* **Note 9**) and further incubate for 30 min at 37°C in dark conditions.
4. Centrifuge the cells (100×*g* for 5 min), wash the pellet once with pre-chilled PBS, and keep it on ice until analysis.
5. For large cell populations the analysis of $\Delta\psi_m$ is performed on a flow cytometer. The loss of transmembrane potential in treated cells is measured as a decrease in DiOC6(3) green fluorescence (*see* **Note 10**).

3.4.3.3. Immunocytochemistry

1. For immunocytochemistry the cells are plated and treated on two-chamber slides.
2. After PDT, and 30 min prior to the staining procedure, add 50 nM of MitoTracker® Red CMXRos (Molecular Probes, Invitrogen, Carlsbad, CA, USA) to the culture medium and incubate at 37°C.
3. Wash the slides carefully with 1 ml of ice-cold PBS.
4. Fix the cells with 1 ml 4% paraformaldehyde diluted in PBS pH 7.4 for 20 min. Aspirate the paraformaldehyde and wash three times for 3 min with 1 ml PBS with gentle shaking.
5. Permeabilize the cells with 1 ml of 0.1% (v/v) Triton X-100 solution in PBS for 10 min. Aspirate the Triton solution and wash three times for 3 min with 1 ml PBS with gentle shaking.
6. Incubate the slides twice with 1 ml 0.1 M glycine solution for 10 min. Glycine will neutralize the ionic charges on

proteins and will prevent unspecific binding of the primary and secondary antibodies.

7. Wash once with 1 ml of PBS with gentle shaking.
8. Block the slides for 20 min with a 1% (ultrapure grade) BSA solution in PBS complemented with 10% serum derived from the host species in which the secondary antibody was raised. This will suppress non-specific binding of IgG during the staining.
9. Blot the excess serum and incubate the chambers with 400 μl of the primary anti-cytochrome *c* antibody, diluted 1:500 in 1% BSA–PBS, supplemented with 10% serum for 1 h.
10. After incubation, aspirate the antibody solution and wash four times for 3 min with 1 ml PBS with gentle shaking.
11. Incubate with 400 μl of the Alexa488-labeled secondary antibody diluted 1:1,000 in 1% BSA–PBS, supplemented with 10% serum for 1 h. After the staining, aspirate the antibody solution and wash four times for 3 min with 1 ml PBS with gentle shaking.
12. Blot all excess liquids and mount the slides with a drop of Prolong Gold antifade reagent containing DAPI (Invitrogen, Carlsbad, CA, USA), cover the slides with a cover glass, and allow curing for 24 h at 4°C. The DAPI in the mounting medium will provide a blue fluorescent counterstaining of the nuclei.
13. Image samples on a fluorescent microscope.

3.5. Transmission Electron Microscopy (TEM) for the Study of Cell Death

Although TEM is time consuming and requires expensive equipment, this technique has been considered a "golden standard" in cell death research. It offers high-resolving power (0.1–0.4 nm), thereby providing much more detailed information about cell morphology as compared to conventional light microscopy. Two of the earliest ultrastructural changes detectable in apoptosis via TEM are formation of uniformly dense masses of chromatin distributed against the nuclear envelope (**Fig. 2.4**) and persistence of a nucleolar structure until the very late stages (13, 14). Apoptotic cells are further characterized by the loss of specialized surface structures, such as microvilli and cell–cell contacts, condensation of cytoplasm, and formation of membrane-bound apoptotic bodies of different sizes containing well preserved but compacted cytoplasm organelles and/or nuclear fragments (**Fig. 2.4**) (13, 15). Necrosis is morphologically distinct from apoptosis and is characterized by a general swelling of the cell (oncosis) and cytoplasmic organelles and rapid loss of plasma membrane integrity (16). The nuclear morphology remains relatively unchanged until later stages, when chromatin condenses into small irregular pieces (**Fig. 2.4**).

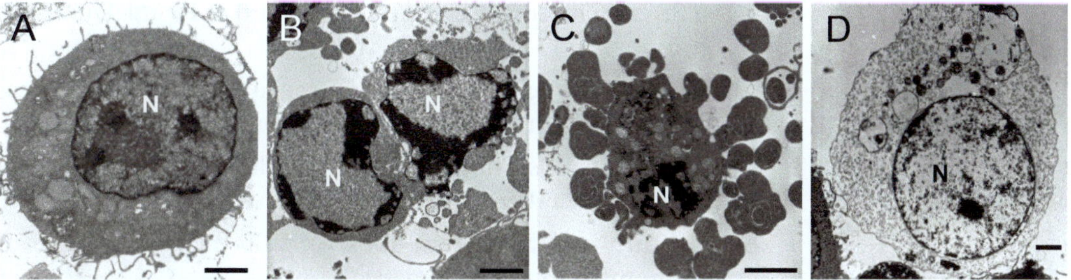

Fig. 2.4. Analysis of cell morphology of apoptotic and necrotic cells by transmission electron microscopy. J774A.1 macrophages were treated with 300 μM spermine NONOate for 3 h. (**a**) Untreated cell showing microvilli protruding from the entire surface, a smoothly outlined nucleus with chromatin in the form of heterochromatin and well-preserved cytoplasmic organelles. (**b**) Two apoptotic cells with sharply delineated masses of condensed chromatin. (**c**) Apoptotic cell with convolution of the cellular surface and formation of apoptotic bodies. (**d**) Necrotic cell containing clumps of chromatin with ill-defined edges, swollen mitochondria, and electron lucent cytosol. Scale bar = 2 μm. N indicates nucleus.

These instructions assume the use of suspension cells (*see* **Note 11**).

1. Centrifuge cells (1–2 × 10^6 cells) at 100×*g* for 5 min.
2. Remove the supernatant and add 4 ml 0.1 M sodium cacodylate-buffered (pH 7.4) 2.5% glutaraldehyde solution to the pellet without resuspending the cells. Allow fixation for 2 h at 4°C.
3. Remove fixative and rinse cell pellet (3 × 10 min) with 5 ml 0.1 M sodium cacodylate-buffered (pH 7.4) 7.5% saccharose without resuspending the cells (*see* **Note 12**).
4. Add 3–4 ml 1% osmium tetroxide (OsO_4) in 0.033 M veronal acetate buffer containing 4% saccharose. Allow postfixation for 2 h at 4°C.
5. Remove OsO_4 solution and rinse cell pellet (3 × 10 min) with 5 ml 0.05 M veronal acetate buffer containing 6% saccharose.
6. Dehydrate cell pellet in an ethanol gradient as follows: 70% ethanol (15 min), 90% ethanol (15 min), 96% ethanol (15 min), and 100% ethanol (5 × 20 min).
7. Treat cell pellet with the following ethanol/Durcupan ACM (Fluka, Bornem, Belgium) mixtures at room temperature: Ethanol/Durcupan ACM (3:1) (1 h), ethanol/Dur cupan ACM (1:1) (1 h), and ethanol/Durcupan ACM (1:3) (1 h).
8. Incubate cell pellet in Durcupan ACM1 containing 10 ml Durcupan component A (embedding substance), 10 ml Durcupan component B (hardener), and 0.15 ml Durcupan component D (plasticizer) at 40°C (2 × 90 min).
9. Incubate cell pellet in Durcupan ACM2 containing 10 ml Durcupan component A, 10 ml Durcupan component B,

0.35 ml Durcupan component C, and 0.15 ml Durcupan component D at 40°C (90 min).

10. Transfer cell pellet into a gelatin capsule, cover with Durcupan ACM2, and allow polymerization at 60°C for 3 days.
11. Cut ultrathin sections (±50 nm thick) with an ultramicrotome using a diamond knife (Element Six, Berkshire, UK).
12. Capture and air-dry sections on 200-mesh copper grids (Canemco, Quebec, Canada).
13. Stain sections with 2% uranyl acetate for 15 min in the dark. Rinse sections with ultrapure water.
14. Stain sections with Reynolds solution pH 12.4 for 10 min. Rinse sections with 0.05 M NaOH Titrisol and CO_2-free ultrapure water (*see* **Note 13**).
15. View samples with a TEM at an accelerating voltage of 80 kV.

3.6. Methods to Monitor Autophagy

At the onset of the process of autophagy, the cytosolic protein LC3 (LC3-I) is lipidated to LC3-phosphatidylethanolamine (LC3-II) and targeted to the autophagosomal membranes. Although the molecular weight of the cytosolic LC3-I is estimated to be 18 kDa and the addition of the PE tail significantly increases its molecular weight, the hydrophobic nature of PE causes a faster migration of the lipoprotein LC3-II during SDS gel electrophoresis resulting in an apparent molecular weight of only 16 kDa. The conversion of LC3-I to LC3-II, which is thought to correlate well with the amount of autophagosomes present in a cellular system, by Western blotting has become an accepted biochemical marker of autophagy (17) as shown in **Fig. 2.5a**. Another well-explored method requires the ectopic expression of a GFP-LC3 chimeric protein followed by fluorescence imaging. Under normal conditions, GFP-LC3 is cytosolic and will display a diffuse pattern of green fluorescence, while upon autophagy stimulation the association of LC3-II to the autophagosomes will increase the concentration of GFP at the autophagosomal membranes, resulting in the visualization of a typical punctuated pattern (**Fig. 2.5b**). Counting the amount of GFP-punctuae per cell provides an excellent method for the quantification of autophagosomes after PDT. Based on the same principle LC3 relocalization can be visualized by immunostaining for the endogenous LC3. However, due to the transient nature of autophagosomes (half-life is 20–30 min) and the basal levels of autophagy as a homeostatic process, an increased LC3 conversion seen on Western blot might indicate either the stimulation of autophagy (increased ON rate) or the inhibition of the degradation of autophagosomes (decreased OFF rate). Only the evaluation of "autophagic flux," the degradation of autophagosomes, and their cargo can distinguish the two events. Pharmacological inhibitors

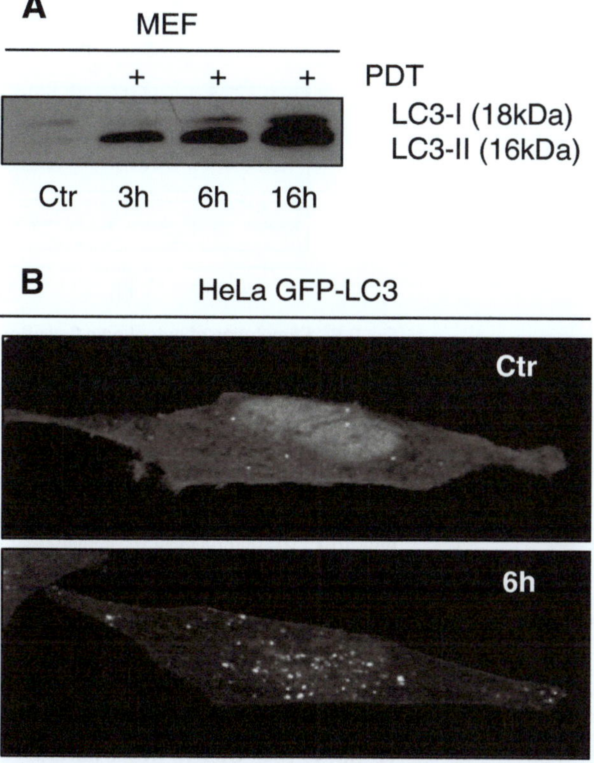

Fig. 2.5. Formation of autophagosomes after hyp-PDT. (**a**) At the indicated time points after irradiation (controls are incubated with hypericin but not irradiated) total protein lysates were made from MEFs and processed for Western blotting according to protocols in **Sections 3.3** and **3.6.1**. Chemiluminescent detection reveals both an induction of LC3-I and a simultaneous conversion to LC3-II, suggesting the formation of autophagosomes after PDT. (**b**) Seventy-two hours before PDT treatment, HeLa cells were transiently transfected with GFP-LC3, according to protocol in **Section 3.6.2**. Six hours after treatment, the cells were visualized on a confocal microscope. The punctuated pattern apparent at the 6 h time point indicates the formation of autophagosomes after hyp-PDT, as also suggested by the Western blot in the *upper panel* (**a**).

of the lysosomal–autophagosomal fusion, such as BafilomycinA1 (BafA1), prevent the formation of autolysosomes and result in the inhibition of LC3-II degradation and autophagic flux. Thus, only if the ON rate of autophagy has been stimulated by PDT, this will result in a superimposed detection of LC3-II caused by the accumulation of autophagosomes. If after co-treatment with BafA1 no increase in LC3-II detection is noticed, one can assume that PDT interferes with the autophagosome–lysosome fusion, limiting the OFF rate. Additionally, in cells transfected with GFP-LC3, GFP is readily separated from LC3-II in the inner membrane during the degradation phase but is very resistant to mammalian hydrolysis. This allows for the monitoring of the accumulation of "free GFP" on Western blot as an accumulating degradation product of autophagy and therefore an event truly representative

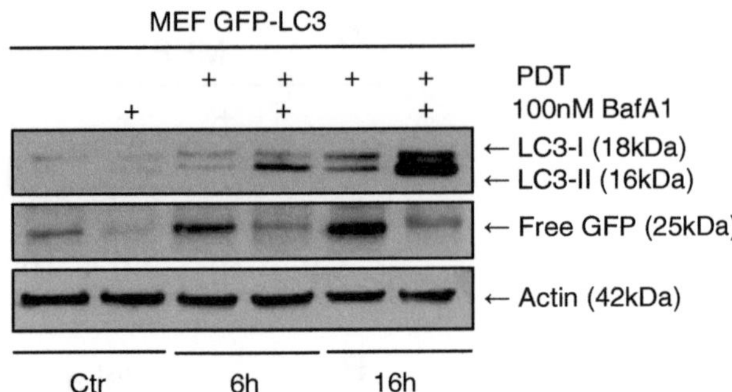

Fig. 2.6. Stimulation of autophagic flux after hyp-PDT. MEFs stably expressing GFP-LC3 were PDT treated and at the indicated time points full protein lysates were made for Western blot application as described in **Sections 3.3** and **3.6.3**. Where indicated 100 nM BafA1 was added to the incubation medium 1 h prior to irradiation. The detection of increasing amounts of "free GFP" indicates the stimulation of autophagic flux which can be inhibited with BafA1. The superimposed detection of LC3-II in the case of BafA1 co-treatment further substantiates the activation of autophagic flux (increased ON rate) after hyp-PDT. Control cells were incubated with hypericin but not irradiated.

for autophagic flux. BafA1 pretreatment inhibits autophagic flux and diminishes the release of "free GFP" (**Fig. 2.6**). Apart from the identification of apoptotic and necrotic cells, TEM analysis remains one of the most sensitive methods to detect the accumulation of autophagic compartments in mammalian cells (**Fig. 2.7**). Autophagosomes are by definition membrane-bound structures that contain cytoplasm (i.e., cytosol and possibly organelles). Structures that do not fulfill this criterion should not be classified as autophagosomes or autophagic vacuoles. Because of the subjective nature of this morphological analysis (*see* **Note 14**), TEM as a method to monitor autophagosomes has to be complemented with other techniques described in this chapter.

3.6.1. LC3 Detection on Western Blot

Total protein lysates are made according to the protocol in **Section 3.2** (*see* **Note 15**). Detection of LC3 on Western blot is carried out according to the protocols described in **Section 3.3**. The LC3 antibody is diluted 1:800 in blocking buffer (*see* **Notes 16** and **17**).

3.6.2. Visualization of Autophagosomes by Overexpressing GFP-LC3 (see Note 18)

1. On day 0, seed HeLa cells at a density of 5×10^5 cells per 10-cm plate. On day 1 transfect cells with GFP-LC3 using FuGENE® HD (Roche Applied Science, Indianapolis, IN, USA):
   a. Replace the medium of the cells with 5 ml antibiotics-free DMEM supplemented with 10% FBS.
   b. Incubate 10 μg vector DNA carrying GFP-LC3 with 15 μl FugeneHD in a total volume of 500 μl DMEM for 15 min at RT.

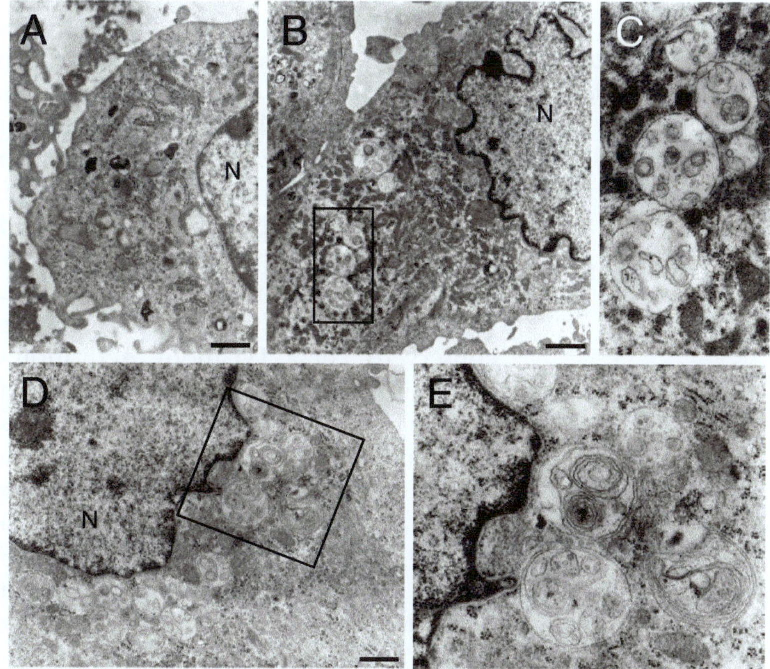

Fig. 2.7. Analysis of cell morphology of autophagic cells by transmission electron microscopy. C2C12 cells were subjected to amino acid deprivation for 12 h. (**a**) Untreated cell showing a normal cell morphology. (**b–e**) Starved cells with numerous autophagic vesicles in the cytosol. (**c**) The *boxed area* in *panels* **b** and **d** is shown at higher magnification in *panels* **c** and **e**, respectively. Scale bar = 1 μm. N indicates nucleus.

c. Add this solution to the cells medium and incubate the plates for 24 h at 37°C.

2. On day 2, replate the transfected cells to a density of 3 × 10^5 cells per 6-cm plate or 5 × 10^4 cells per chamber on a chamber slide. This ensures equal expression (*see* **Note 19**) of GFP-LC3 in all conditions tested.
3. Incubate plates for at least 48 h, or up to 72 h, before analysis on the microscope (*see* **Note 20**).

3.6.3. Autophagic Flux

1. One hour prior to irradiation, 100 nm of BafA1 is added to the medium (*see* **Note 21**).
2. The following steps are carried out according to the protocol described in **Section 3.6.1** for LC3 detection or combined with **Section 3.6.2** if the cells are transfected with GFP-LC3.

3.6.4. Detection of Autophagosomes by TEM

See **Section 3.5**.

3.7. Methods to Monitor MAPK and Akt-mTOR-Signaling Cascades

Signaling pathways governed by the Ser/Thr protein kinases MAPKs and Akt (also known as protein kinase B, PKB) regulate both apoptosis and autophagy. In mammalian cells the three major MAPK family members include the extracellular signal-regulated kinases (ERK 1 and 2), which are typically stimulated in response to growth and differentiation signals, the c-Jun amino-terminal kinases (JNK 1, 2, and 3), and the p38 MAPKs (p38 $\alpha/\beta/\gamma$ and δ), which are activated by a diverse array of stress signals (18). Common for all family members of the MAPKs is the activation by an upstream MAP2K through phosphorylation on a conserverd Thr-X-Tyr motif. Activation of the different MAPKs results in either pro- or anti-apoptotic effects depending on the cellular background and the type of stress.

Cytosolic Akt is recruited to the plasma membrane following the generation of phosphatidylinositol (3,4,5)-trisphosphate (PIP3) by the growth factor-mediated activation of class I PI3 kinase (PI3K), where it becomes phosphorylated on Thr308 and Ser473 by 3-phosphoinositide-dependent kinase-1 (PDK1) and by PDK2, respectively, resulting in its activation (19). Akt activation not only leads to the suppression of apoptosis, a well-studied functional outcome of this pleiotropic pathway, but also of autophagy through the activation of the mammalian target of rapamycin (mTOR). mTOR is a Ser/Thr kinase which, upon activation, leads to inhibition of autophagy while favoring anabolic pathways, such as mRNA translation via the activation of its direct downstream target p70-S6 kinase (20). Whereas the role of MAPKs in PDT has been abundantly scrutinized (2, 21), the role of the Akt-mTOR pathway is still largely unexplored.

Since the activation mechanism of these kinases and often of their downstream kinase substrates entails the phosphorylation of specific residues, a convenient method to monitor the activation status of these signaling cascades after PDT relies on Western blot analysis with antibodies that specifically recognize either the phosphorylated/active or non-phosphorylated/inactive forms of these kinases. If possible, detection of the activation status is performed preferentially by infrared (IR) fluorescence detection with the Odyssey® Imaging System (LiCor Biosciences, Lincoln, NE, USA). This detection method offers several advantages over the classical chemiluminescent method. The use of infrared wavelengths dramatically reduces autofluorescence and light scatter conferring a clean background, high signal-to-noise ratio, and sensitivity. The presence of two different infrared channels allows for probing two separate targets in the same experiment simultaneously (multiplex detection), which makes normalization easy and eliminates errors introduced by stripping and reprobing or by comparison of separate blots. In this way, both the phosphorylated form and the total amount of a given protein (kinase) can be detected at the same time (two-color Western), with the only requirement being the availability of phospho- and total protein-directed antibodies from two different sources (i.e., rabbit and mouse). Additionally, the wide linear dynamic range and accompanying software makes fast and accurate quantification possible. For example, the activation status of mTOR can be monitored indirectly by assessing the phosphorylation status of p70-S6 kinase and its substrate the S6 ribosomal protein. Additionally, kinase immunoprecipitation followed by in vitro kinase assays using specific model substrates has been employed in previous studies (8).

In general, kinetic experiments in PDT exposed cells should be initially performed due to the dynamic regulation of these kinases by (de-)phosphorylation events.

Preparation of lysates and Western blot procedures are performed according to the protocols detailed in **Sections 3.2** and **3.3**, respectively (*see* **Note 22**).

3.7.1. ECL as Detection Method

1. Incubate the membrane with phospho-specific primary antibody diluted in 5% BSA in TBS-T, ON at 4°C with gentle shaking (**Fig. 2.8a**).
2. Proceed for ECL detection of phosphorylated protein as described in Step 9 of protocol in **Section 3.3**.
3. After detection, incubate the membrane in 50 ml stripping buffer for 15 min at 65°C.
4. Wash the membrane several times with fresh TBS-T to remove all traces of β-mercaptoethanol.
5. Incubate the membrane in blocking buffer for 1 h at RT with gentle shaking.
6. Incubate the membrane with the primary antibody for the detection of the total protein diluted in 5% BSA in TBS-T, ON at 4°C with gentle shaking.
7. Proceed for ECL detection of total protein as described in Step 9 of protocol in **Section 3.3**.

3.7.2. Odyssey as Detection Method

1. Because Tween emits IR fluorescence that is detected in the 700 nm channel of the Odyssey, block the membranes in 5% BSA dissolved in TBS without Tween for 1 h at RT with gentle shaking (**Fig. 2.8b**).
2. Incubate the membrane with both phospho-specific and total protein primary antibodies diluted in 5% BSA in TBS-T, ON at 4°C with gentle shaking (*see* **Note 23**).
3. Wash the membrane three times for 15 min in an excess amount of TBS-T.

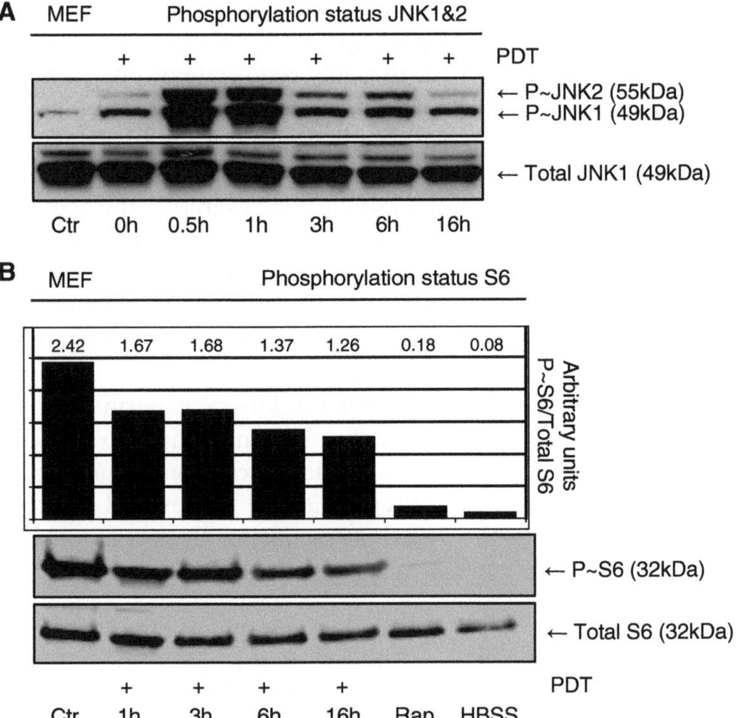

Fig. 2.8. Monitoring the activation status of phosphoproteins. At the indicated time points after PDT, full protein lysates were made for Western blot detection according to the protocols in **Sections 3.2** and **3.3**. Determination of phosphorylation status was performed according to protocol in **Section 3.7.1**. (**a**) *ECL as a detection method* – After the detection of phospho-JNK1 and 2, the membrane was stripped, blocked, and reprobed for the detection of total JNK1. (**b**) *Odyssey as detection method* – Phospho-ribosomal protein S6 (P-S6) and total ribosomal protein S6 (S6) were simultaneously monitored on the Odyssey IR Imager. The graph represents the quantification of the Western blot and is expressed as the level phospho-S6 normalized to the total amount for each time point. Where indicated, samples were treated with 100 nM rapamycin (Rap) or a 2 h starvation in Hank's balanced salt solution (HBSS), two known inducers of autophagy. In all experiments, control cells were incubated with hypericin but not irradiated.

4. Incubate the membrane with both IR-labeled secondary antibodies, diluted 1:5,000 in 5% BSA dissolved in TBS-T for 1 h at RT with gentle shaking.
5. Wash the membrane in subdued light conditions two times for 15 min in an excess amount of TBS-T and once for 15 min with TBS.
6. Scan the membranes on the Odyssey IR Imager for simultaneous detection of phospho- and total protein levels.
7. Use Odyssey software to quantify phospho- and total protein levels and plot the phospho-/total protein ratio.

4. Notes

1. Preliminary experiments with appropriate activity assays should be carried out to define the optimal pre-incubation time for every compound. Generally a pre-incubation time of 1 h at 37°C suffices, when cell permeable compounds are used.
2. The proper amount of protein to load and the dilution range of the primary antibody to use should be assessed in advance in order to establish a linear range of immunodetection for each antibody/antigen pair.
3. If there is too much background staining after visualization, the blocking step can also be performed in 5% BSA solution in TBS±T.
4. Based on the known sequence specificity of the cleavage site for different caspase members, specific substrates have been developed and include Ac-DEVD-AMC for caspases 3 and 7, Ac-LEHD-AMC for caspase 5, Ac-YVAD-AMC for caspases 1 and 4, Ac-IETD-AMC for caspases 8 and 6, and Ac-WEHD-AMC for caspases 1,4, and 5. It should be mentioned, however, that the commercially available substrates, and related FMK inhibitors, do not display restricted specificity. Therefore it is always advisable to combine Western blot assays, for the detection of procaspase processing, with activity assay.
5. In order to detect caspase activity in their natural environment, new tools including activity-based probes, such as CaspACE™ FITC-VAD-FMK In Situ Marker from Promega (Madison, WI, USA), have been developed, which avoid the preparation of lysates and allow a readout of caspase activity state after PDT with minimal interference (Noemi Rubio, personal communication).
6. For quantification of DNA fragmentation during apoptosis a miniaturized (96-well plate format) immunoassays based on the principle of the ELISA (enzyme-linked immunosorbent assay) can also be used. Such assays are commercially available and ensure a high degree of sensitivity. For example, determination of cytoplasmic histone-associated DNA fragments (mono- and oligonucleosomes) using Cell Death Detection ELISA^{PLUS} (Roche Applied Science, Indianapolis, IN, USA) is a useful technique to quantify apoptotic cell death after PDT.
7. The choice of the DNA binding dye is restricted by the absorption and emission spectra of the photosensitizer utilized, which should not overlap.

8. As an alternative method to this Step 3, lysis of the plasma membrane can also be performed with Streptolysin O. Streptolysin O is a bacterial protein that will permeabilize the plasma membrane by binding to cholesterol. Due to the lower abundance of cholesterol in the membranes of organelles, the intracellular membranes will retain their integrity. In this case, resuspend the pellet in 150 μl of stabilization buffer with 200 units of Streptolysin O and transfer to fresh eppendorfs. Vortex shortly and incubate the eppendorfs for 30 min at 37°C. Vortex shortly after incubation and centrifuge for 30 min at 700×g at 4°C.
9. Essential for the protocol is the use of DiOC6(3) in the range of 30–40 nM concentration. At higher concentrations the dye will accumulate also in the membranes of the Golgi apparatus and the endoplasmic reticulum, and it is therefore not longer displaying a specific mitochondrial localization.
10. It should be mentioned that the measurement of $\Delta\psi_m$ may not always be a reliable indicator of IM permeabilization, since a drop in $\Delta\psi_m$ can result from inhibited respiration or from transient openings of the permeability transition pore complex (PTPC), which are not necessarily followed by IM permeabilization. The best technique is the calcein quenching method, which can be employed to measure transient IM permeabilization events. This method relies on the loading of the cells with the fluorescent probe calcein, in its acetoxymethyl ester form, as well as with its quencher, cobalt (Co^{2+}) (22). Calcein diffuses to all subcellular compartments, including mitochondria, whereas Co^{2+} ions are excluded from the mitochondrial matrix because the IM is impermeable to these ions. Therefore, functional mitochondria in healthy cells will be visualized by a punctuate fluorescence signal after confocal fluorescence microscopy, whereas upon transient or permanent IM permeabilization, as observed in different PDT paradigms (4), Co^{2+} enters the mitochondrial matrix and quenches the calcein fluorescence (22).
11. Adherent cells can be trypsinized. However, this procedure should be kept as short as possible as it may cause damage to the original morphology of the cells. One method that helps to circumvent this problem is growing adherent cells on plastic coverslips. A major drawback of the latter approach is that only a small amount of cells per section can be analyzed.
12. After fixation with glutaraldehyde, samples can be stored in 0.1 M sodium cacodylate-buffered (pH 7.4) 7.5% saccharose at 4°C for several days.

13. Reynolds solution should be free of carbon dioxide to prevent formation of $PbCO_3$ deposits. Therefore, always use carbon dioxide-free water and sodium hydroxide (Titrisol). Carbon dioxide-free water is prepared by boiling ultrapure water. After transfer of the boiling water in a separating funnel, a carbon dioxide trap filled with soda lime is connected to the outlet on top of the separating funnel to prevent re-infiltration of fresh carbon dioxide.
14. Interpreting electron microscopy is subjective and it can be difficult to distinguish autophagosomes from lysosomes, endosomes, or other structures in the cell. For example, if mitochondria are swollen or contain precipitates, they can be misinterpreted as autophagosomes. Lipid droplets as well as electron lucent or empty vacuoles are also sometimes incorrectly called autophagic vacuoles. Because these vacuoles have no contents, it is not possible to say whether they are autophagic compartments or some other kind of vacuoles. An additional complication is that maturation of mammalian autophagosomes involves a transition to single-membrane structures (i.e., amphisomes and autolysosomes). Therefore, the presence of a double limiting membrane should not be used as a criterion for the identification of autophagosomes. Sometimes, the limiting membrane of autophagic compartments may not have contrast at all, probably due to lipid extraction during sample preparation.
15. LC3-I is highly susceptible to degradation in the lysis buffer, especially during freeze–thaw cycles. Samples with loading buffer should be made as soon as possible after lysis to prevent degradation of LC3-I.
16. The endogenous expression of LC3 might vary notably between cells of different origin. In our experience it is easier to detect LC3 with the commercially available antibody in cells of murine origin than of human origin. The amount of protein and/or concentration of the antibody used might have to be adapted accordingly.
17. The majority of the antibodies for LC3 detection have a higher affinity for LC3-II. This is probably due to the hydrophobic nature of the protein.
18. If overexpression of GFP-LC3 is contraindicated (e.g., transfection problems or another vector carrying a GFP tag), autophagosomes can also be visualized by immunocytochemical staining for endogenous LC3 (use 1–10 μg/ml ab diluted in 1% BSA with 10% serum).
19. GFP-LC3 tends to aggregate in the cell when expressed at high levels, forming "punctuae" independent of the induction of autophagy. Untreated cells and rapamycin-treated

cells as positive controls should be included in the assay. Furthermore, for the visualization of the GFP-LC3 punctuae a mild expression level of the chimeric construct will generate the best results as it will prevent the GFP-LC3-II punctuae from "fading away" in a strong cytoplasmic staining of LC3-I.

20. To detect the specific removal of PDT-damaged organelles by autophagy, a LC3 co-localization analysis can be performed. Either a fluorescent organelle "tracker" or a marker protein, which is specifically targeted to an organelle, can be used for co-localization studies. The latter case requires that the primary antibodies against the marker protein and LC3 have been raised in a different species and that the corresponding secondary antibodies are labeled with different fluorochromes but raised in the same species to prevent crossreactivity. It is also important to make sure that their absorption and excitation spectra do not overlap with those of hypericin or other photosensitizers used. Alternatively hypericin can be washed out during the staining procedure when using 100% ice-cold methanol as a permeabilization agent instead of Triton X-100.
21. When using BafA1 as an inhibitor of autophagy one has to take into account that BafA1 has apoptosis-inducing effects.
22. When monitoring phosphoproteins by Western blotting, replacement of the blocking buffer by 5% BSA in TBS±T is recommended. BSA will repress the crossreactivity of the phospho-specific antibodies with the phosphoproteins present in the milk powder, resulting in a lower background and an enhanced reactivity of the antibodies with their target proteins.
23. While it is essential to remove Tween from the blocking buffer, it does not confer detection problems if added to the incubation buffer for the antibodies. All traces of Tween will be removed in the final washing step (Step 5) with TBS without Tween.

Acknowledgments

The work in author's laboratory is supported by OT/06/49 grant of the Catholic University of Leuven, by F.W.O grants G.0492.05 and G.0661.09. This chapter presents research results of the IAP6/18, funded by the Interuniversity Attraction Poles

Programme, initiated by the Belgian State, Science Policy Office. Michael Dewaele's research is funded by a Ph.D. grant of the Institute for the Promotion of Innovation through Science and Technology in Flanders (IWT-Vlaanderen). Dr. Wim Martinet is a postdoctoral fellow of the F.W.O. Flanders.

References

1. Kroemer, G., Galluzzi, L., Vandenabeele, P., Abrams, J., Alnemri, E. S. et al. (2008) Classification of cell death: recommendations of the Nomenclature Committee on Cell Death 2009. *Cell Death Differ*, **16**, 3–11.
2. Oleinick, N. L., Morris, R. L., and Belichenko, I. (2002) The role of apoptosis in response to photodynamic therapy: what, where, why, and how. *Photochem Photobiol Sci*, **1**(1), 1–21.
3. Dolmans, D. E., Fukumura, D., and Jain, R. K. (2003) Photodynamic therapy for cancer. *Nat Rev Cancer*, **3**(5), 380–387.
4. Buytaert, E., Dewaele, M., and Agostinis, P. (2007) Molecular effectors of multiple cell death pathways initiated by photodynamic therapy. *Biochim Biophys Acta*, **1776**(1), 86–107.
5. Yorimitsu, T. and Klionsky, D. J. (2007) Eating the endoplasmic reticulum: quality control by autophagy. *Trends Cell Biol*, **17**(6), 279–285.
6. Mizushima, N., Levine, B., Cuervo, A. M., and Klionsky, D. J. (2008) Autophagy fights disease through cellular self-digestion. *Nature*, **451**(7182), 1069–1075.
7. Falk, H., Meyer, J., and Oberreiter, M. (1993) A convenient semisynthetic route to hypericin. *Monatshefte fur Chemie*, **124**(3), 339–341.
8. Assefa, Z., Vantieghem, A., Declercq, W., Vandenabeele, P., Vandenheede, J. R. et al. (1999) The activation of the c-Jun N-terminal kinase and p38 mitogen-activated protein kinase signaling pathways protects HeLa cells from apoptosis following photodynamic therapy with hypericin. *J Biol Chem*, **274**(13), 8788–8796.
9. Agostinis, P., Vantieghem, A., Merlevede, W., and De Witte, P. A. (2002) Hypericin in cancer treatment: more light on the way. *Int J Biochem Cell Biol*, **34**(3), 221–241.
10. Buytaert, E., Callewaert, G., Hendrickx, N., Scorrano, L., Hartmann, D. et al. (2006) Role of endoplasmic reticulum depletion and multidomain proapoptotic BAX and BAK proteins in shaping cell death after hypericin-mediated photodynamic therapy. *FASEB J*, **20**(6), 756–758.
11. Salvesen, G. S. and Riedl, S. J. (2008) Caspase mechanisms. *Adv Exp Med Biol*, **615**, 13–23.
12. van Loo, G., Saelens, X., van Gurp, M., MacFarlane, M., Martin, S. J. et al. (2002) The role of mitochondrial factors in apoptosis: a Russian roulette with more than one bullet. *Cell Death Differ*, **9**(10), 1031–1042.
13. Cummings, M. C., Winterford, C. M., and Walker, N. I. (1997) Apoptosis. *Am J Surg Pathol*, **21**(1), 88–101.
14. Falcieri, E., Gobbi, P., Cataldi, A., Zamai, L., Faenza, I. et al. (1994) Nuclear pores in the apoptotic cell. *Histochem J*, **26**(9), 754–763.
15. Kerr, J. F., Winterford, C. M., and Harmon, B. V. (1994) Apoptosis. Its significance in cancer and cancer therapy. *Cancer*, **73**(8), 2013–2026.
16. Clarke, P. G. (1990) Developmental cell death: morphological diversity and multiple mechanisms. *Anat Embryol (Berl)*, **181**(3), 195–213.
17. Klionsky, D. J., Abeliovich, H., Agostinis, P., Agrawal, D. K., Aliev, G. et al. (2007) Guidelines for the use and interpretation of assays for monitoring autophagy in higher eukaryotes. *Autophagy*, **4**(2), 139–140.
18. Chang, L. and Karin, M. (2001) Mammalian MAP kinase signalling cascades. *Nature*, **410**(6824), 37–40.
19. Woodgett, J. R. (2005) Recent advances in the protein kinase B signaling pathway. *Curr Opin Cell Biol*, **17**(2), 150–157.
20. Hay, N. (2005) The Akt-mTOR tango and its relevance to cancer. *Cancer Cell*, **8**(3), 179–183.
21. Agostinis, P., Buytaert, E., Breyssens, H., and Hendrickx, N. (2004) Regulatory pathways in photodynamic therapy induced apoptosis. *Photochem Photobiol Sci*, **3**(8), 721–729.
22. Bernardi, P., Scorrano, L., Colonna, R., Petronilli, V., and Di, L. F. (1999) Mitochondria and cell death. Mechanistic aspects and methodological issues. *Eur J Biochem*, **264**(3), 687–701.

Chapter 3

Photodynamic Therapy and Cell Death Pathways

David Kessel and Nancy L. Oleinick

Abstract

Photodynamic therapy (PDT) is the term used to describe the irradiation of photosensitized cells or tissue with phototoxic consequences. This process can result in the rapid initiation of not only apoptosis, an irreversible death pathway, but also autophagy. The procedures described here are designed to characterize the correlation between the PDT dose vs. survival of cells in vitro, the apoptotic effects of photodamage, and the extent of an autophagic response. These are assessed by clonogenic assays, observation of condensed chromatin characteristic of apoptosis, activation of "executioner" caspases, and the autophagic flux as indicated by comparing accumulation of the LC3-II protein under conditions where processing of autophagosomes is retarded vs. is not retarded.

Key words: Apoptosis, autophagy, Bcl-2, Bid, Bax, photosensitization, photodynamic therapy.

1. Introduction

Photodynamic therapy (PDT) is a procedure for cancer control based on the selective localization of photosensitizing agents (often porphyrins or its analogs) in malignant cells and tissues (1). When photosensitized cells are irradiated with light at a wavelength corresponding to the absorbance band of the photosensitizing agent, this leads to two distinct phenomena: fluorescence and an energy transfer process. The latter can convert dissolved oxygen ($^3O_2$) in cells or tissues into a highly reactive intermediate termed "singlet oxygen" ($^1O_2$). Once formed, $^1O_2$ immediately reacts with biological systems, usually nearby lipids and proteins. If sufficient drug and light are provided, this results in a selective means for oxidative stress and tumor eradication. Additional

C.J. Gomer (ed.), *Photodynamic Therapy*, Methods in Molecular Biology 635,
DOI 10.1007/978-1-60761-697-9_3, © Springer Science+Business Media, LLC 2010

reactive oxygen species may also be formed, but the immediate precursor is believed to be $^1O_2$ in most cases.

This report will deal with procedures for identifying the immediate consequences of PDT in cell culture: apoptosis and autophagy. The former results from photodamage to Bcl-2/Bcl-xL and/or lysosomes (2–8), while the latter can be both a repair process and a death mode (9–13). Subsequent biochemical processes in dying cells can evoke a variety of stress responses, upregulation of heat-shock proteins, and similar phenomena. These will be discussed elsewhere in this volume.

Several photosensitizing agents have been approved for clinical use, and many others are in clinical and pre-clinical trials. These agents are not always commercially available. Common porphyrins and phthalocyanines can be obtained from the major suppliers, e.g., Sigma-Aldrich. A large selection of porphyrins, phthalocyanines, and related compounds is available from Frontier Science, PO Box 31, Logan, Utah 84323-0031 (www.info@frontiersci.com). Frontier Science can carry out a custom preparation of any agent whose structure and synthetic route has been published. In this report, we will discuss the procedures utilized for a product that can be purchased from VWR, the benzoporphyrin derivative (BPD, Verteporfin). This photosensitizer is approved by the United States Food and Drug Administration for the treatment of age-related macular degeneration.

The report is also written for study of L1210 mouse leukemia cells, which grow in suspension. It should be noted that many workers use cell lines that are derived from human carcinomas representative of the type of cancers treated with PDT. Such lines grow attached to a tissue culture flask or dish, and some procedures described below differ when applied to these cultures.

2. Materials

2.1. Cell Culture and Photosensitization

1. The "alpha" modification of minimum essential Eagle's medium (Sigma-Aldrich, St Louis, MO) supplemented with 10% horse serum (Atlanta Biologicals, Norcross, GA) + 2.2 g/l of $NaHCO_3$ and 10 mg/l gentamicin (Invitrogen) as an antibiotic, although others can be employed (*see* **Note 1**).
2. Fisher's medium with 10% horse serum (FHS): $NaHCO_3$ is omitted from the medium and is replaced with 20 mM HEPES buffer, pH 7.0. This permits short-term maintenance of high-density cell cultures at a neutral pH.

3. Benzoporphyrin derivative (BPD; VWR, Westchester, PA) dissolved in DMSO at a concentration of 7.12 mg/ml (10 mM and further diluted to 1 mM with DMSO (*see* **Note 2**)).

2.2. Irradiation System

1. A 700-W Oriel quartz-halogen light source or an equivalent capable of producing 1–10 mW/cm^2 of light at wavelengths between 600 and 750 nm, with a bandwidth of 10 nm. Diode lasers can also accomplish this purpose (Intense, Inc., North Brunswick, NJ) (*see* **Note 3**).
2. Interference filters: For BPD, a filter with a center wavelength of 690 nm and a bandwidth of 10 nm can be obtained from Oriel (Newport Corporation, Stratford, CT). It is also possible to use a filter system with a broader bandwidth, but the pertinent light dose needs to be calculated at wavelengths for which there is an absorbance band.
3. Water filter (10 cm of water in the light path): This reduces the contribution of infrared radiation and can also be obtained from Newport/Oriel.
4. Power density monitor (ScienTech H 10 or equivalent; Scientech, Inc., Boulder, CO (*see* **Note 4**)).

2.3. DEVDase Assays

1. Phosphate-buffered saline (PBS): 130 mM NaCl, 20 mM sodium phosphate, pH 7.
2. Insect lysis buffer (BD Biosciences, San Jose CA).
3. EnzChek caspase 3 assay kit #2 from Invitrogen. This relies on a fluorogenic interaction between caspase activity and DEVD-rhodamine 110, releasing the free rhodamine dye.
4. Protein assay system: Biuret reagent (Sigma-Aldrich); Folin–Ciocalteau phenol reagent (Sigma-Aldrich).

2.4. Fluorescence Microscopy

1. Hoechst dye HO3342 (Sigma-Aldrich).
2. Fluorescence microscope with an appropriate filter cube for HO342 fluorescence (excitation 350–380 nm, emission >400 nm (*see* **Note 5**)).
3. CoolSnap CCD camera (Photometrics, Tucson, AZ) and MetaMorph software (Molecular Devices) or equivalent image-capturing system and processing software.

2.5. Western Blots for Autophagy

1. Insect lysis buffer (BD Biosciences, San Jose, CA).
2. SDS buffer: 2X Tris-glycine SDS sample buffer (Invitrogen, Carlsbad, CA).
3. 4–20% Tris-glycine gels (Invitrogen).
4. 5% blocking buffer (Amersham division/GE, Buckinghamshire, UK).

5. PVDF membrane (Invitrogen).
6. TBS-T (20 mM Tris–HCl, pH 7.6, 137 mM NaCl, 0.1% Tween 20) and add an antibody to the autophagy-associated protein LC3 (Proteintech Group, Inc., Chicago, IL) (*see* **Note 6**).
7. Secondary antibody: Anti-Rabbit IgG, alkaline phosphatase-linked whole antibody (Amersham).
8. ECF substrate Amersham/GE Western blotting reagent pack.
9. Novex mini-cell electrophoresis chamber.

2.6. Clonogenic Assays for L1210 Cells

1. Agar (Sigma-Aldrich).
2. Thiazolium salt (Sigma-Aldrich).
3. 96-well plates NUNC, Roskilde, Denmark.

2.7. Clonogenic Assays for Adherent Cells

1. 0.25% trypsin (1X) solution with EDTA (Hyclone Laboratories, Inc., Logan, UT).
2. 60-mm tissue culture Petri dishes (Becton Dickinson Labware, Franklin Lakes, NJ).
3. 0.1% crystal violet (Fisher Scientific) in 20% ethanol.

3. Methods

3.1. Photosensitization of Cells

1. Exponentially growing L1210 cells are collected by centrifugation (500×*g*, 10 min), then resuspended in FHS at a density of 7 mg/ml (wet weight). This corresponds to a cell count of 2.5×10^6/ml.
2. Portions of 1 ml each are placed in glass tubes and treated with a 1 mM solution of BPD in DMSO (final concentration = 2 μM).
3. Incubate cells for 30 min at 37°C, then collect by centrifugation (100×*g*, 30 s) using a mini-centrifuge.
4. Resuspend the cell pellets in cold FHS and irradiate in a chamber that maintains the temperature at 10°C (*see* **Note 7**).
5. At this point, the cells can be used for evaluation of immediate photodamage or incubated for 30–60 min to follow the time course of apoptosis and autophagy.

3.2. DEVDase Assay

1. Using control cells and cells treated with varying PDT doses, wash 7 mg cell pellets in phosphate-buffered saline (PBS,

130 mM NaCl + 20 mM sodium phosphate, pH 7), then disperse in 110 μl of insect lysis buffer at 4°C.

2. Vortex this mixture at 10 min intervals for 1 h.
3. Spin down the debris (2,500 rpm, 4°C, 1 min), then take two 50 μl samples of the supernatant fluid for duplicate determinations of caspase 3/7 activity.
4. Prepare a working solution composed of 590 μl of water, 400 μl of reaction buffer, 10 μl of 1 M DTT, and 10 μl of 5 mM z-DEVD-R110 substrate. These components are contained in the assay kit.
5. Pipette the 50 μl aliquots (in duplicate) of samples into wells of a 96-well plate designed for fluorescence measurements (*see* **Note 8**).
6. Add 50 μl of working solution to each well and start the program.
7. Monitor appearance of fluorescence with a fluorescence plate reader. A typical result is shown in **Fig. 3.1**. Wells A1 and A2 are controls. Other samples received different PDT doses or reflect the presence of caspase inhibitors. The highest PDT dose was given to the sample shown in well C1.

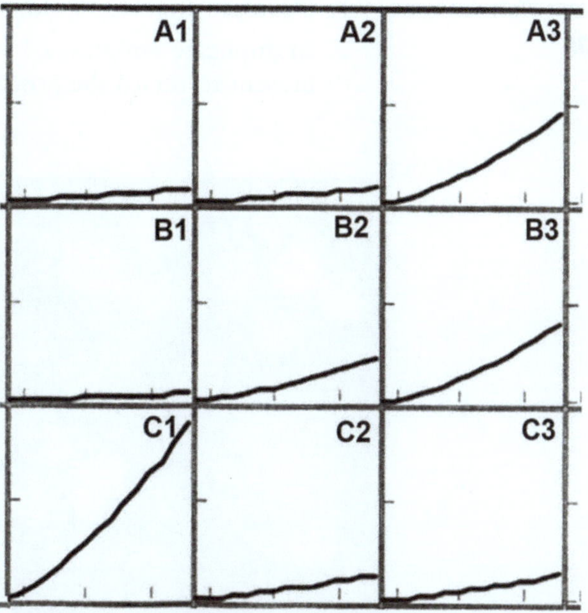

Fig. 3.1. Fluorogenic effects of PDT in the caspase 3/7 assay system. Numbers in each cell reflect the position of the sample in the 96-well plate. A1 and B1 are controls; other samples received different PDT doses.

8. Using a sample of R110 provided in the kit, determine the fluorescence intensity of a series of different concentrations. From this and the acquired data, the rate of the enzyme reaction can be calculated in terms of nanomole substrate hydrolyzed per minute.
9. Determine the protein concentration in an aliquot of the cell extracts so that caspase activity can be calculated (nmol/mg protein/min).

3.3. Fluorescence Microscopy

1. After irradiation, incubate cells (7 mg/ml in FHS) for 60 min at 37°C, adding 2 μM Höchst dye 33342 (HO342) during the final 5 min.
2. Collect cells by centrifugation at 100×*g* for 30 s, then resuspend in 5 μl of growth medium.
3. Examine patterns of HO342 fluorescence using fluorescence microscopy.
4. Apoptotic chromatin patterns can be detected by noting relative numbers of fragmented nuclei (*see* **Note 9**). Typical images are shown in **Fig. 3.2**, with the figure to the left showing normal chromatin and the image on the right reflecting the apoptotic response to an LD_{90} PDT dose. Approximately 50% of the cells were apoptotic 60 min after irradiation.

3.4. Western Blots for Autophagy

1. Photosensitize and irradiate cells as specified above.
2. In duplicate samples, a 15 mM concentration of NH_4Cl is present to retard the processing of autophagosomes.

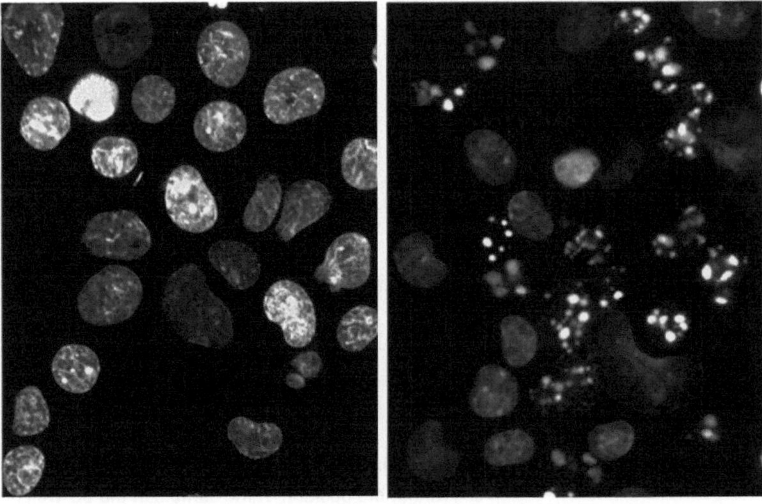

Fig. 3.2. Typical patterns of chromatin labeled with H0342. *Left*, control L1210 cells; *right*, 60 min after an LD_{90} PDT dose using BPD.

3. Prepare lysates by mixing 7 mg cell pellets in 110 μl of Insect cell lysis buffer.
4. Incubate the lysates on ice for 30–60 min.
5. Centrifuge at 2,500×*g* for 1 min at 5°C. Discard debris.
6. Use a 10 μl portion of the lysate for determination of protein concentration.
7. Dilute lysates 1:1 with 2X Tris-glycine SDS sample buffer. Heat to 80°C for 5 min in stoppered tubes. Then cool. These samples can be stored at –70°C before electrophoresis.
8. Based on the protein concentration, determine the amount of samples to be used for electrophoresis. We generally use 40 μg of protein/well.
9. Apply samples to a 4–20% gradient gel.
10. Electrophoresis is carried out at room temperature using a potential of 25 V for 1–1.5 h.
11. Transfer proteins from the gel to a PVDF membrane in a chilled chamber for 1 h.
12. Block membrane with 5% blocking buffer for 1 h at room temperature or overnight at 4°C.
13. Rinse membrane with TBS-T (20 mM Tris-HCl, pH 7.6, 137 mM NaCl, 0.1% Tween 20) and add an LC3 antibody at 1:1,000 dilution. Incubate at room temperature with gentle agitation for 1 h or overnight at 4°C.
14. Wash membrane three times with TBS-T for 5 min each.
15. Apply the secondary antibody: Anti-rabbit IgG alkaline phosphatase-linked whole antibody at 1:10,000 in TBS-T.
16. Incubate at room temperature with gentle agitation for 1 h.
17. Wash three times using TBS-T for 5 min each.
18. Drain membrane and then apply the ECF substrate (Amersham/GE Western blotting reagent pack) to the protein side using 24 μl/cm^2. Remove all air bubbles and incubate for 5 min at room temperature.
19. Assess fluorescence on the membrane using blue wavelength excitation and a 570-nm emission filter (STORM 840 system, Molecular Dynamics, Sunnyvale, CA). **Figure 3.3** demonstrates the conversion of LC3-I to LC3-II, an index of autophagy. The effects of ammonium chloride can readily be seen: this retards the processing of autophagosomes providing an indication of the autophagic flux (13, 14).
20. Membranes can be stored dry at 2–8°C for re-probing if necessary (*see* **Notes 6** and **10**).

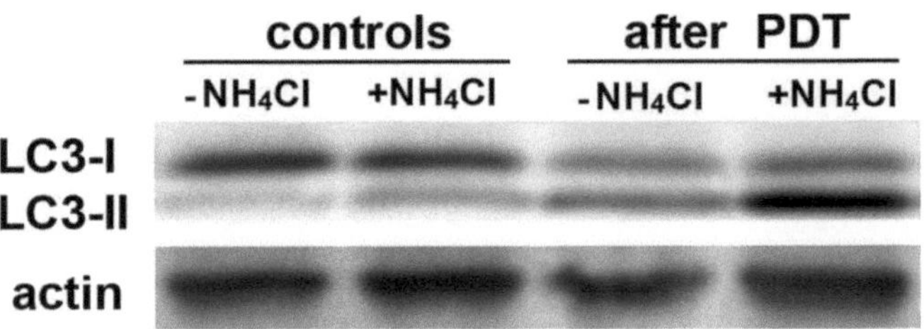

Fig. 3.3. Conversion of LC3-I to LC3-II during PDT. Cells were treated with BPD and given a 25 mJ/cm^2 light dose. Lysates were prepared for Western blots 15 min later. Where shown, 15 mM ammonium chloride was present during all incubations. A probe for actin was used to confirm that equal levels of protein were applied to each lane.

3.5. Clonogenic Assays

1. Using sterile conditions, prepare a 30% solution of agar in water, heat to 60°C to dissolve, then dilute 1:10 with growth medium. This solution is poured into 60-mm diameter plates and allowed to cool.

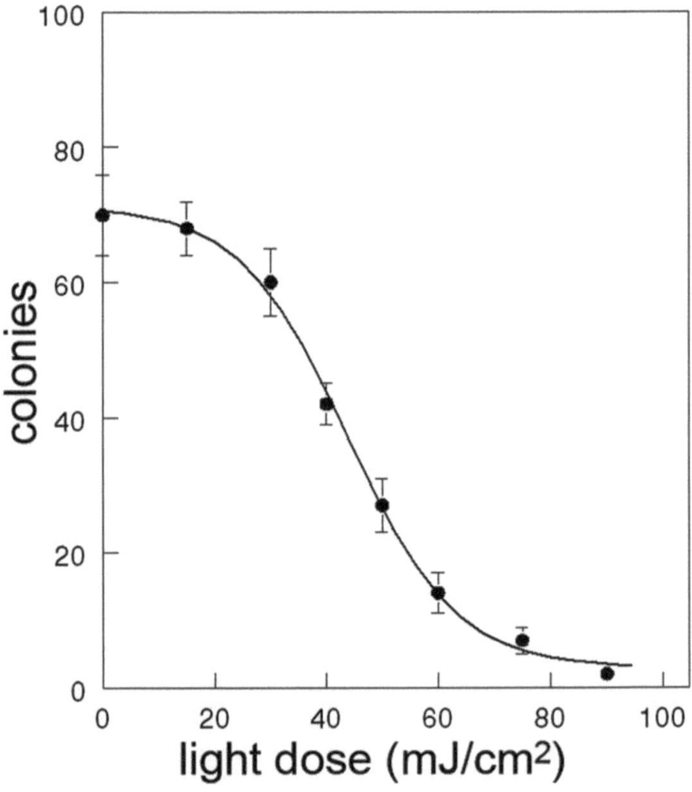

Fig. 3.4. Dose–response curve for L1210 cells using BPD and 690 ± 10 nm light. Cells were incubated with 2 μM BPD for 30 min, then irradiated as described in the text. Data indicate numbers of colonies/plate after 10 days. Approximately 100 cells were plated using light doses of 0–50 mJ/cm^2 and 1,000 cells for greater light doses.

2. Using a cell counter, dilute cultures of treated (photosensitized and irradiated) and control cells so that 100–10,000 cells are placed on each plate (*see* **Note 11**).
3. For PDT-treated cells provide other dilutions, since some protocols will kill 90–99% of the cells. We normally plate several dilutions. The cell suspensions (20 μl) are added to the plates and spread over the surface with a sterile rod.
4. Incubate the plates in a humidified CO_2 incubator at 37°C (5% CO_2) for several days until distinct micro-colonies are seen.
5. Add 0.5 ml of 0.1% thiazolyl blue tetrazolium bromide (Sigma) to each plate. After 3–24 h, the colonies are counted using an inverted microscope (×10 magnification). The dose–response curve obtained with L1210 cells and BPD at different light doses is shown in **Fig. 3.4**.

4. Notes

1. For growth of murine leukemia L1210 cells, we supplement this medium so as to approximate the composition of Fisher's medium, which is no longer available. We add 45 mg/l $MgCl_2$, 75 mg/l methionine, 30 mg/l phenylalanine, 30 mg/l valine, and 9 mg/l folic acid.

   Other cells that we have used in studies of PDT-induced cell death include several human carcinoma cell lines, such as the human breast cancer MCF-7 cells and human prostate DU145 and PC-3 cells, and human skin cancer A431 cells. They require different media (RPMI 1640 or Eagle's minimal essential medium with 10% fetal bovine serum). Furthermore, since these cells grow attached to the substratum, procedures for studying them must be modified slightly. For example, we use trypsin–EDTA to release the cells from the monolayer and gentle pipetting to break cell clumps into single cells before counting and replating.
2. There are dozens of compounds with photosensitizing capacity. In this report, use of BPD is illustrated since, unlike many of the others, this is readily available from a laboratory supply company and can be used without any special solubilization or formulation process. However, if another photosensitizer is used, it may be necessary to dissolve it in different medium. Many of the photosensitizers are hydrophobic, so use of DMSO, DMF, or ethanol is often employed. When these solvents are used, it is important to prepare a sufficiently concentrated stock solution

so that the amount of the organic solvent added to the cultures never exceeds 0.1%, or if more is needed, it must be determined that none of the responses to be studied is affected by the solvent.

3. The fiber optic output from these diodes can deliver light at doses up to 250–500 mW, but these devices are essentially confined to single wavelengths. Varying the temperature of the diode can change this but only by a few nanometer. A lamp system that can be configured to deliver a 2′ diameter circle of light will permit the irradiation of several wells or small tubes. The diode system is excellent for irradiation of single tubes or cell samples in a cuvette where something else is being monitored. Quantum Devices can fabricate large arrays of LEDs at specified wavelengths for irradiation of multiple wells or tubes. These can deliver several 100 mW/cm^2.
4. The light dose is calculated in terms of the photons actually absorbed by the photosensitizing agent. Investigators often report the total light dose over a broad wavelength range, where only a small portion of the total dose will be pertinent to PDT effects.
5. We have successfully used a Nikon Eclipse E600 scope fitter with Nikon Plan Fluor objectives. We have also employed a water immersion objective (60X Plan Apo VC) for acquiring a series of images acquired with a "z" drive. There is less drag with this objective than with an oil immersion system so that a series of images acquired using a "z" drive will show better registration. Such a series, coupled with an image-processing program, can be used to show enhanced lysosomal expression during autophagy.
6. The general procedure for Western blots can also be used to monitor the levels and changes in levels of any protein for which an antibody is available. For example, antibodies to apoptosis-associated proteins, such as Bcl-2 family members, caspases, and apoptosis-initiating factor, are available from several different suppliers. For each primary antibody, the secondary antibody must recognize the IgG of the specie in which the primary antibody was raised.
7. By manipulating the temperature of irradiation, it is possible to alter the immediate consequences. After Bcl-2 photodamage, insertion of Bax into mitochondria occurs only when the temperature is greater than 15°C (15). It is therefore possible to carry out irradiation at a temperature <15°C so as to prevent the initiation of apoptosis, so that localization and certain other studies can be carried out before any additional effects occur. With adherent human carcinoma cells in culture, all of the metabolic responses

occur more slowly than in leukemic cells at equally toxic PDT doses. As a result, as long as the dose is lethal but not supralethal (e.g., killing no more than 90% of the cells), the early steps in apoptosis will be delayed for several minutes to hours without maintaining low temperatures. For these cells, photoirradiation is accomplished by placing the flask or dish in which the cells are growing directly on a glass plate above a suitable light source. After irradiation, the cells can be recovered immediately for measurement of initial photodynamic damage or the flasks can be returned to the incubator and recovered at later times for monitoring of delayed responses.

8. We employ the Fluoroskan Ascent plate reader (Thermo Scientific) using excitation at 485 nm and emission at 538 nm; settings appropriate for fluorescein. This is done at 2 min intervals over 30 min at room temperature. The maximum slope of the resulting fluorescence intensity curve is acquired and compared with standards provided in the kit.
9. It is also feasible to collect a series of planes using a Z-drive system (Prior Scientific Instruments, Folbourn, Cambridge, UK). These can be processed for maximum signal strength or maximum focus, using MetaMorph software or with the AutoQuant software (Media Cybernetics, Bethesda, MD). The latter is a system said to save rather than discard the out-of-focus pixels. This process produces images comparable with confocal fluorescence microscopy.
10. We have recently been exploring use of the Snap ID gel apparatus (Millipore). This uses a vacuum system to speed processing of gels and can cut 1 day off of the time involved. The results appear to be equivalent to the procedure outlined above.
11. The plating efficiency of L1210 cells is 60–70%, so that control plates will contain 60–70 colonies. Depending on the degree of cell kill, plating 100 cells could result in a plate containing 6–7 cells (LD_{90} conditions) or less. In order to deal with such an outcome, we normally plate between 1,000 and 10,000 photosensitized and irradiated cells. Under LD_{99} conditions, plating 10,000 cells will result in the appearance of 60–70 colonies. All such studies are done in triplicate. For human carcinoma cells, the cells must be released from the monolayer with 0.25% trypsin-EDTA, counted, and then plated at appropriate numbers in 60-mm Petri dishes without agar. After 10–14 days, colonies are stained with 0.1% crystal violet and counted. Plating efficiencies of human carcinoma cells are generally lower than for rodent cells, usually <50%; therefore, more cells must be plated to obtain a suitable number of colonies.

Acknowledgments

The authors' research is supported by NIH grant CA 23378 (to DK) and NIH grant CA 106491 (to NLO) from the National Cancer Institute, DHHS and by the State of Ohio Biomedical Research and Technology Transfer Trust TECH 05-063 (to NLO).

References

1. Dougherty, T. J., Gomer, C. J., Henderson, B. W., Jori, G., Kesse, L. D., Korbelik, M., Moan, J., and Peng, Q. (1998) Photodynamic therapy. *J Natl Cancer Inst*, **90**, 889–905.
2. Kim, H. R., Luo, Y., Li, G., and Kessel, D. (1999) Enhanced apoptotic response to photodynamic therapy after Bcl-2 transfection. *Cancer Res*, **59**, 3429–3432.
3. Kessel, D. and Castelli, M. (2001) Evidence that Bcl-2 is the target of three photosensitizers that induce a rapid apoptotic response. *Photochem Photobiol*, **74**, 318–322.
4. Xue, L. Y., Chiu, S. M., and Oleinick, N. L. (2001) Photochemical destruction of the Bcl-2 oncoprotein during photodynamic therapy with the phthalocyanine photosensitizer Pc 4. *Oncogene*, **20**, 3420–3427.
5. Xue, L. Y., Chiu, S. M., Fiebig, A., Andrews, D. W., and Oleinick, N. L. (2003) Photodamage to multiple Bcl-xL isoforms by photodynamic therapy with the phthalocyanine photosensitizer Pc 4. *Oncogene*, **22**, 9197–9204.
6. Kessel, D. and Reiners, J. J., Jr. (2007) Apoptosis and autophagy after mitochondrial or endoplasmic reticulum photodamage. *Photochem Photobiol*, **83**, 1024–1028.
7. Reiners, J. J., Jr., Caruso., J. A., Mathieu, P., Chelladurai, B., Yin, X. M., and Kessel, D. (2002) Release of cytochrome c and activation of pro-caspase-9 following lysosomal photodamage involves Bid cleavage. *Cell Death Differ*, **9**, 934–944.
8. Rodriguez, M. E., Azizuddin, K., Chiu, S. M., Xue, L. Y., Zhang, P., Lam, M., Kenney, M. E., Nieminen, A. L., and Oleinick, N. L. (2009) Structural factors and mechanisms underlying the improved photodynamic cell killing with silicon phthalocyanine photosensitizers directed to lysosomes vs. mitochondria. *Photochem Photobiol*, **85**, 1189–1200.
9. Buytaert, E., Callewaert, G., Hendrickx, N., Scorrano, L., Hartmann, D., Missiaen, L., Vandenheede, J. R., Heirman, I., Grooten, J., and Agostinis, P. (2006) Role of endoplasmic reticulum depletion and multidomain proapoptotic BAX and BAK proteins in shaping cell death after hypericin-mediated photodynamic therapy. *FASEB J*, **20**, 756–758.
10. Kessel, D. and Arroyo, A. S. (2007) Apoptotic and autophagic responses to Bcl-2 inhibition and photodamage. *Photochem Photobiol Sci*, **6**, 1290–1295.
11. Kessel, D., Vicente, M. G., and Reiners, J. J., Jr. (2006) Initiation of apoptosis and autophagy by photodynamic therapy. *Lasers Surg Med*, **38**, 482–488.
12. Xue, L. Y., Chiu, S. M., Azizuddin, K., Joseph, S., and Oleinick, N. L. (2007) The death of human cancer cells following photodynamic therapy: apoptosis competence is necessary for Bcl-2 protection but not for induction of autophagy. *Photochem Photobiol*, **83**, 1016–1023.
13. Klionsky, D. et al. (2008) Guidelines for the use and interpretation of assays for monitoring autophagy in higher eukaryotes. *Autophagy*, **4**, 151–175.
14. Mizushima, N. and Yoshimori, T. (2007) How to interpret LC3 immunoblotting. *Autophagy*, **3**, 542–545.
15. Pryde, J. G., Walker, A., Rossi, A. G., Hannah, S., and Haslett, C. (2000) Temperature-dependent arrest of neutrophil apoptosis. Failure of Bax insertion into mitochondria at 15 degrees C prevents the release of cytochrome c. *J Biol Chem*, **275**, 33574–33584.
16. Iwai-Kanai, E., Yuan, H., Huang, C., Sayen, M. R., Perry-Garza, C. N., Kim, L., and Gottlieb, R. A. (2008) A method to measure cardiac autophagic flux in vivo. *Autophagy*, **4**, 322–329.

Chapter 4

Identification of MAP Kinase Pathways Involved in COX-2 Expression Following Photofrin Photodynamic Therapy

Marian Luna, Angela Ferrario, Sam Wong, and Charles J. Gomer

Abstract

Photodynamic therapy (PDT) using the photosensitizer Photofrin is approved for the clinical treatment of solid tumors. PDT causes cytotoxic oxidative stress, but additionally induces prosurvival molecules such as cyclooxygenase-2 (COX-2). Combining PDT with COX-2 inhibitors increases the efficacy of in vivo treatment. Understanding mechanisms leading to prosurvival molecule induction is relevant to the design of more effective treatments. Using COX-2 promoter constructs, transcription factor-binding assays, identification of protein kinase activation, and inhibitors of transcription factor binding we were able to determine that COX-2 expression following PDT involves the p38 MAP kinase pathway.

Key words: Photofrin (PH), photodynamic therapy (PDT), oxidative stress, p38MAP kinase, p44/42MAP kinase, JNK, NFκB, cyclooxygenase-2 (COX-2).

1. Introduction

PDT using Photofrin, a FDA-approved photosensitizer together with targeted non-thermal light, generates cytotoxic reactive oxygen species within the defined treatment field (1). Initial treatment responses are positive; however, recurrences can occur and methods to improve the efficacy of PDT are needed (2). Additionally PDT induces expression of a number of angiogenic and prosurvival molecules including vascular endothelial growth factor (VEGF), cyclooxygenase-2 (COX-2), matrix metalloproteinases, and survivin (3–9). Preclinical studies have shown that targeting these molecules in combination protocols with PDT increases the treatment efficacy (3, 4, 7–9).

C.J. Gomer (ed.), *Photodynamic Therapy*, Methods in Molecular Biology 635,
DOI 10.1007/978-1-60761-697-9_4, © Springer Science+Business Media, LLC 2010

We evaluated the signaling pathways involved with PH-PDT-mediated COX-2 expression in a mouse fibrosarcoma cell line. COX-2 is an inducible early response gene involved in inflammation, mitogenesis, and tumor progression (10, 11). Following PDT, strong upregulation of COX-2 transcription and translation is observed (3–6). We evaluated COX-2 promoter constructs containing either the wild-type promoter sequence or a sequence with mutated transcription elements. Cells containing constructs with a mutated cyclic-AMP response element 2 (CRE-2), CCAAT/enhancer-binding protein (C/EBP) element, activator-binding protein-1 (AP-1), and nuclear factor kappa B (NFκB) element showed inhibition of luciferase activity induction following PDT. Next we evaluated kinase phosphorylation upstream of COX-2 following PDT and examined the effect of the kinase inhibitors on the induction of COX-2 post-PDT. Although stress-activated protein kinase/c-jun (SAPK/JNK) and c-jun were phosphorylated, the SAPK/JNK inhibitor SP600125 failed to block PDT-induced COX-2 expression. In contrast, p38 mitogen-activated kinase (p38MAPK), an activator of CRE binding, was not only phosphorylated but the p38MAPK inhibitors SB203580 and SB202190 were effective in blocking the induction of COX-2 post-PDT. Another activator of CRE binding, extracellular signal-regulated kinase (ERK1/2) was high in untreated cells dropped immediately following PDT then rapidly increased. Inhibitors of MEK1/2, immediately upstream of ERK1/2, either failed to attenuate or only partially decreased COX-2 expression. An inhibitor to NFκB had no effect on COX-2 expression. These results indicate that the p38 MAPK signaling pathway and CRE-2 binding are involved in COX-2 expression following PDT (12).

2. Materials

2.1. Cell Culture and Photosensitization Reactions

1. Mouse radiation-induced fibrosarcoma (RIF) cells (13).
2. RPMI-1640 culture media (Mediatech, Inc., Manassa, VA) supplemented with 15% fetal bovine serum (Omega Scientific, Tarzana, CA), 100 U/ml penicillin, and 100 μg/ml streptomycin (Gibco, Grand Island, NY).
3. Phosphate-buffered saline (PBS): 0.137 M NaCl, 2.7 mM KCl, 4.3 mM Na_2HPO_4, 1.47 mM KP_2PO_4, pH 7.2.
4. Trypsin solution: 0.05% (w/v) trypsin, 0.53 mM EDTA, dissolved in PBS, pH 7.2.
5. Photofrin: Axcan Scandipharm, Inc. (Birmingham, AL). The photosensitizer is dissolved in 5% dextrose in water at 2.5 mg/ml and stored at –20°C.

6. Light source for cell treatments: Visible red light (570–650 nm, 0.35 mW/cm^2) generated by a parallel series of 30-W fluorescent bulbs filtered with a red mylar film.
7. p38 MAP kinase inhibitors SB-203580 and SB-202190, A.G. Scientific, Inc. (San Diego, CA), dissolved in DMSO.
8. MEK1 inhibitor PD98059 and MEK1/2 inhibitor U0126, Cell Signaling Technology (Beverly, MA), dissolved in DMSO.
9. JNK inhibitor SP600125, Calbiochem (La Jolla, CA), dissolved in DMSO.
10. NFκB inhibitor SN50, Calbiochem (La Jolla, CA), dissolved in H_2O.

2.2. mRNA Isolation

1. 2 M Sodium acetate.
2. Water-saturated phenol.
3. Denaturing solution: 4 M guanidinium thiocyanate, 25 mM sodium citrate, pH 7.0, 0.5% sarcosyl, 0.1 M 2-mercaptoethanol (*see* **Note 1**).
4. Chloroform:isoamyl alcohol mixture (49:1).
5. 15-ml Polypropylene tubes (Falcon cat. no. 2059).
6. Isopropanol.
7. 75% Ethanol.
8. 10X DNase buffer: 200 mM Tris–HCl, pH 8.4, 20 mM $MgCl_2$, 500 mM KCL.
9. 0.1% Diethyl pyrocarbonate (DEPC)-treated water.

2.3. Northern Analysis

1. Oligo-labeling buffer (OLB): made from solutions A:B:C in a ratio of 100:250:150 (store OLB at –80°C). (a) Solution A: 1 ml (1.25 M Tris–HCl, 0.125 M $MgCl_2$, pH 8.0) plus 8 μl 2-mercaptoethanol, 5 μl dCTP, 5 μl dGTP, and 5 μl dTTP (each triphosphate previously dissolved in TE, pH 7.0) at a concentration of 0.1 M. (b) Solution B: 2 M HEPES, pH 6.6. (c) Solution C: hexadeoxyribonucleotides in TE at 90 U/ml.
2. Bovine serum albumin (BSA): 10 mg/ml.
3. ^{32}P-dCTP, specific activity 3,000 Ci/mmol (DuPont-NEN, Wilmington, DE).
4. Klenow DNA polymerase I: 2 U/μl (Boehringer, Mannheim).
5. Stopping solution: 20 mM NaCl, 30 mM Tris–HCl, pH 7.5, 2 mM EDTA, 0.2% sodium dodecyl sulfate (SDS), 1 μM dCTP.

6. 10X MOPS (3-[*N*-morpholino]propanesulfonic acid) buffer: 0.2 M MOPS, 0.05 M sodium acetate, 0.01 M EDTA.
7. 37% Formaldehyde solution.
8. Loading buffer: 0.72 ml formamide, 0.16 ml 10X MOPS buffer, 0.26 ml 37% formaldehyde, 0.18 ml H_2O, 0.1 80% glycerol, 0.08-ml saturated bromophenol blue solution.
9. 1% Denaturing agarose gel: 1 g agarose, 10 ml 10X MOPS buffer, 85 ml H_2O. (Heat in microwave to dissolve agarose, cool to 50°C, add 5.4 ml 37% formaldehyde, swirl to mix, position comb, and pour gel [pour gel in hood to minimize exposure to formaldehyde fumes]).
10. Nylon filter; Nytran Plus (Schleicher and Schuell, Keene, NH).
11. UV light or vacuum oven for cross-linking RNA to nylon filter.
11. Hybridization buffer: 1 M NaCl, 50 mM Tris, pH 7.5, 10% dextran sulfate, 1% SDS, 0.2 mg/ml salmon sperm DNA (boiled) and 50% formamide.
12. Wash solutions: 1X SSC (150 mM NaCl, 15 mM sodium citrate), 0.1% SDS.

2.4. Plasmid Transfection

1. Effectene enhancer reagent, enhancer, EC buffer (Qiagen, Chatsworth, CA).
2. 60-mm Tissue culture dishes.
3. Plasmids containing COX-2 promoter with or without various mutations and the luciferase reporter gene (pGL2 C2-1, pGL2 C2-m1, pGL2 C2-m2, pGL2 C2-m4, pGL2 C2-m5, pGL2 C2-m8, and pGL2 C2-m9 gifts from Yoshiyuki Hakedea, Sakado, Japan) dissolved in TE buffer, pH 7.4.
4. pMC1neo plasmid (Stratagene, La Jolla, CA).

2.5. Luciferase Activity

1. Luciferase assay system (luciferase assay substrate, luciferase assay buffer, and luciferase cell culture lysis reagent (5X); Promega Corporation, Madison, WI).
2. Luminometer (Lumat LB950: Berthoid Analytical Instruments, Inc., Nashua, NH).
3. Luminometer tubes.

2.6. Transcription Factor-Binding Assays

1. TransAM transcription factor assay kit for NFκB, c-fos, phospho-c-jun, and phospho-CREB (active motif). These kits contain reagents for preparation of nuclear extracts.
2. Bio-Rad protein assay dye reagent (Bio-Rad Laboratories, Inc., Hercules, CA).

3. Protein standard 2 mg BSA (Sigma), reconstituted with 5 ml of ddH_2O and stored at 4°C.
4. DU-65 spectrophotometer from Beckman (Fullerton, CA).
5. MR 600 microplate spectrophotometer from Dynatech Laboratories (Chantilly, VA).

2.7. Western Immunoblot Analysis

1. 10% Tris-glycine precast polyacrylamide gel, 1.5 mm × 10 well (Invitrogen).
2. 1× Electrode running buffer: 0.25 M Tris base, 192 mM glycine, 0.1 SDS, pH 8.6–8.8.
3. 4X – XT sample buffer (Bio-Rad Laboratories, Inc., Hercules, CA). With β-mercaptoethanol added 8/100 μl buffer.
4. Transfer blotting buffer: 0.03 M Tris, pH 8.3, 150 mM glycine, 20% methanol.
5. Transfer nitrocellulose paper, Optitran BA-S 83 reinforced NC (Whatman GmbH, Dassel, Germany).
6. Protein transfer unit (Hoefer Scientific Instruments).
7. TBS (Tris-buffered saline) buffer: 100 mM Tris, 0.9% NaCl, pH 7.5.
8. TTBS (Tween Tris-buffered saline): 0.1% Tween 20 in TBS.
9. ECL Western blotting detection reagents (GE Healthcare, Buckinghamshire, UK).
10. Antibodies (mouse monoclonal anti-COX-2 (clone 33; BD Transduction Laboratories, San Diego, CA), ERK1/2 kinase (Thr202/Tyr204) antibody, p38 MAP kinase (Thr 180/Tyr182) antibody, pSAPK/JNK (Thr 183/Try 185) antibody, pMSK1 (Ser376) antibody, pATF-2 (Thr71) antibody (Cell Signaling Technology; Beverly, MA), anti-actin antibody (clone C-4) from MP Biomedicals, Inc. (Aurora OH), anti-mouse peroxidase conjugate (Sigma, St. Louis, MO), and anti-rabbit (Cell Signaling Technology, Beverly, MA)).
11. Premium Clear Blue X-ray film (Bioland Research Products, La Palma, CA).

2.8. Kinase Assays

1. Sonifier, Virsonic 300 (Virtis, Gardiner, NY).
2. Phenylmethylsulfonyl fluoride (PMSF) (Sigma, St. Louis, MO).
3. p38 Map kinase assay kit (immobilized phospho-p38 MAPK (Thr180/Tyr 182) mouse monoclonal antibody, ATF-2 fusion protein, kinase buffer (10X), cell lysis buffer (10°C), ATP (10 mM), anti-rabbit IgG, HRP-linked antibody,

biotinylated protein ladder detection pack, 20X LumiGLO reagent and 20X peroxide, and phospho-ATF-2 Ab; Cell Signaling Technology, Beverly, MA).

4. p44/42 MAP kinase assay kit (immobilized phospho-p44/42 MAPK (Erk1/2) (Thr202/Tyr204) mouse mAb, phospho-Elk-1 (Ser383) antibody, Elk-1 fusion protein, kinase buffer (10X), cell lysis buffer (10X), ATP (10 mM), anti-rabbit IgG, HRP-linked antibody, anti-biotin, HRP-linked antibody, biotinylated protein ladder detection pack, 20X LumiGLO reagent and 20X peroxide, and active p42 MAP kinase (10 ng/μl); Cell Signaling Technology, Beverly, MA).

2.9. Kinase Inhibitor Studies

1. Materials include those for cell culture and photosensitization reactions, **Section 2.1**, mRNA isolation and Northern blot analysis, **Sections 2.2** and **2.3**, and Western immunoblot analysis, **Section 2.7**.
2. p38 MAP kinase inhibitors SB-203580 and SB-202190; A.G. Scientific, Inc. (San Diego, CA), stock solutions 1 mM in DMSO, stored at –20°C.
3. MEK1 inhibitor PD98059 and MEK1/2 inhibitor U0126; Cell Signaling Technology (Beverly, MA), stock solutions 1 mM in DMSO, stored at –20°C.
4. JNK inhibitor SP600125; Calbiochem (La Jolla, CA), stock solution 1 mM in DMSO, stored at –20°C.
5. NFκB inhibitor SN50; Calbiochem (La Jolla, CA), 1 mM in H_2O, stored at –20°C.

3. Methods

Cells and tissues exposed to photosensitizers remain light sensitive even after removal of the photosensitizer. As a consequence, in order to obtain consistent results it is imperative that all work with PH or cells exposed to PH be performed in a darkened room. Photographic safe lights in the red range provide the adequate light. Alternatively low-intensity fluorescent lights covered with a ruby red Mylar filter may be used.

The active, phosphorylated forms of the MAPK proteins are inherently liable due to the protein phosphatase activities within cells. Therefore it is important to work quickly to terminate these activities when harvesting protein. Samples are immediately placed on ice and the phosphatase inhibitor PMSF is added to the lysis buffer. Protein samples are frozen in aliquots to avoid repeated freeze/thaw cycles.

3.1. Cell Culture and Photosensitization Reactions

1. RIF cells are maintained as a monolayer culture on RPMI-1640 media containing 15% FCS and antibiotics (complete growth media). Cells are grown in a humidified incubator at 37°C with 5% CO_2.
2. Exponentially growing cells are removed from T-75 plastic tissue culture flasks by trypsinization (remove culture media, rinse once with PBS, add 2.0 ml of trypsin solution, incubate at 37°C for 5 min, and inactivate trypsin by adding 10 ml of complete growth media).
3. Pipet cell mixture vigorously to obtain a single cell suspension and count cells with a Coulter counter.
4. Cells, 10^6 or 2×10^5, are replated in 100-mm or 60-mm plastic tissue culture dishes and incubated at 37°C for 24 h to allow for attachment.
5. Replace growth media with RPMI media-containing Photofrin (25 μg/ml) and 5% FCS, incubate for 16 h, rinse with RPMI-containing 0% FBS, incubate with growth media ± inhibitors for 30 min. Remove growth media.
6. Expose dishes to 315 J/m^2 red light, feed with growth media ± various inhibitors for various times.

3.2. Isolation of Total RNA from Mouse Cells

1. Culture control and PDT-treated cells in 100-mm dishes.
2. To harvest RNA rinse cells with PBS and add 2 ml of denaturing solution. (Harvest 6 h post-PDT for COX-2 mRNA or a variety of times following PDT ranging from 0 min to 2 h to observe phosphorylation levels of various kinases.)
3. Swirl until cells are completely dissolved.
4. Scrape flask and place solution of denatured cells in 15-ml polypropylene tubes.
5. Add sequentially: 0.2 ml of 2 M sodium acetate pH 4.0, 2 ml phenol, 0.4 ml chloroform–isoamyl alcohol (mix after each addition).
6. Shake mixture vigorously for 10 s and cool on ice for 15 min.
7. Centrifuge samples at 10,000×*g* for 20 min at 4°C.
8. Transfer the aqueous phase (upper layer) to new tube and add 2 ml isopropanol and mix.
9. Precipitate RNA by incubating at –20°C for 1 h.
10. Centrifuge sample at 10,000×*g* for 20 min at 4°C to obtain RNA pellet.
11. Resuspend the RNA pellet in 0.3-ml denaturing solution and transfer to a 1.5-ml eppendorf tube.

12. Precipitate RNA by adding 1 volume of isopropanol and incubating at –20°C for 1 h.
13. Spin down RNA in microfuge for 10 min at 4°C.
14. Rinse RNA pellet with 75% ethanol and air-dry.
15. Resuspend RNA in DEPC-treated water for Northern analysis. Read OD at 260/280 nm to determine RNA concentration.
16 Aliquot RNA in several small volumes, store at –80°C, do not subject to repeated freeze/thaw cycles as this leads to RNA degradation.

Adapted from the Procedure by Chomeznski and Sacchi (14.

3.3. Northern Analysis

1. Place 10 μl RNA in eppendorf tube with RNA loading buffer (2–4 μl RNA plus 14 μl RNA loading buffer) and heat to 60°C for 5 min.
2. Load RNA sample on a denaturing 1% agarose gel containing 0.66 M formaldehyde, 1X MOPS buffer.
3. Separate RNA using 100 V until bromophenol blue dye migrates three-fourths of the way down the gel.
4. Transfer separated RNA to nylon filter (capillary method or with an electro-transfer apparatus).
5. Cross-link RNA to nylon filter by exposure to UV light or by baking in a vacuum oven at 80°C for 2 h.
6. Set up radioisotope-labeling reaction for cDNA probe with 10 μl OLB, 2 μl BSA, cDNA probe (up to 31.5 μl and between 20 and 200 ng cDNA), 5 μl [^{32}P]dCTP, 1 μl of appropriate T12MN primer, water to bring the final reaction volume to 50 and 1 μl Klenow.
7. Run labeling reaction at room temperature overnight.
8. Add 200 μl stop solution when reaction is complete. The probe is ready to use for Northern blot analysis.
9. Boil probe for 10 min to denature ^{32}P-labeled cDNA prior to hybridization.
10. Hybridize labeled probe with filter in 5-ml hybridization buffer at 42°C overnight.
11. Wash filter at room temperature in 1X SSC, 0.1% SDS for 15 min, followed by 2–42°C washes in 0.2X SSC, 0.1% SDS for 15–30 min each. An additional wash at 55°C in 0.2X SSC, 0.1% SDS for 15 min may be necessary if radioactivity of filter is high.

12. Expose the filter, using an intensifying screen, to Kodak XAR-5 film at –80°C (overnight to 1 week) to visualize mRNA levels.

3.4. Plasmid Transfection

Cells were transfected with plasmids containing either the wild-type COX-2 promoter (–959 to +39) ligated into pGL2 basic luciferase or COX-2 promoters containing site mutations on one of the putative transcriptional regulatory elements, CRE-1, NFκB, C/EBP, AP-1, CRE-2, and E-Box.

1. Seed 2×10^5 cells in 5 ml complete growth media in 60-mm dishes, place in 37°C incubator with 5% CO_2, and incubate for 24 h for cell attachment. The cells should be 40–80% confluent on the day of the transfection.
2. Combine up to 150 μl EC buffer (DNA condensation buffer) with 1.2 μg COX-2 promoter plasmid of interest, 0.3 μg pMC1neo, and 8 μl Effectine. Mix by vortexing for 1 s. (For plasmid DNA concentrations of 1 μg/μl, place 1.2 μl COX-2 promoter plasmid, 0.3 μl pMC1, and 8 μl enhancer in 140.5 μl EC buffer.) (*see* **Note 1**).
3. Incubate the DNA enhancer solution for 2–5 min at room temperature. Spin briefly in centrifuge to insure that the entire sample is at the bottom of the tube.
4. Add 25 μl of effectene reagent to DNA enhancer solution by pipetting five times or vortexing for 10 s.
5. Incubate the samples for 5–10 min at room temperature to allow for complex formation.
6. While complex formation takes place, gently aspirate the growth medium from the plate and wash cells once with PBS. Add 4 ml of fresh growth medium (with serum and antibiotics) to the cells.
7. Add 1 ml of cell growth medium to the tube containing the transfection complexes. Mix by pipetting and immediately add the transfection complexes drop-wise onto the cells in the 60-mm dishes. Gently rock the dish to ensure uniform distribution of the complexes.
8. Incubate cells with the complexes at 37°C in 5% CO_2 to allow for gene expression.
9. 24–48 h post-transfection pass the cells 1:5 in growth medium containing G418 (800 μg/ml) and select for 10 days.
10. Pool positive colonies for each promoter construct. Grow cells in selective media until the number of cells required to perform a PDT experiment are obtained.
11. Use transfected cells to set up a PDT experiment as described in **Section 3.1**.

3.5. Luciferase Activity

1. PDT experiments are performed with cells in 60-mm dishes.
2. Prior to harvesting and lysing cells prepare 1X lysis buffer from the 5X luciferase cell culture lysis reagent (Luciferase Assay System, Promega) by adding four volumes of water to one volume stock solution.
3. Remove media from cells 6 h after PDT.
4. Carefully rinse cells with 5-ml PBS. Tilt dishes slightly to allow residual PBS to drain to one side, carefully remove PBS using a pipet.
5. Add 400 μl 1X lysis buffer to the plate. Rock the plate gently to insure that all of the cells are covered with the buffer.
6. Subject cells to one freeze/thaw cycle to insure the lysis of cells. Dishes are placed at –80°C for 30 min then thawed at room temperature.
7. Scrape cells from the dishes, transfer cells and liquid to a microcentrifuge tube, and place on ice.
8. Vortex microcentrifuge tube 10–15 s, then centrifuge at 12,000×*g* for 2 min at 4°C.
9. Transfer supernatant to fresh microfuge tube. Store at –70°C until luciferase assay is performed.
10. The Lumat LB950 is a manual luminometer. Place 100 μl of the luciferase assay reagent into luminometer tubes, one tube per sample.
11. Program the luminometer to perform a 2 s measurement delay followed by a 10 s measurement read for luciferase activity.
12. Add 20 μl of cell lysate to a luminometer tube containing the luciferase assay reagent. Mix by pipetting two to three times.
13. Place the tube in the luminometer and initiate reading. Print or record reading.
14. Calculations to determine relative luciferase activity are determined by the ratio of the PDT-treated samples over the control samples for each COX-2 promoter/luciferase construct. By comparing the ratio obtained from the cells containing the wild-type construct with those obtained for the cells containing the mutated constructs, the promoter elements that are affected by the treatment can be determined (**Fig. 4.1**) (*see* **Note 2**).

3.6. Transcription Factor-Binding Assays

1. Plate and treat cells with PDT as described in **Section 3.1**.

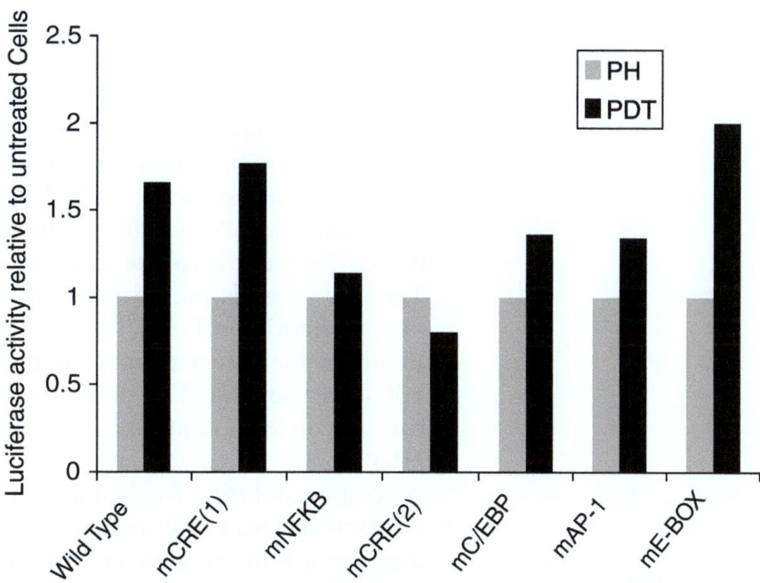

Fig. 4.1. COX-2 promoter site mutation analysis following PH-PDT. A series of pGL2 basic luciferase vectors containing the full length murine COX-2 promoter (–959 to +39 bp) mutated at specific transcriptional regulatory elements were stably transfected into RIF-1 cells. Cells were either incubated with PH or treated with PH-PDT. Six hours later samples were collected and assayed for luciferase activity and total protein levels. The normalized luciferase activities from the various transfected cell lines were directly compared with the luciferase activity obtained from PH-PDT-treated cells containing COX-2 wild-type promoter.

2. Obtain nuclear extract from treated and control cells by following manufacturer's instructions in the TransAM Kit. Wash and collect treated cells (15, 30, 45, 60, 90, and 120 min after PDT) and controls (120 min) in ice-cold PBS. Transfer the cells into pre-chilled 15-ml tube and spin at 300×*g* for 5 min at 4°C. Resuspend the pellet in 1 ml of ice-cold hypotonic buffer and transfer the cells to pre-chilled 1.5-ml tube. Let cells swell on ice for 15 min, then add 50 μl of 10% Nonidet P-40. Centrifuge at 4°C and resuspend the nuclear pellet in 50 μl of complete lysis buffer and shake the tube at 4°C on a rocking platform. Centrifuge for 10 min at 14,000×*g* at 4°C and save aliquoted supernatants at –80°C.
3. Determine protein concentration of the extracts by using the Bio-Rad protein protocol. Briefly, dilute 2 μl of the supernatant into 798 μl of ddH$_2$O. Add 200 μl of dye reagent concentrate. Transfer each sample to a clear cuvette and read absorption at 595 nm. Use a standard curve generated by plotting OD values for known concentrations of BSA to obtain protein concentrations of each sample.

4. Prepare the complete binding buffer, 1X wash buffer, and 1X antibody-binding buffer as described in the kit manual.
5. Perform TransAM binding assay as per manufacturer's protocol. Dilute samples containing 10 μg of protein to 50 μl with complete binding buffer in microcentrifuge tubes (test each sample in triplicate). Add 1 pmol of biotinylated probe to each nuclear extract diluted to 50 μl in complete binding buffer. Mix and incubate at room temperature for 30 min. Transfer to wells pre-coated with a consensus binding site oligonucleotide of the indicated nuclear binding factor. Incubate for 3 h with mild agitation and, after wash, add 100 μl of the diluted antibody to the factor of interest. Incubate for another hour and, after wash, add 100 μl diluted HRP-conjugated secondary antibody. Wash and add 100 μl developing solution for 15 min in the dark. Add 100 μl stop solution and read at absorbance on a microplate spectrophotometer at 450 nm with a reference of 655 nm.
6. Plot treated samples' binding levels of c-fos, phospho-c-jun, phospho-CREB, and NFκB relative to constitutive control values (**Fig. 4.2**).

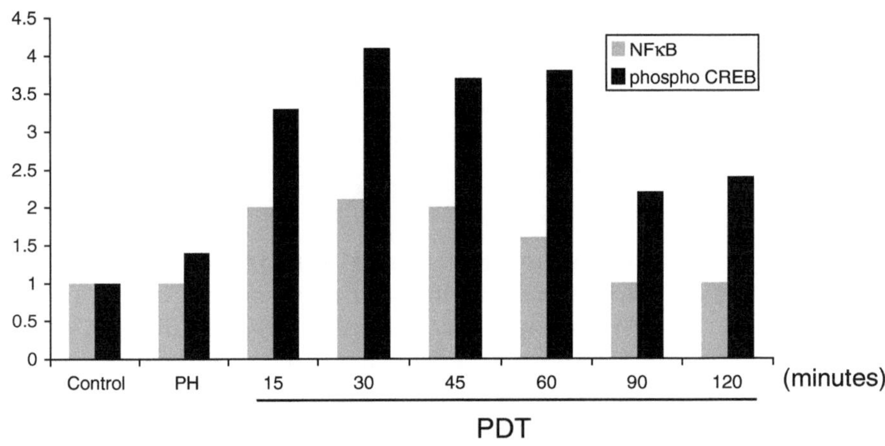

Fig. 4.2. Transcription factor-binding activity to COX-2 promoter following PH-PDT. Nuclear protein-binding activity to transcription regulatory elements in the COX-2 promoter was measured by spectrophotometry using the commercial TransAM kits for NFκB and phospho-CREB. PDT-treated and control RIF-1 cells were collected, processed, and assayed for NFκB and phospho-CREB binding activity to the COX-2 promoter at the indicated time points. All spectrophotometric readings of PH- and PDT-treated cells were plotted relative to constitutive control values.

3.7. Western Immunoblot Analysis

1. Plate 10^6 cells in 100-mm tissue culture plates, treat cells with PDT as described in **Section 3.1**.
2. Prepare 1X lysis buffer. Dilute 10X lysis buffer 1:10 in Milli-Q or equivalently purified water. Dissolve 17.4 mg PMSF in 1 ml ethanol to prepare 100X. 1 M PMSF stock. Add PMSF to 1X cell lysis buffer to bring the final concentration of PMSF to 1 mM (1–100 dilution).

3. Harvest and lyse cells at 0, 5, 15, 30, 60, 120, 240, or 360 min post-PDT in subdued light. (Because of the presence of photosensitizer in the cell lysate continue to work in subdued light until samples have been loaded onto the gel.)
4. Remove tape and comb from polyacrylamide gel. Clean the wells of the gel by squirting 1X running buffer into each well and then pour the buffer out. Repeat three times. Insert 10% discontinuous polyacrylamide gel into gel apparatus.
5. Fill apparatus with 1X electrode running buffer.
6. Pipet 50 μg protein per sample into 1.5-ml microfuge tubes. Add 4X XT sample buffer to protein. Heat samples to 95°C for 3 min.
7. Load the samples onto the gel. Load first or last lane with molecular weight markers.
8. Run gel at 150 V at 4°C for about 2.5 h until blue dye reaches the bottom of the gel.
9. Remove gel from apparatus and pry the plastic plates apart with a spatula, be careful not to tear gel.
10. Set up the transfer cassette: Fill transfer unit with blotting buffer and keep unit at 4°C while running. Place the remainder of the blotting buffer in a large flat tray along with plastic transfer cassette, sponges, blotting paper, and nitrocellulose (cut to the size of the gel). Assemble the cassette: place one side of the plastic cassette on the bottom of the tray, layer a sponge, then one piece of blotting paper, the gel, the nitrocellulose, another piece of blotting paper, another sponge, and the other side of the plastic cassette. Roll all air bubbles out from between each layer as it is placed on top of the last with a glass rod. Carefully secure the two sides of the plastic cassette, making sure the gel and nitrocellulose remain exactly aligned.
11. Place the cassette in the transfer apparatus and secure lid. Run at 20 V overnight. Orient the cassette so that the nitrocellulose is between the gel and the anode.
12. Remove the nitrocellulose from the transfer apparatus and wash the filter in TBS then incubate the filter with 5% nonfat dry milk in TBS for 1 h at room temperature with constant rocking.
13. Wash the nitrocellulose three times with TTBS and then incubate the nitrocellulose with the primary antibody of choice overnight at 4°C. The phospho-antibodies were diluted 1:1,000 in TTBS containing 5% BSA.
14. Wash nitrocellulose with TTBS 3X for 5 min each wash.

15. Incubate nitrocellulose filter with either anti-mouse or anti-rabbit peroxidase conjugate diluted 1/10,000 in TTBS for 1 h at room temperature.
16. Wash nitrocellulose with TTBS 3X for 5 min each wash.
17. Visualize the resulting complexes with enhanced chemiluminescence autoradiography: Mix 1 ml solution "1" with 1 ml solution "2" of the detections reagents and pour evenly over the nitrocellulose filter, incubate for 1 min, drain detection reagent from the filter. Wrap in plastic film, place in an autoradiography cassette, and expose to blue X-ray film for between 1 min and 2 h depending on the antibody. Develop film (**Fig. 4.3**).

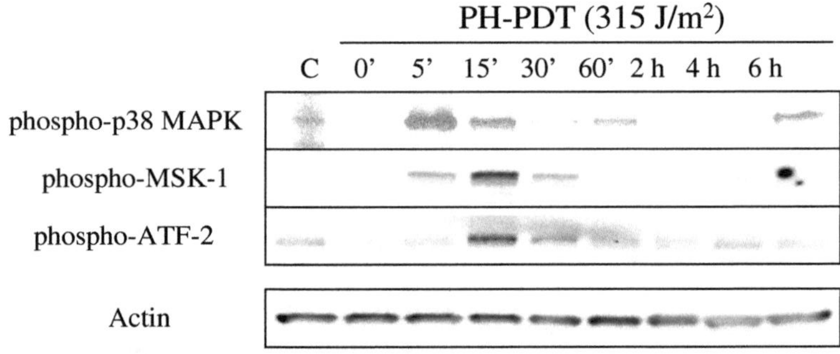

Fig. 4.3. Analysis of p38 MAP kinase signaling pathway following PH-PDT. Control and PDT-treated RIF-1 cells were harvested at various time intervals after treatment and analyzed by Western blotting using anti-phospho-p38 MAPK to document PDT-mediated phosphorylation of p38 MAPK, anti-phospho-MSK-1 and ATF-2 to document phosphorylation of downstream substrates of activated p38 MAPK, and anti-actin to document protein loading.

3.8. Kinase Assays

1. Plate 10^6 cells in 100-mm tissue culture plates, treat cells with PDT as described in **Section 2.2**.
2. Prepare 1X lysis buffer. Dilute 10X lysis buffer 1:10 in Milli-Q or equivalently purified water. Dissolve 17.4 mg PMSF in 1 ml ethanol to prepare 100X 1 M PMSF stock. Add PMSF to 1X cell lysis buffer to bring the final concentration of PMSF to 1 mM (1–100 dilution).
3. Harvest and lyse cells at 0, 5, 15, 30, 60, 120, 240, and 360 min post-PDT in subdued light. (Because of the presence of photosensitizer in the cell lysate continue to work in subdued light until all reactions involving enzymatic reactions have been completed.)
4. Aspirate media from dish-containing cells and wash cells with ice-cold PBS.

5. Remove PBS and add 0.5 ml 1X ice-cold cell lysis buffer containing 1 mM PMSF to each plate and set plates on ice for 5 min.
6. Scrape cells off the plates and transfer buffer-containing cells to microcentrifuge tubes. Keep tubes on ice.
7. Sonicate samples on ice four times for 5 s each. (Set the output control on the sonifier at "5" or the microprobe limit.)
8. Microfuge samples for 10 min on maximum speed at 4°C. Transfer supernatant to a new microfuge tube and store lysate at –80°C.
9. Pipet 200 μl cell lysate into a new tube, add 20 μl immobilized antibody (either immobilized phospho-p38 MAPK (Thr180/Tyr182) or immobilized p44/42 MAPK (ERK1/2) (Thr202/Tyr204)), and incubate in the dark (wrap in foil) with gentle rocking overnight at 4°C.
10. Microfuge samples for 30 s at 4°C. Wash pellet two times with ice-cold 1X cell lysis buffer. Keep on ice and in subdued light during the washes.
11. Wash pellet two additional times with 500 μl of 1X kinase buffer and then place on ice.
12. Suspend pellet in 50 μl of 1X kinase buffer supplemented with 200 μM ATP and 2 μg of ATF-2 for p38 MAPK activity or ELK-1 for ERK1/2 activity.
13. Incubate for 30 min at 30°C.
14. Terminate reaction with 25 μl of 3X SDS sample buffer. Vortex, then microfuge for 30 s.
15. Samples are heated to 95°C for 3 min then loaded on a 10% polyacrylamide gel for Western analysis. (Follow the protocol in Section **3.7**, Step 4.)
16. Antibodies against phospho-ATF-2 and phospho-ELK-1 are used to detect phosphorylated forms of ATF-2 or ELK-1, which indicate the level of kinase activity within the samples (**Fig. 4.4**).

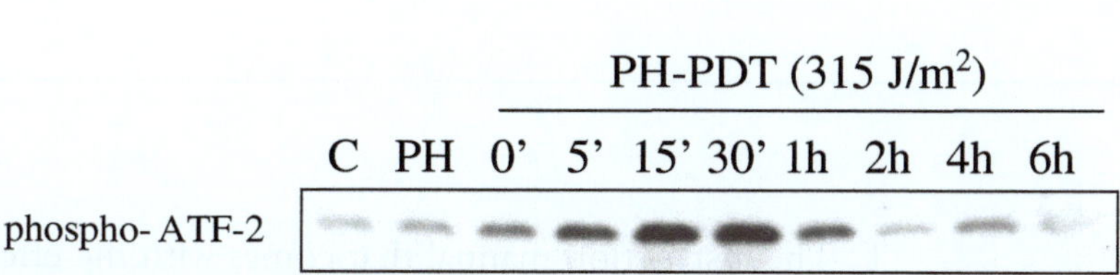

Fig. 4.4. p38 MAP kinase activity assay following PH-PDT. PDT-treated RIF-1 cells were collected at various time intervals and processed for p38 MAP kinase activity using a commercial kinase assay kit. Processed samples were run on acrylamide gels and assayed for phospho-ATF-2 (Thr71) by Western immunoblot analysis.

3.9. Kinase Inhibitor Studies

1. Cells were plated and treated as described in **Section 3.1**.
2. Inhibitors are added as indicated in **Section 3.1**, Step 5. The MAP kinase inhibitors SB203580 and SB202190 are added at concentrations of 12 and 25 μM and 1 and 10 μM, respectively. The concentrations of MEK1 inhibitors U0126 and PD98059 are 1 and 10 μM, respectively. The concentrations of the JNK inhibitor SP600125 are added at 20, 2, and 0.2 μM. The concentration for the NFκB inhibitor SN50 is 50 μM. Inhibitors are present both 30 min prior to light irradiation and then following PDT until the point at which the cells are harvested for RNA or protein.
3. RNA from the samples are subjected to Northern analysis for COX-2 as described in **Section 3.3** and proteins are subjected to Western analysis as described in **Section 3.7** (**Fig. 4.5**).

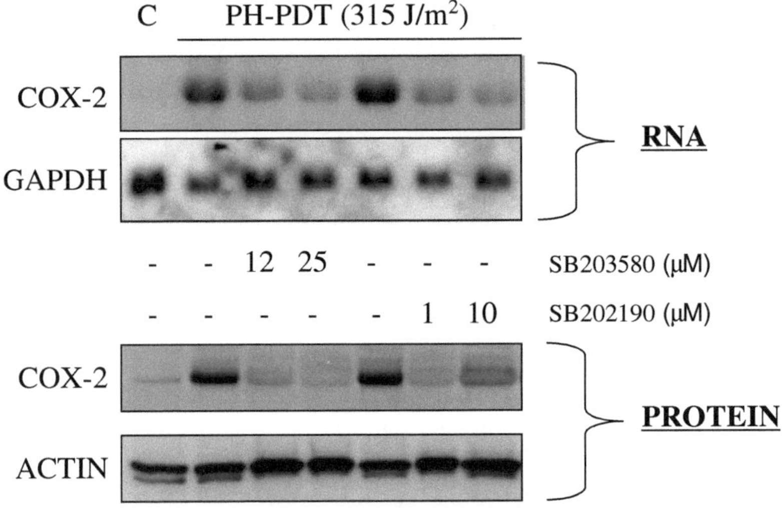

Fig. 4.5. Effect of p38 MAPK inhibitors on COX-2 mRNA and protein expression following PH-PDT. RIF-1 cells were incubated with either inhibitor of p38 MAP kinase cascade SB203580 (12–25 μM) or SB202190 (1–10 μM) for 30 min prior to PH-PDT and for an additional 6 h post-PH-PDT. Cells were then collected for analysis of COX-2 mRNA and protein expression profiles.

4. Notes

1. The instruction manual that comes with the effectene transfection reagent contains information on titrating for the optimal effectene and plasmid concentrations in order to achieve high transfection efficiency.

2. Depending on the wavelength of the photosensitizer used, there may be interference between the luciferase reading and the photosensitizer. To compensate for this interference, the PDT-treated cell readings are compared with readings from cells that have been exposed to the photosensitizer but not light.

References

1. Dougherty, T. J., Gomer, C. J., Henderson, B. W., Jori, G., Kessel, D., Korbelik, M., Moan, J., and Peng, Q. (1998) Photodynamic therapy. *J Natl Cancer Inst*, **90**, 889–905.
2. Triesscheijn, M., Bass, P., Schellens, J. H. M., and Stewart, F. A. (2006) Photodynamic therapy in oncology. *Oncologist*, **11**, 1034–1044.
3. Ferrario, A., von Tiehl, K., Wong, S., Luna, M., and Gomer, C. J. (2002) Cyclooxygenase-2 inhibitor treatment enhances photodynamic therapy mediated tumor response. *Cancer Res*, **62**, 3956–3961.
4. Ferrario, A., Fisher, A. M., Rucker, N., and Gomer, C. J. (2005) Celecoxib and NS-398 enhance photodynamic therapy by increasing in vitro apoptosis and decreasing in vivo inflammatory and angiogenic factors. *Cancer Res*, **65**, 9473–9479.
5. Hendrickx, N., Volanti, C., Moens, U., Seternes, O. M., de Witte, P., Vandenheede, R. J., Piette, J., and Agostinis, P. (2003) Up-regulation of cyclooxygenase-2 and apoptosis resistance by p38 MAPK in hypericin-mediated photodynamic therapy of human cancer cells. *J Biol Chem*, **278**, 52231–52239.
6. Volanti, C., Hendrickx, N., Van Lint, J., Matroule, J.-Y., Agostinis, P., and Piette, J. (2005) Distinct transduction mechanisms of cyclooxygenase-2 gene activation in tumour cells after photodynamic therapy. *Oncogene*, **24**, 2981–2991.
7. Ferrario, A., von Tiehl, K. F., Wong, S., Rucker, N., Schwartz, M. A., Gill, P. S., and Gomer, C. J. (2000) Anti-angiogenic treatment enhances photodynamic therapy responsiveness in a mouse mammary carcinoma. *Cancer Res*, **60**, 4066–4069.
8. Ferrario, A., Chantrain, C. F., von Tiehl, K. F., Buckley, S., Rucker, N., Shalinsky, D. R., Shimada, H., DeClerck, Y. A., and Gomer, C. J. (2004) The matrix metalloproteinase inhibitor Prinomastat enhances photodynamic therapy responsiveness in a mouse tumor model. *Cancer Res*, **64**, 2328–2332.
9. Ferrario, A., Rucker, N., Wong, S., Luna, M., and Gomer, C. J. (2007) Survivin, a member of the inhibitor of apoptosis family, is induced by photodynamic therapy and is a target for improving treatment response. *Cancer Res*, **67**, 4989–4995.
10. Subbaramaiah, K. and Dannenberg, A. J. (2003) Cyclooxygenase-2: a molecular target for cancer prevention and treatment. *Trends Pharmacol Sci*, **24**, 96–102.
11. Pyo, H., Choy, H., Amorino, G. P., Kim, J., Cao, Q., Hercules, S. K., and DuBois, R. N. (2001) A selective cyclooxygenase-2 inhibitor, NS-398, enhances the effect of radiation in vitro and in vivo preferentially on the cells that express cyclooxygenase-2. *Clin Cancer Res*, **7**, 2998–3005.
12. Luna, M., Wong, S., Ferrario, A., and Gomer, C. J. (2008) Cyclooxygenase-2 expression induced by Photofrin photodynamic therapy involves the p38 MAPK pathway. *Photochem Photobiol*, **84**, 509–514.
13. Luna, M. C., Ferrario, A., Wong, S., Fisher, A. M. R., and Gomer, C. J. (2000) Photodynamic therapy mediated oxidative stress as a molecular switch for the temporal expression of genes ligated to the human heat shock promoter. *Cancer Res*, **60**, 1637–1644.
14. Chomczynski, P. and Sacchi, N. (1987) Single-step method of RNA isolation by acid Guanidinium Thiocyanate-Phenol-Chloroform extraction. *Anal Biochem*, **162**, 156–159.

Chapter 5

Metronomic PDT and Cell Death Pathways

Gurmit Singh, Omar Alqawi, and Myrna Espiritu

Abstract

The term "metronomic" was recently introduced to describe continuous low-dose administration of chemotherapeutics following the discovery that this causes minimal side effects (Hanahan et al. 2000, J Clin Invest, 105(8), 1045–1047; Bisland et al. 2004, Photochem Photobiol, 80, 22–30). Metronomic dosing in PDT is proposed by analogy and the rationale is as a means to improve the tumor-specific response through cell death by apoptosis. We investigated the molecular mechanisms associated with apoptosis following ALA-PDT treatment in two brain glioma cell lines, namely U87 (human) and CNS-1 (rat) cells. We used the high energy of light at a short time (acute PDT) and the low energy of light at a long time of exposure (metronomic PDT) to treat both cell lines. To identify potential cell death pathways associated with metronomic PDT, microarray analysis of gene expression was conducted on RNA from glioblastoma cells with metronomic ALA-PDT. The apoptosis mechanism for metronomic ALA-PDT occurred via the inhibition of LTβR and the transcription factor NF-κB. This inhibition was ALA concentration dependent.

Key words: Metronomic PDT, gliomas, LTβR, NFB, apoptosis, microarrays.

1. Introduction

PDT affects several different signaling pathways, some of which lead to cell death whereas others mediate cell survival (1–4). The cell death response to PDT depends on experimental conditions, such as the concentration of the photosensitizer, the subcellular localization of the photosensitizer, and the magnitude of the light exposure (4). PDT kills tumor cells via apoptosis or necrosis (or both) in vivo and in vitro (5). Mitochondrial damage has been suggested as an early event in PDT-mediated apoptosis, which results in the release of apoptotic factors like cytochrome *c*,

C.J. Gomer (ed.), *Photodynamic Therapy*, Methods in Molecular Biology 635,
DOI 10.1007/978-1-60761-697-9_5,

which activates the downstream targets in the apoptotic pathways (6). Bcl-2 family members of proteins are critical regulators of the apoptotic pathway. Bcl-2, an antiapoptotic member of Bcl-2 family inhibits the release of cytochrome *c* from mitochondria whereas Bax and Bid proteins are pro-apoptotic members and have been shown to release cytochrome *c* from mitochondria and enhance apoptotic response (7–9). PDT-mediated apoptosis by the expression of Bcl-2 family members (intrinsic pathway) has been demonstrated using several photosensitizers in different cell lines (10–12). Apoptosis can also be induced via the extrinsic apoptotic pathway, which is mediated through the activation of cell surface death receptors independent of p53, which leads to the activation of the intracellular adapter molecule, Fas-associated death domain (FADD). The adapter molecule recruits caspases 8 and 10 to the death receptor, forming the death-inducing signal complex (DISC), where they are cleaved and activated (13–15).

The initiating signal is sufficient to cleave and activate the terminal executioner molecules, caspases 3, 6, and 7 in some cells; however, other cells require activation of mitochondrial-based apoptosis to amplify the death receptor signal (16). The intrinsic signals for apoptosis are mediated by a group of death receptors within the tumor necrosis factor receptor super family (TNFRS). These death receptors are characterized by similar

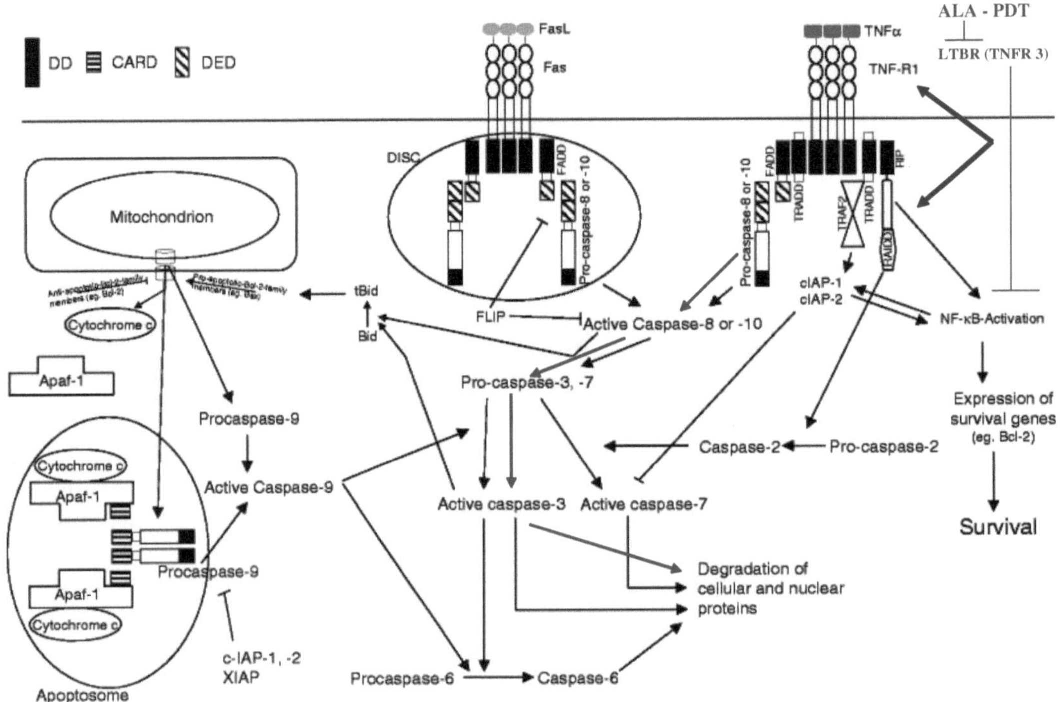

Fig. 5.1. Apoptosis pathways.

cysteine-rich extracellular domains as well as by a conserved cytoplasm sequence called the "death domain" (17). They include DR1, DR2,. . ., DR6, EDAR, and NGFR. The lack of a functional death domain prevents the receptors from recruiting the cytoplasmic adapter proteins required to initiate apoptosis and known as decoy receptors such as DcR1 and DcR2.

We have demonstrated that metronomic ALA-based photodynamic therapy induces apoptosis by the expression of TNF receptor super family members as well as Bcl-2-related proteins. Acute ALA-based photodynamic therapy induces more necrosis in brain cancer cells as a response to the treatment. Hence the idea of activating TNF receptor super family members via metronomic PDT which initiates the subsequent apoptotic pathways to destroy cancer cells is desirable as it limits toxicity from collateral damage (*see* **Fig. 5.1**).

2. Materials

2.1. Cell Lines and Reagents

1. The U87 human glioblastoma cell line and CNS-1 rat glioblastoma cell line were obtained from American Type Culture Collection (ATCC, Maryland, USA).
2. RPMI 1640 medium (Invitrogen, Inc.), supplemented with 10% fetal bovine serum and 1% penicillin and streptomycin (Gibco/BRL).
3. 5-Aminolevulinic acid (ALA) (Sigma Chemical Co., St. Louis, Mo). A stock of 25 mM ALA is prepared in Dulbecco's phosphate-buffered saline (PBS) (Invitrogen), sterilized by filtering in 0.45-μm Acrodisc® syringe filter (PALL, Life Science), and stored in aliquots (2 ml) at –20°C in the dark. Serum-free RPMI 1640 with L-glutamine medium is used to dilute the drug to desired concentrations.
4. A 10X trypsin/ethylenediaminetetraacetic acid (T/EDTA) (Gibco/BRL, Mississauga, Canada), diluted at a concentration of 2.5X with sterile PBS, stored in aliquots (10 ml) at –20°C.

2.2. SDS-Polyacrylamide Gel Electrophoresis (SDS-PAGE) Reagents

1. Gel resolving buffer (4X): 1.5 M Tris–HCl, pH 8.8, 0.4% SDS. Store at room temperature.
2. Gel stacking buffer (4X): 0.5 M Tris–HCl, pH 6.8, 0.4% SDS. Store at room temperature.
3. Polymerizing solution: tetramethylethylenediamine (TEM ED, Invitrogen, Canada). Store at 4°C.

4. Stock A: running buffer (10X) – 250 mM Tris–HCl, 1.9 M glycine, and 0.5% sodium dodecyl sulfate (SDS). Solutions are stored at room temperature.
5. Stock B: transfer buffer (10X) – 500 mM Tris–HCl, 390 mM glycine, and 0.4% sodium dodecyl sulfate (SDS). Solutions are stored at room temperature.
6. Stock C: dilution and washing buffer (10X) – 807 mM NaCl, 99 mM Tris–HCl, pH 8.0 (TBS). Make a 1X solution in 0.1% Tween 20 (TBS-T). Solutions are stored at room temperature.
7. 30% acrylamide/bis solution (37.5:1 with 2.6% C), care should be observed when using the unpolymerized acrylamide which is neurotoxic, and *N,N,N,N′*-tetramethylethylenediamine (TEMED, BioRad).
8. Prestained protein molecular weight marker (Gibco/BRL).
9. Ammonium persulfate: freshly prepared 10% solution in sterile distilled water.

2.3. Western Blotting Reagents

1. Cell lysis buffer: 50 mM Tris–HCl, pH 8.0, 150 mM NaCl, and 1% Nonidet P-40 (Sigma/Aldrich). Store at 4°C. A protease inhibitor tablet (ROCHE) is dissolved in 1.0-ml sterile distilled water, store in aliquots (0.1 ml) at –20°C. A 0.1 ml of the protease inhibitor is added per milliliter of the lysis buffer during use.
2. Cell scrapers Teflon spatula (Fisher).
3. BioRad protein assay reagent (BioRad).
4. 6X sample loading buffer: 1.3 M β-mercaptoethanol, 0.6 M Tris–HCl, pH 6.8, 26% sodium dodecyl sulfate (SDS), 30% glycerol, and add a drop of dye bromophenol blue solution (to give a dark blue colored loading buffer). Store at room temperature.
5. Blotting paper (VWR International, Canada) and a 0.45-μm nitrocellulose membrane Hybond-HCl (Amersham Bioscience, Canada).
6. Blocking buffer: 3% (w/v) BSA fraction V (Sigma/Aldrich, Canada) in TBS-T.
7. Primary antibodies: LTβR, NFRSF-6B, TNFRSF12A, and TNFRSF10B (Cedarlane/Abcam, Canada) diluted (1:5,000) in TBS-T.
8. Secondary antibodies: anti-mouse IgG, anti-goat IgG, and ant-rabbit IgG are conjugated to horse radish peroxidase (Santa Cruz, CA) diluted (1:10,000) in TBS-T.

9. Detection kit: enhanced chemiluminescent (ECL) reagents (VWR/GE Health Care).
10. Kodak Biomax Film.

2.4. Probe Stripping Reagents

1. Stripping buffer: 62.5 mM Tris–HCl, pH 6.8, 2% (w/v) SDS. Warm to 60°C and add 100 mM β-mercaptoethanol upon use.
2. Sterile distilled water for rinsing β-mercaptoethanol from blot.
3. Equilibrating wash buffer: TBS-T.

2.5. Microarray Reagents for Human Apoptosis Genes

1. RNeasy Kit (Qiagen, Canada): cell RNA extraction.
2. Oligo GEArray for human apoptosis microarrays OHS-012 (SuperArray, Frederick, USA).
3. True Labeling-AMP Linear RNA amplification kit (SuperArray, Frederick, USA).
4. Biotin-16 UTP (Roche) for detection probe.
5. ArrayGrade cRNA cleanup kit (Qiagen).
6. Alkaline phosphatase-conjugated streptavidin and CDP-Star substrate.
7. ReactionReady First Strand cDNA synthesis kit.
8. Oligo-dT primers for LTβR, NFRSF6B, TNFRSF10B, TNFRSF12A (174, 192, 182, and 181 bp, respectively), kits, and reagents above were obtained from SuperArray, Frederick, USA; others specified.

3. Methods

3.1. Cell Culture and Harvesting

1. The U87 human glioblastoma and CNS-1 rat glioblastoma cells should be handled in an aseptic laminar flow hood, cells are cultured in a 75-cm^2 T-flask as monolayers in RPMI 1640 with L-glutamine medium, supplemented with 10% FBS, 1% penicillin and streptomycin, and 10 mM HEPES buffer, maintain at 37°C, 90% humidified incubator with 5% CO_2 (*see* **Note 1**).
2. The doubling time of U87 and CNS-1 cells is 22 h, plating efficiency of 35 and 40%, respectively. Cells that are used for experiments must be at their highest logarithmic growth phase.

3. Detach cells by incubating with 3 ml of 2.5X T/EDTA for 5 min at 37°C, 10 ml of supplemented medium is added to cells, collected in a culture tube, centrifuge at 257 × *g* for 5 min at room temperature.
4. Cell pellets are resuspended in a warm supplemented medium; determine cell numbers by counting on a Neubauer hemocytometer with the aid of a standard light microscope.

3.2. Colony-Forming Assay for Acute and Metronomic PDT

1. In order to maintain the initial number of cells for experiments, it is important to know the doubling time of the cells. The cells (U87 and CNS-1) are seeded late in the afternoon, incubated overnight with photosensitizer, and treated with light the following day (*see* **Note 2**).
2. The control experimental conditions for both acute and metronomic PDT are (a) no drug and no light, (b) drug and no light, and (c) drug with light. Each condition is repeated in triplicate (*see* **Note 9**).
3. 5×10^4 cells/2 ml are plated in a 24-well plate and incubated overnight prior to exposing to photosensitizer and light treatment.
4. In subdued light, remove medium aseptically by vacuum aspiration; 2 ml of drug ALA (0.25 mM) in serum-free medium are added to cells; control cells are in serum-free medium only; incubate for 4 h at 37°C.
5. Replenish cells with 2-ml warm serum-free medium, subject cells to acute or metronomic PDT treatments. A light-emitting diode (LED) box with fixed (635 nm) wavelength is used for light treatment (*see* **Note 3**). Cells are maintained in an incubator at 37°C. Fluency rates of 21 and 0.21 mW/cm^2/s are used for acute and metronomic PDT, respectively.
6. Cells are treated with varying light doses of 1.25, 2.5, and 5.0 J/cm^2/s for both acute and metronomic PDT. Following the treatment, cells are supplemented with media containing 200 μl of serum, approximate serum concentration is 10%, and cells are incubated for approximately 2 h at 37°C prior to harvesting.
7. Floating cells are collected in a 15-ml culture tube. Adherent cells are detached from plate with 1 ml of 2.5X T/EDTA. Cell pellets are resuspended in 10-ml supplemented medium; 1 ml from the cell suspensions is further diluted into 9 ml of medium and dispense 1 ml into wells of 6-well plates containing 3 ml of fresh supplemented medium.

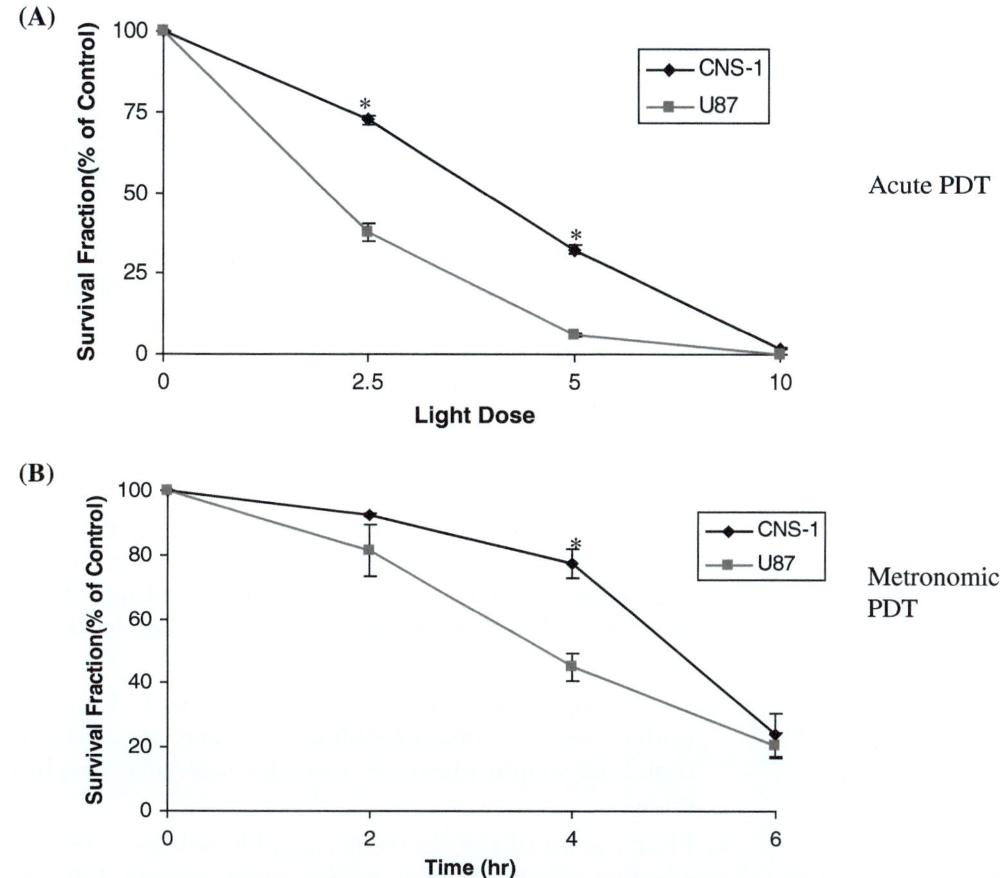

Fig. 5.2. Effects of acute and metronomic PDT on survival of CNS-1 and U87 cells. (**a**) Acute PDT: cells were incubated with ALA (0.25 mM) for 4 h and then irradiated with varying light doses (2.5, 5, and 10 J). (**b**) Metronomic PDT: cells were incubated with ALA (0.25 mM) for varying times (2, 4, and 6 h) and irradiated with 5 J at the same time. Cell survival was measured using a colony-forming assay. $*p < 0.05$.

8. Cells are incubated undisturbed at 37°C for 10 days in the dark for colony formation; colonies are fixed and stained with 0.05% methylene blue in 70% methanol, air-dry cell plates. Colonies are counted under a light microscope equipped with gridded stage. The percentage of cell survival is determined. An example of this is shown in **Fig. 5.2**.

3.3. Electrophoresis Assembly

1. A mini-Protean II gel system is used for the electrophoresis of proteins. The gel glass plates and glass spacers are washed in bactericidal detergent, rinsed with distilled water, wiped with a 95% ethanol, and air-dried. The clean plates and glass spacer's sandwich slide gently into the clamp assembly and secure into the casting stand. The plates' clamp assembly is rested on the rubber gasket to prevent leakage.

2. 12% resolving gel is prepared accordingly: 4.84 ml of sterile distilled water, 6 ml of 30% acrylamide, 4.0 ml of 1.5 M Tris–HCl, pH 8.8, 0.15 ml of 10% ammonium persulfate, and 15 μl of TEMED (*see* **Note 4**). Fill sandwich plates with the gel solution using a rubber dropper and a Pasteur pipette, leaving a space for the 4.5% stacking gel. The gel solution will polarize within 30 min.
3. 4.5% stacking gel is prepared accordingly: 3.46 ml of sterile distilled water, 0.9 ml of 30% acrylamide, 1.5 ml of 0.5 M Tris–HCl, pH 6.8, 0.06 μl of ammonium persulfate, and 6 μl of TEMED. Rinse the top of the gel with sterile distilled water, insert a 1.5-mm thick comb in a slanting position on top slot of the plates, and fill with the stacking solution up to the top of the plates, press comb down horizontally and gel solution polymerizes within 30 min.
4. Remove the comb when the gel solution is polymerized and gently rinse the wells with the 1X running buffer. The sandwich plate assembly is removed from the casting stand and snaps onto the electrode assembly and place inside the buffer tank.
5. Fill the upper and the lower chambers with 1X running buffer, load denatured protein samples, and add a prestained molecular weight marker in a well for molecular weight reference.
6. Place the lid of the electrode assembly unit and connect to a power supply, 45 V is set for approximately 1 h run in the stacking gel and the marker dye to reach the interphase between stacking gel and resolving gel prior to changing the current to 100 V, and run for 3 h in the resolving gel.

3.4. Western Blot for TNFRSF

1. 1×10^6/10 ml cells are plated in 100 × 20 mm culture dishes (Corning); experimental conditions, treatments, and cell collection as above.
2. 18 h following PDT treatments, cells are rinsed once with 5-ml cold PBS, decanted, and add back 1-ml PBS into cell plates; scrape monolayer cells with Teflon scraper and collect into 15-ml culture tubes containing 5-ml cold PBS, centrifuge.
3. Cell pellets are lysed in 200 μl of lysis buffer and transferred into a sterile eppendorf tube, aspirate at least 10 times in a 1-ml syringe with a 21-gauge needle. Lysed cells are allowed to stand for 30 min on ice and centrifuged at 257×*g* force for 5 min at 4°C.
4. The supernatants are retrieved into a fresh sterile eppendorf tubes, avoiding cell debris. BioRad protein assay method is used to determine the protein concentration.

5. A 20-μg protein aliquot in 20-μl volume is added to 20 μl of 2X sample loading buffer (1:1 ratio) and denatured at 95°C for 7 min. This is loaded on a (1.5-mm thick gel) 4.5% stacking/12% resolving SDS-polyacrylamide gel for electrophoresis at 100 V for 1 h.
6. The resolved proteins are electrophoretically transferred to nitrocellulose membranes for 3 h at 80 V. Membranes are rinsed in 3X TBS-T 5 min each and blocked with 3% BSA fraction V in TBS-T for 1 h. Finally it is rinsed three times with TBS-T.
8. Incubate with diluted primary antibodies LTβR (1:4,000), TNFRSF6B (1:4,000), NFRSF10B (1:6,000), TNFRSF12A (1:6,000), caspase 3 (1:4,000), and B-actin (1:10,000) in TBS-T; incubate in the cold with gentle shaking overnight.
9. Membranes are rinsed three times in TBS-T, incubated for 1 h with diluted secondary antibodies: (secondary antibody should be complementary with the primary antibody species) anti-goat IgG, mouse IgG, and rabbit IgG that are conjugated to horse radish peroxidase (1:5,000) in TBS-T. Rinse 3X in TBS-T.
10. Detection of protein bands with enhanced chemiluminescence kit, following manufacturer's instructions. The secondary antibody conjugated to horse radish peroxidase catalyzed the oxidation of luminol in alkaline conditions and triggers emission of chemiluminescent that is captured when the membrane is exposed to film for 5–10 min (decays in 60 min). Density of the protein bands is measured using quantitative software for densitometry (*see* **Note 5**).

3.5. Quantification of Apoptotic Cell Death

1. 2.5 × 10^4 cells/4 ml are seeded in a 60 × 15 mm culture dishes, incubated overnight prior to incubation with photosensitizer and light treatment using experimental conditions as above.
2. This procedure is done at 4°C to minimize cell activity. Cells are harvested 18 h following PDT treatment (*see* **Note 6**). Cell pellets are washed once with 5 ml of cold supplemented medium, centrifuge at 4°C at 257×*g* force (g) for 5 min.
3. Cell pellets are resuspended in 0.5-ml cold binding buffer supplied in the Annexin V-FITC/propidium iodide (PI) detection kit as per the manufacturer's instructions.
4. Cells are analyzed using a flow cytometer with excitation wavelength of 488 nm and emission wavelength at 530 nm. The Annexin V-FITC/PI is used to quantitatively determine the percentage of cells undergoing apoptosis.

5. Apoptotic cells lose their membrane asymmetry. Membrane phospholipid phosphotidylserine is translocated from the inner leaflet of the plasma membrane to the outer leaflet, and Annexin V specifically binds it. Viable cells with intact membranes exclude PI, whereas dead cells are permeable to PI. Cells that are negative for both Annexin V and PI staining are viable and not undergoing apoptosis. Cells that stain positive with Annexin V are apoptotic cells. Cells that stain positive for both Annexin V and PI are either in the later stages of apoptosis or necrotic. An example of this is shown in **Fig. 5.3**.

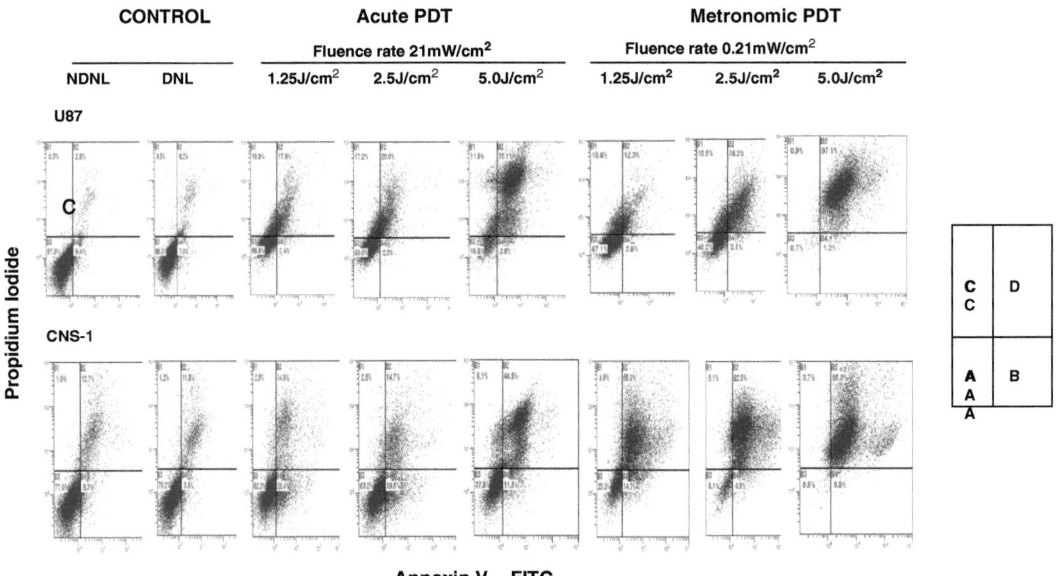

Fig. 5.3. Flow cytometric analysis. ALA-PDT-induced apoptosis in U87 and CNS-1 cells using Annexin V-FITC. U87 and CNS-1 cells treated with acute PDT (1.25, 2.5, and 5 J/cm^2; using fluence rate 21 mW/cm^2) or metronomic PDT (1.25, 2.5, and 5.0 J/cm^2; using fluence rate 0.21 mW/cm^2). Annexin V-FITC positive staining indicates apoptotic cells, while propidium iodide staining indicates necrotic cells. The legend box on the *right side* define the panels (**a**) is for survival fraction, (**b**) is early apoptosis, (**c**) is necrosis/late apoptosis, and (**d**) is intermediate apoptosis.

3.6. Microarray Analysis

1. Cells seeded are harvested 18 h following PDT treatment for both acute and metronomic PDT.
2. Total RNA is extracted using RNeasy kit; the extracted RNA from control and treated cells is purified with the ArrayGrade mRNA purification kit as per the manufacturer's instructions (*see* **Note 7**).
3. RNA is amplified using the True Labeling-AMP Linear RNA amplification kit. The mRNA is reversely transcribed to obtain cDNA and converted into biotin-labeled cRNA using biotin-16-UTP by in vitro transcription.

4. Prior to hybridization, the cRNA probes are purified with the ArrayGrade cRNA cleanup kit. The purified cRNA probes are then hybridized to the pretreated oligo GEArray for human apoptosis microarrays, which covers 112 apoptosis-related genes.
5. Following several washing steps, array spots-binding cRNA is detected using alkaline phosphatase-conjugated streptavidin and CDP-Star as chemiluminescent substrate.
6. Chemiluminescence is detected by exposing the blots to Kodak Biomax film. The image data are transformed into numerical data using software called ScanAlyze v2.50. The numerical data are then further evaluated.
7. Data evaluation includes background correction and median normalization. Data filtering criteria are as follows: at least one of the spot intensities to be compared has to be more than twice the background intensity, and the spot intensity ratios have to be higher than 1.5 (for upregulation) or lower than –1.5 (for downregulation) (*see* **Note 8**). An example of this is shown in **Fig. 5.4**.

3.7. Validation by Real-Time PCR

1. 1 × 10^6 cells are seeded in a 60 × 15 mm culture dish, incubated overnight, and treated. Total RNA is isolated from cells with the RNeasy mini kit. This RNA is used for real-time quantitative RT-PCR.

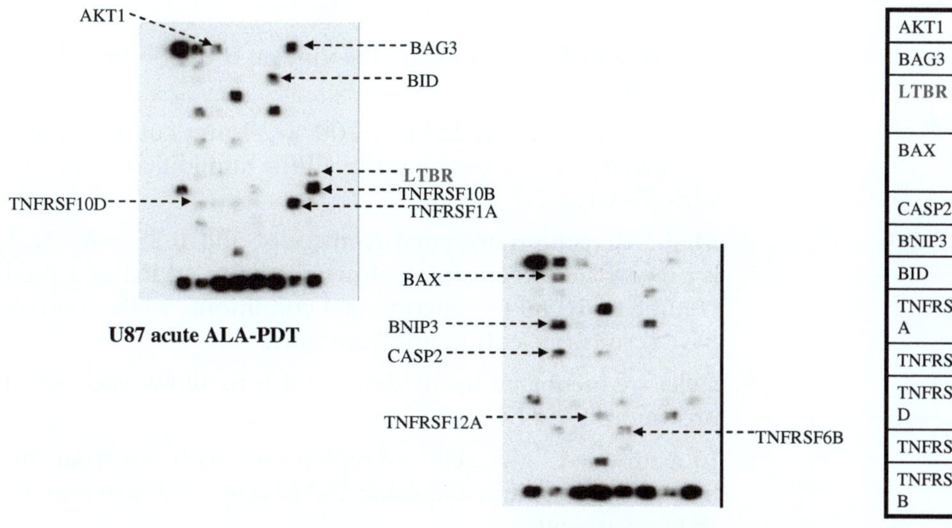

AKT1	-1.6
BAG3	-6
LTBR	-9
BAX	+4
CASP2	+4.5
BNIP3	+2..3
BID	-1.8
TNFRSF12A	+4
TNFRSF6B	+9
TNFRSF10D	-3.5
TNFRSF1A	-2
TNFRSF10B	-4.5

Fig. 5.4. Microarray analysis of U87 cells. Cells were treated with acute or metronomic ALA-PDT and total RNA was extracted and subjected to Oligo GEArray human apoptosis microarray as described in **Section 2**. Data were analyzed by Affymetrix microarray analysis (SuperArray BioScience, MD).

2. The RNA samples are reversely transcribed using the ReactionReady First Strand cDNA Synthesis Kit as per the manufacturer's instructions.
3. Oligo-dT primers are used for priming the reverse transcription of TNF receptors expressed in U87 during acute or metronomic ALA-PDT. The primers are specific for LTβR, NFRSF6B, TNFRSF10B, and TNFRSF12A. The expected PCR products are 174, 192, 182, and 181 bp, respectively.
4. Glyceraldehyde-3-phosphate dehydrogenase (GAPDH) is chosen as the reference gene for normalization of the results.
5. The real-time PCR is performed in a BioRad iCycler using SYBR Green I as the detection system.
6. The results are analyzed using the BioRad iCycler Software 3.0. PCR primers are designed by SuperArray. The PCR products are analyzed by melt-curve analysis and agarose gel electrophoresis to determine product size and to confirm that no by-products are formed.

3.8. Intracellular Accumulation of PpIX

1. U87 and CNS-1 cells are seeded at 25 × 10^4 cells/4 ml in 60 × 15 mm culture dishes, incubated overnight. Media is removed and photosensitizer is added (ALA 0.25 mM) and prepared in serum-free medium for various time periods (0.5–24 h). Cells are detached by 2.5X trypsin/EDTA, centrifuged, cell pellets are rinsed once with 10-ml cold PBS, and resuspended in 1.0-ml cold PBS. The fluorescence intensities of cell suspensions are measured at excitation wavelengths of 635 and 488 nm on a flow cytometer.

3.9. Acute and Metronomic Photodynamic Treatments

1. Experimental conditions are the same as those of the colony-forming assay.
2. 1 × 10^6 cells are seeded in a 100 × 20 mm culture dishes, incubated at 37°C overnight in a 90% humidified incubator with 5% CO_2.
3. Media is vacuum aspirated from cells, and 0.25 mM ALA is prepared in serum-free culture medium, added in a total volume of 10 ml to experimental conditions, while controls have serum-free culture medium only.
4. Cells are incubated in the dark for 4 h to allow synthesis of protoporphyrin IX.
5. In a subdued light, cells are replenished with warm serum-free culture medium and subjected to acute and metronomic PDT treatment.
6. Metronomic PDT treatment fluency rate used is 0.21 $mW/cm^2/s$ and light doses used are 1.25, 2.5, and 5.0 J (2, 4, and 6 h, respectively). Acute PDT treatment fluency rate used is 21 $mW/cm^2/s$ and light doses are 1.25, 2.5 and 5.0 J (1, 2 and 4 min, respectively).

7. After the acute and metronomic PDT treatments, a 1.1 ml of 100% FBS is added to medium of cells and 18 h post-PDT treatments, lysates are prepared as above for protein determination and Western blotting.

4. Notes

1. The U87 and CNS-1 cells should be acclimatized from the freezer for at least one passage prior to use. Also make sure that the passage number remains low as the cell characteristics change with time.
2. For colony-forming assay make sure that appropriate number of cells is plated. For acute PDT and metronomic PDT at higher doses plate a higher proportion of cells as fewer colonies will be formed.
3. It is critical that appropriate light doses are calibrated at the beginning of every experiment as there is fluctuation in the fluence with the age of the bank of lights.
4. TEMED is best stored at room temperature in a desiccator. This reagent declines with age after opening the bottle and it takes longer for gel to polymerize.
5. Chemiluminescent signals should be standardized when doing densitometer as various kits will give different values.
6. Ensure that all cells are kept on ice to reduce artifacts in apoptotic death while doing flow cytometry.
7. Use of RNeasy kits cuts down on the integrity of RNA especially for students who are new to the procedure.
8. The genes identified on the SuperArray must be confirmed at least three times and further confirmed both by RT-PCR and by Western blotting to ensure change in gene profile following acute or metronomic PDT.
9. Every experiment should have several controls including (i) no light no light, (ii) drug no light, and (iii) no drug and light. The number of controls can be reduced by only using highest drug concentration and highest light used in the experiments.

Acknowledgments

This work was supported by PO1 CA043892-16.

References

1. Oltvai, Z. N. and Korsmeyer, S. J. (1994) Checkpoints of dueling dimers foil death wishes. *Cell*, **79**, 189–192.
2. Reed, J. C. (1995) Regulation of apoptosis by bcl-2 family proteins and its role in cancer and chemo resistance. *Curr Opin Oncol*, **7**, 541–546.
3. Korsmeyer, S. J. (1999) BCL-2 gene family and the regulation of programmed cell death. *Cancer Res*, **59**, 1693s–1700s.
4. Srivastava, M., Ahmad, N., Gupta, S., and Mukhtar, H. (2001) Involvement of Bcl-2 and Bax in photodynamic therapy-mediated apoptosis. Antisense Bcl-2 oligonucleotide sensitizes RIF 1 cells to photodynamic therapy apoptosis. *J Biol Chem*, **276**, 15481–15488.
5. Shen, X. Y., Zacal, N., Singh, G., and Rainbow, A. J. (2005) Alterations in mitochondrial and apoptosis-regulating gene expression in photodynamic therapy-resistant variants of HT29 colon carcinoma cells. *Photochem Photobiol*, **81**, 306–313.
6. Chiu, S. M., Xue, L. Y., Azizuddin, K., and Oleinick, N. L. (2005) Photodynamic therapy-induced death of HCT 116 cells: apoptosis with or without Bax expression. *Apoptosis*, **10**, 1357–1368.
7. Barnhart, B. C., Alappat, E. C., and Peter, M. E. (2003) The CD95 type I/type II model. *Semin Immunol*, **15**, 185–193.
8. Micheau, O. and Tschopp, J. (2003) Induction of TNF receptor I-mediated apoptosis via two sequential signaling complexes. *Cell*, **114**, 181–190.
9. Varfolomeev, E. E. and Ashkenazi, A. (2004) Tumor necrosis factor: an apoptosis JuNKie? *Cell*, **116**, 491–497.
10. Wang, S. and El Deiry, W. S. (2003) TRAIL and apoptosis induction by TNF-family death receptors. *Oncogene*, **22**, 8628–8633.
11. Ashkenazi, A. (2002) Targeting death and decoy receptors of the tumour-necrosis factor superfamily. *Nat Rev Cancer*, **2**, 420–430.
12. Xue, L. Y., Chiu, S. M., and Oleinick, N. L. (2001) Photodynamic therapy-induced death of MCF-7 human breast cancer cells: a role for caspase-3 in the late steps of apoptosis but not for the critical lethal event. *Exp Cell Res*, **263**, 145–155.
13. Eleouet, S., Rousset, N., Carre, J., Bourre, L., Vonarx, V., Lajat, L., Beijersbergen, G. M., Henegouwen, V., and Patrice, T. (2000) In vitro fluorescence, toxicity and phototoxicity induced by delta-aminolevulinic acid (ALA) or ALA-esters. *Photochem Photobiol*, **71**, 447–454.
14. Stummer, W., Stocker, S., Novotny, A., Heimann, A., Sauer, O., Kempski, O., Plesnila, N., Wietzorrek, J., and Reulen, H. J. (1998) In vitro and in vivo porphyrin accumulation by C6 glioma cells after exposure to 5-aminolevulinic acid. *J Photochem Photobiol B*, **45**, 160–169.
15. Wilson, C. and Browning, J. (2002) Death of HT-29 adenocarcinoma cells induced by TNF family receptor activation is caspase-independent and displays features of both apoptosis and necrosis. *Cell Death Differ*, **9**, 1321–1333.
16. Wajant, H., Gerspach, J., and Pfizenmaier, K. (2005) Tumor therapeutics by design: targeting and activation of death receptors. *Cytokine Growth Factor Rev*, **16**, 55–76.
17. Tamada, K. and Chen, L. (2006) Renewed interest in cancer immunotherapy with the tumor necrosis factor superfamily molecules. *Cancer Immunol Immunother*, **55**, 355–362.

Chapter 6

How to Monitor NF-κB Activation After Photodynamic Therapy

Isabelle Coupienne, Jacques Piette, and Sébastien Bontems

Abstract

The nuclear factor-kappa B (NF-κB) is a multipotent factor involved in many cellular processes such as inflammation, immune response and embryonic development and it can be activated by a large number of stimuli. Consequently, this transcription factor plays a pivotal role in many natural processes but also in different pathologies. For several years, photodynamic therapy (PDT) has emerged as an attractive alternative approach for the treatment of different affections involving various forms of cancer and an increasing number of reports have highlighted the activation of the NF-κB following PDT treatment. Furthermore, it has been shown that the mechanism of activation of the NF-κB as well as its target genes depends on the nature of the photosensitizers and the cell type used. As this transcription factor is known to be a key regulator of the immune response but also controls cell survival and proliferation, it is important to assess its activation status and its impact on the target genes. In this review, we will present different techniques allowing identification of the activation status of this factor, from the degradation of its inhibitor in the cytoplasm to its ability to induce the expression of a reporter gene under the control of a target promoter. As a working model we will present results obtained from a 5-aminolevulinic acid-PDT treatment on cervix adenocarcinoma cells.

Key words: Nuclear factor-kappa B (NF-κB), photodynamic therapy (PDT), 5-aminolevulinic acid (5-ALA), Western blotting, electromobility shift assay (EMSA), supershift, luciferase assay.

1. Introduction

Since its discovery in the late 1980s, a tremendous number of reports have been published concerning the role of the nuclear factor-kappa B (NF-κB) and its implication in a wide variety of physiological processes such as organ development but also cell survival, proliferation and migration (1) This transcription factor

C.J. Gomer (ed.), *Photodynamic Therapy*, Methods in Molecular Biology 635,
DOI 10.1007/978-1-60761-697-9_6, © Springer Science+Business Media, LLC 2010

is also an important factor in the innate and immune response (2). Furthermore, it can be activated by a large number of different stimuli such as cytokines, bacterial or viral compounds, oxidative stress, DNA damage, etc. (3), emphasizing its implication in a variety of physiological events as well as in several diseases and cancers (4). The NF-κB family is composed of five members (RelA or p65, RelB, c-Rel, p50 and p52 processed forms of the p105 and p100 proteins, respectively). They all share a Rel homology domain required for their dimerization, the interaction with the IκB (Inhibitor of κB) inhibitor, their nuclear localization and the interaction with DNA. The most common NF-κB heterodimer is the p65 (RelA)/p50 complex, which is maintained as an inactive form in the cytoplasm by the IκBα protein. However, different homo- or heterodimers may be formed depending on the stimulus, each possessing a different affinity and transduction ability of its target genes. Stimulation of the "classical" pathway (i.e. with TNF-α) leads to the activation of a complex of kinases, the IKK (IκB kinase) complex, which is able to phosphorylate the IκBα protein on the Ser32 and Ser36 residues. The phosphorylation of IκBα leads to its subsequent ubiquitination and degradation by the 26S proteasome, allowing the release of the NF-κB complex and its migration to the nucleus where it can stimulate the expression of target genes (**Fig. 6.1**). The "alternative" pathway is mainly activated upon LTβ, BAFF and CD40L stimulation, mostly during B-cell maturation, and plays an important role in the development of the adaptive immune response (2). We propose to focus this review on the description of several techniques highlighting the activation of the NF-κB upon a 5-ALA-PDT treatment, from the degradation of its specific inhibitor (IκBα) in the cytoplasm to its ability to stimulate the expression of target genes. Several reports have already underlined the important role played by this transcription factor in PDT using different photosensitizers. Ryter et al. have shown for the first time that NF-κB can be activated following irradiation of Photofrin-treated mouse leukaemia cells (5). Another example from our lab was the demonstration that this transcription factor is activated following an APP (aminopyropheophorbide)- or a PPME (pyropheophorbide-a-methylester)-PDT treatment in HCT116 colon cancer cells or in HMEC-1 endothelial cells, respectively (6, 7). Granville et al. have also proved the activation of NF-κB in a promyelocytic leukaemia cell line after photodynamic therapy using verteprofin as photosensitizer (8). However, the exact mechanism underlying the NF-κB activation seems to depend on the photosensitizer as well as the cell type used (9, 10); it could indeed result from a direct effect of the ROS production (11) or from a ROS-independent mechanism involving, for example, the IL-1 receptor and the acidic sphingomyelinase, as observed in PPME-treated colon cancer cells (12).

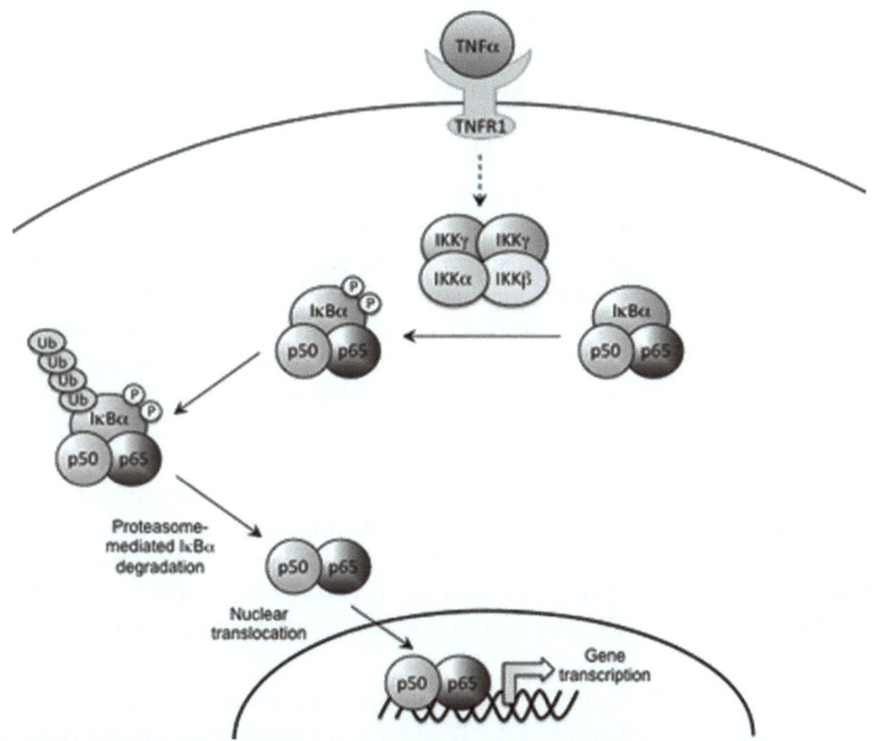

Fig. 6.1. Schematic representation of the NF-κB "classical" activation pathway upon TNF-α stimulation.

2. Materials

2.1. Cell Culture and Photosensitizer Preparation

1. HeLa cells (ATCC number CCL-2) are grown in EMEM (Eagle's minimum essential medium; Lonza, Switzerland) supplemented with 2 mM L-glutamine, non-essential amino acids (Gibco, USA) and antibiotics (penicillin 100 U/ml and streptomycin 100 μg/ml; Gibco, USA).
2. Stock solutions of 5-aminolevulinic acid (5-ALA, 150 mM) (Sigma-Aldrich, USA) are prepared in PBS (140 mM NaCl, 2.7 mM KCl, 8 mM Na_2HPO_4, 1.8 mM KH_2PO_4, pH 7.4) and stored at –20°C for up to 6 months.

2.2. Protein Extraction and Sample Preparation

1. Cytoplasmic proteins are extracted using the following buffer: 10 mM HEPES–KOH (pH 7.9), 2 mM $MgCl_2$, 0.1 mM EDTA, 10 mM KCl, 0.1% Igepal, 1 mM DTT, 1 mM PMSF, Complete (Roche, Germany), 3.3 mM NaF, 1 mM Na_3VO_4, 25 mM β-glycerophosphate, 10 mM nitrophenyl phosphate (*see* **Note 1**). Nuclear proteins were isolated using nuclear extraction buffer: 50 mM HEPES–KOH

(pH 7.9), 50 mM $MgCl_2$, 0.1 mM EDTA, 10 mM KCl, 300 mM NaCl, 1 mM DTT, 1 mM PMSF, Complete (Roche, Germany), 3.3 mM NaF, 1 mM Na_3VO_4, 25 mM β-glycerophosphate, 10 mM nitrophenyl phosphate (*see* **Note 1**). All reagents are purchased from Sigma-Aldrich (Germany) except when noted.

2. Protein concentration is determined by the Bradford method using the Bio-Rad Protein Assay reagent (Bio-Rad GmbH, Germany). The absorbance is measured at 595 nm with a 96-well plate reader spectrophotometer (Multiskan MS, Labsystem, Finland). The standard curve is achieved using bovine serum albumin (BSA; Sigma-Aldrich, Germany).

2.3. SDS-Polyacrylamide Gel Electrophoresis (SDS-PAGE) and Western Blotting

1. Separating solution (10% acrylamide/bisacrylamide): for 1 mini-gel: 37.5:3.11 ml acrylamide/bisacrylamide (ICN Biomedicals, USA), 1.3 ml of 1.5 M Tris–HCl (pH 8.8) (MBI, Fermentas), 120 μl of 10% SDS, 5.7 ml H_2O, 5 μl TEMED, 60 μl of 10% ammonium persulfate solubilized in water.
2. Concentration solution (4% acrylamide/bisacrylamide): for 1 mini-gel: 37.5:3.11 ml acrylamide/bisacrylamide (ICN Biomedicals, USA), 519 μl of 0.5 M Tris–HCl (pH 6.8) (MBI, Fermentas), 50 μl of 10% SDS, 3.2 ml H_2O, 5 μl TEMED, 50 μl of 10% ammonium persulfate solubilized in water.
3. Samples loading buffer: 10 mM Tris–HCl (pH 6.8), 1% SDS, 25% glycerol, 0.1 mM β-mercaptoethanol, 0.003% bromophenol blue.
4. Migration buffer: 20 mM Tris–HCl (pH 8.8) (MBI, Fermentas), 200 mM glycine (MBI, Fermentas), 10% SDS.

   All reagents are purchased from Sigma-Aldrich (Germany) except when noted.
5. Transfer buffer: 25 mM Tris–HCl, 192 mM glycine, 10% methanol.
6. Washing buffer: PBS (*see* **Section 2.2**), 0.1% Tween 20 (Sigma-Aldrich, Germany).
7. Milk blocking solution: PBS (*see* **Section 2.2**), 0.1% Tween 20 (Sigma-Aldrich, Germany), 5% dry non-fat milk.
8. Stripping solution: 2% SDS (w/v), 62.5 mM Tris–HCl (pH 6.7), 100 mM β-mercaptoethanol.

2.4. Antibodies

1. Goat polyclonal anti-p65 antibody (Santa Cruz, USA, ref SC-372; 1:1,000 dilution for the detection by Western blotting).

2. Rabbit polyclonal anti-p65x antibody (Santa Cruz, USA, ref SC-109 X; for Supershift experiments).
3. Goat polyclonal anti-p50x (Santa Cruz, USA, ref SC-1191 X; for supershift experiments).
4. Rabbit polyclonal anti-IκBα (Santa Cruz, USA, ref SC-371; 1:500 dilution for the detection by Western blotting).
5. Mouse monoclonal anti-phospho-IκBα (Ser32, Ser36) (Cell Signaling, USA, ref 9246; 1:500 dilution for the detection by Western blotting).
6. Mouse monoclonal anti-NBS-1 (Becton Dickinson, ref SC-611870; 1:1,000 dilution for the detection by Western blotting).
7. Mouse monoclonal anti-HSP60 (Stressgen, ref SPA-806; 1:2000 dilution for the detection by Western blotting).
8. Secondary antibodies are anti-mouse, anti-goat or anti-rabbit antibodies coupled to horseradish peroxidase (HRP) (Dako, Denmark; 1:1,000 dilution for the detection by Western blotting).

2.5. Electromobility Shift Assay (EMSA) and Supershift Gel Preparation

1. The sequence of the NF-κB probe is as follows: first strand 5′-GGTTACAAGGGACTTTCCGCTG-3′ and the second strand: 5′-TGGCAGCGGAAAGTCCCTTGT-3′ (Eurogentec, Belgium).
2. Klenow polymerization buffer (10×): 0.5 M Tris–HCl (pH 7.6), 0.1 mM $MgCl_2$.
3. Non-denaturing polyacrylamide/bisacrylamide 6% gel for EMSA: 6 ml of 29.1 acrylamide/bisacrylamide (ICN Biochemicals, USA), 24 ml H_2O, 10 ml Tris–borate–EDTA buffer (TBE: 10 mM Tris–HCl, 10 mM boric acid, 10 mM EDTA), 280 μl of 10% ammonium persulfate, 36 μl TEMED.
4. Non-denaturing polyacrylamide/bisacrylamide 4% gel for supershift: 4 ml acrylamide/bisacrylamide (ICN Biochemicals, USA), 26 ml H_2O, 10 ml Tris–borate–EDTA buffer (TBE: 10 mM Tris–HCl, 10 mM boric acid, 10 mM EDTA), 280 μl of 10% ammonium persulfate, 36 μl TEMED.
5. EMSA loading buffer: 30% glycerol, 0.25% bromophenol blue.
6. TNE buffer: 100 mM Tris–HCl (pH 8), 1 mM EDTA, 100 mM NaCl.
7. Binding buffer (10×): 200 mM HEPES–KOH (pH 7.9), 50% glycerol, 10 mM EDTA, 5 mM $MgCl_2$ and add 10 mM DTT extemporaneously.

3. Methods

Monitoring NF-κB activation after a PDT treatment can be achieved using several techniques that have been set up for many years and broadly used for the detection of this transcription factor in different cellular contexts, for example, after a TNF-α stimulation. Nevertheless, the important point to keep in mind when these experiments are performed after a PDT treatment is that NF-κB can be rapidly activated following illumination of the photosensitizer (PS). It is therefore very important to handle the cells in dark from the moment the PS is added until the end of the cellular extraction to avoid artefactual NF-κB activation.

As mentioned in **Section 1**, it is possible to monitor NF-κB at different stages of its activation process. In this review, we will focus on its activation in HeLa cell (epithelial cells from an adenocarcinoma) after a 5-ALA-PDT treatment. We will check that the NF-κB inhibitor (IκBα) is properly degraded and that the main NF-κB subunits, p50 and p65, are able to translocate to the nucleus to bind a consensus NF-κB site on a synthetic probe. Finally, we will show that this transcription factor is able to stimulate the expression of a reporter gene upon a PDT treatment.

It is also important to mention that the time and the duration of the NF-κB activation may depend on the cell type studied as well as the photosensitizer used. Therefore, we suggest performing some kinetics to define the best time points.

3.1. Cell Culture, Treatment and Photosensitization

To illustrate the activation of NF-κB by PDT, we decided to show some results obtained in HeLa cells treated with 5-aminolevulinic acid (5-ALA). 5-ALA is not a photosensitizer by itself but a precursor in the biosynthesis cycle of heme which partly occurs in the mitochondria. In cancer cells, its conversion leads to the accumulation of protoporphyrin IX (PPIX) rather than heme. This is possibly due to the lack of ferrochelatase, the enzyme that converts PPIX into heme, in these cells. The photosensitizing and tumour-localizing properties of this porphyrin derivative have been largely explored in photodynamic detection (PDD) but are also of great interest as a putative way to eradicate tumour cells. Indeed, irradiation of porphyrins can lead to the generation of reactive oxygen species (ROS) that can cause important cellular damage and may lead to cell death.

1. HeLa cells are cultured in 80-cm^2 flasks by successive passages using trypsin/EDTA. For the different experiments, HeLa cells are grown either in 25-cm^2 flasks or in 6-well plates; 250,000 and 100,000 cells are seeded, respectively, the day before the experiment takes place.

2. 5-ALA is added to the culture medium at a final concentration of 1 mM 3 h prior to illumination. Cells are kept in the dark during this period in an incubator at 37°C, 5% CO_2.
3. Illumination is performed using an illumination system composed of four neon tubes (15 W each) of white light (Aquarelle, Philips) plus a red filter. The measured fluence rate was about 23 W/m^2. Cells are rinsed once with PBS to remove the red-phenol compound present in the growth medium. As mentioned above, the irradiation is performed in PBS, then cells are placed back into the incubator with complete growth medium. Rinsed but non-illuminated, treated or untreated cells are always used as negative controls. TNF-α (200 U) (Pierce) is also used in these experiments as a positive control for NF-κB activation and is added to the medium 15 min before collecting cells.

3.2. Protein Extraction and Sample Preparation

The first experiment we performed to monitor NF-κB activation was the control of the NF-κB inhibitor IκBα phosphorylation on Ser32 and Ser36 by Western blotting analysis and its degradation by the proteasome machinery after the PDT treatment. This step is a prerequisite to NF-κB nuclear translocation (that can also be studied by the same technique). To carry this out, cells were treated with 5-ALA (1 mM) and then irradiated for 15 min (2.1 J/cm^2). Cells were then collected at several times post-irradiation in order to perform kinetics of NF-κB activation (*see* **Note 2**).

1. These experiments were performed using 25-cm^2 flasks of irradiated and non-irradiated cells in order to get large amounts of material for the detection of the different proteins of interest. Cells were collected 1, 2, 4 and 24 h post-irradiation. In order to do so, cells were rinsed twice with PBS, scrapped and centrifuged for 5 min at 1,000×*g*. The supernatants were discarded and 100 μl of cold cytoplasmic extraction buffer was added. The pellets were gently resuspended and placed immediately on ice for 20 min. Next, they were vortexed shortly and centrifuged for 5 min at 4,000×*g*. The supernatants containing the cytoplasmic fraction were then collected and kept on ice if shortly used or stored at –80°C. Thirty microlitres of cold nuclear extraction buffer was added and placed on ice for 30 min. They were centrifuged for 20 min at 22,000×*g*. The supernatants containing the nuclear fractions were collected and kept on ice if shortly used or stored at –80°C. After determination of protein concentration in the samples, 30 μg of cytoplasmic proteins or 10 μg of nuclear proteins were collected in annotated microcentrifuge tubes. After that, an equal volume of loading buffer was added to the proteins and the whole was boiled for 2 min.

3.3. Western Blotting for the Detection of IκBα Degradation and p65 Nuclear Translocation

1. *Gel preparation*: The following procedure is suitable for most mini-gel systems. However, please refer to the manufacturer's instructions for a detailed description of the assembling of the apparatus. Make sure that the glass plates used are clean and dry. For this, wash them once with 70% ethanol and rinse them with distilled water. The thickness of the gel will also depend on the volume of the sample to load. The following description is suitable for one 1.5 mm gel placed in a Bio-Rad device (Germany). Prepare a concentration solution and add ammonium persulfate and TEMED extemporaneously. Pour the separating gel leaving space for the stacking one and overlay it with ethanol. Polymerization occurs within about 30 min. Meanwhile, prepare the stacking gel solution and add ammonium persulfate and TEMED extemporaneously. Discard the ethanol, rinse once with distilled water, pour the stacking gel solution and insert a comb. Polymerization of the stacking gel takes place after about 30 min.
2. Prepare 1 l of running solution. When the gel has polymerized, remove the comb. Rinse the wells once with distilled water, then mount it on the device and add the running solution in both compartments (upper and lower chambers). In the first well, load 5 μl of a pre-stained molecular weight marker (Fermentas, Life Sciences), then carefully add the samples in the other wells. Connect the assembly unit to a power supply. Gel migration is usually performed during 1–2 h at 120 V. You can easily visualize the migration of the samples, thanks to the blue dye front.
3. After separation during the migration step, proteins are transferred from the gel to a polyvinylidene difluoride (PVDF) membrane (Amersham). For this, prepare 1 l of transfer buffer, 1 piece of PVDF membrane having the same size as the gel and four sheets of Whatman paper (Whatman Ltd, England) with a size slightly larger than the gel size. Before application, the PVDF sheet has to be placed in methanol for 1 min, rinsed for 1 min with distilled water and then submerged with the transfer buffer. The Whatman sheets must also be placed in the transfer buffer. Transfer of the proteins on the PVDF is achieved using a transfer apparatus containing a transfer cassette and two pieces of foam (Bio-Rad, Germany). Wet the two pieces of foam with the transfer buffer and place one of them on the top of the transfer cassette. Add two sheets of papers on the foam. Disconnect the gel unit from the power supply and disassemble it. Remove and discard the stacking gel, then carefully place the running gel on the sheets of Whatman paper. Then, on the top of the PVDF membrane, add

successively the two remaining sheets of paper and the second piece of foam. Be very careful that no air bubble is trapped between the different layers of the system. Place the cassette in the transfer tank in such a way that the PVDF membrane is placed between the gel and the anode. Allow the transfer to take place at 4°C either overnight at 30 mA or for 2 h at 250 mA. Use a stirrer to ensure a homogenized temperature of the buffer in the tank. Once the transfer is complete, disassemble the unit, discard the sheets of paper and the gel, then place the PVDF membrane in 50 ml of milk blocking solution for 1 h at room temperature or overnight at 4°C. You should be able to visualize the coloured molecular weight marker on the membrane as control of the transfer. Gently shake the membrane during the incubation period.

4. It is possible to cut the PVDF membrane using the molecular weight marker as reference in order to detect different proteins on the same membrane. This procedure is extensively used to detect a specific protein (i.e. NF-κB p65 subunit) and a loading control (i.e. NBS). In the experiments presented here we have detected IκBα and IκBα (Ser32, Ser36) with the HSP60 protein as loading control of the cytoplasmic extracts and also p65 and NBS as loading control of the nuclear extracts.

   Discard the blocking solution and replace it by the antibodies diluted in a fresh milk blocking solution. All the antibodies used in these experiments have been incubated overnight at 4°C with gentle rocking. After incubation, the membranes are rinsed three times with PBS–Tween for 10 min. Secondary antibodies coupled to HRP are also diluted in PBS–Tween and added for 1 h with gentle shaking. After this incubation period, the membranes are rinsed three times with PBS–Tween for 10 min.

5. For the detection of the proteins we used ECL (enhanced chemiluminescence) reagents. Please refer to the manufacturer's instructions for a detailed description of the procedure. Briefly, after the final wash, the membranes are dried with soft papers, then the membranes are soaked with a mixture of two ECL reagents for 1 min. Membranes are then dried again and placed in an X-ray cassette with a suitable film in a dark room (Fuji, X-Ray, Belgium). Exposure length depends on the antibodies used and is usually between 1 and 20 min. The revelation is performed with an automatic developer.

6. It is also possible to strip the membrane to remove the attached antibodies and then to reprobe it with another antibody. This technique is strongly recommended for

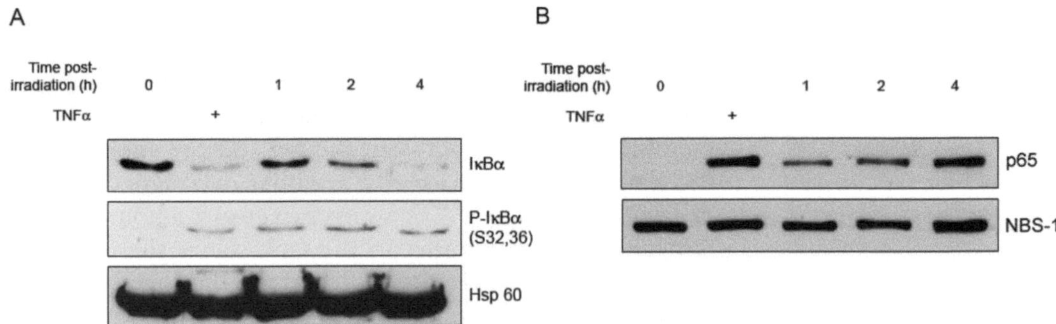

Fig. 6.2. (**a**) Detection of IκBα and phospho IκBα (Ser32, Ser36) by Western-blotting in cytoplasmic extracts of 5-ALA treated and irradiated or unirradiated HeLa cells. TNF-α is used as positive control and HSP60 detection is the loading control. (**b**) Detection of the NF-κB p65 subunit in nuclear extracts of 5-ALA treated and irradiated or unirradiated HeLa cells. TNF-α is used as positive control and NBS detection is the loading control.

the simultaneous detection of a protein and its modified form, for example IκBα and IκBα phosphorylated on Ser32 and Ser 36. After the first detection, the membrane is incubated in the stripping buffer for 30 min at 65°C. Next, it is extensively washed with PBS–Tween (6 × 10 min) and then blocked again in the milk blocking solution.

7. *Results*: As presented in **Fig. 6.2a**, IκBα is heavily present in an unphosphorylated form in untreated and unirradiated cells. TNF-α treatment leads to an important decrease of the IκBα level concomitant to its phosphorylation. As we can observe in this picture, 5-ALA-PDT treatment of these cells also induces a progressive phosphorylation of this inhibitor, leading to its degradation. HSP60 level ensures that the loading of the proteins on the membrane is similar for each condition. Concerning the NF-κB p65 subunit, this protein is clearly absent from the nucleus in normal conditions, whereas both TNF-α and as 5-ALA-PDT treatments lead to its nuclear translocation (**Fig. 6.2b**). The NBS protein level is similar in each condition. These results clearly demonstrate the activation and the nuclear translocation of the NF-κB after a 5-ALA-PDT treatment.

3.4. Specific NF-κB Binding Demonstrated by Electromobility Shift Assay (EMSA) and Supershift Experiments

Next, it is important to determine whether the translocated NF-κB subunits are able to bind DNA on its consensus sequence, which is of course a prerequisite to its transactivation potential. This can be achieved using a synthetic probe labelled with radioactive ^{32}P and by testing the ability of the nuclear NF-κB to bind to it, causing a delayed migration on an acrylamide/bisacrylamide gel. The nature of the NF-κB subunits bound to this probe can also be investigated using some specific antibodies to induce a supershift of the complex previously formed.

1. *Probe labelling and purification*: For these experiments, we used a probe encompassing the consensus sequence (5′-GGGACTTTCC) for the NF-κB binding present in the HIV-1 long terminal repeat (LTR) region (*see* **Note 3**). Double-stranded oligonucleotides are annealed for 15 min at 65°C and then let cooled for 90 min at room temperature. This oligonucleotide probe has sticky ends that can be labelled at the 3′ terminus by incorporation of [α-^{32}P]-dATP and [α-^{32}P]-dCTP using the Klenow fragment of *Escherichia coli* DNA polymerase I (*see* **Note 4**). The polymerization procedure is as follows: dilute the probe to a 100 ng/μl concentration, mix 1 μl of probe with 2 μl of Klenow polymerization buffer (10×), 3 μl of [α-^{32}P]-dATP (3,000 Ci/mmol), 3 μl of [α-^{32}P]-dCTP (3,000 Ci/mmol) and 10 μl of H_2O. Add 1 μl of Klenow (Roche, Germany), let the reaction to take place for 15 min at room temperature, then add another microlitre of Klenow and wait 15 min more. The excess of unbound labelled nucleotides must be removed by purification of the probe using a G25 quick spin column (exclusion limit < 10 bp) following the manufacturer's instructions (Roche, Germany). Briefly, vigorously resuspend the Sephadex in the column, remove the upper cap and let the buffer flow, centrifuge the column for 2 min at 500×*g* and discard the supernatant, pour 20 μl of labelled probe previously mixed with 30 μl of TNE buffer on the top of the column. Centrifuge for 4 min at 500×*g*, collect the supernatant and measure the specific activity of the probe using a scintillation counter (1409 DSA; Perkin Elmer, USA) (the specific activity must be >10^8 cpm/μg of probe). Dilute the probe two times in TNE buffer to have a final concentration of 1 ng/μl and keep it at –20°C.

2. *Gel preparation*: The following procedure is suitable to most large gel systems (i.e. Bio-Rad, Germany). However, please refer to the manufacturer's instructions for detailed description of the assembling of the apparatus. Make sure that the glass plates used are clean and dry. For this, wash them once with 70% ethanol and rinse them with distilled water before assembling. Prepare a non-denaturing polyacrylamide/bisacrylamide 6% gel and add the TEMED and the ammonium persulfate extemporaneously and pour it. Avoid trapping bubbles in the gel, because it would prevent a correct migration of the samples. Place the comb and let the gel polymerize for about 1 h. After this, remove the comb and place the gel in the electrophoresis tank. Add the TBE buffer (0.25×) in the upper and lower parts of the tank and

rinse the wells with a needle. Connect to a cooling system and pre-run the gel for 30 min at 180 V.

3. *Binding reaction and loading of the samples*: First, dilute the labelled probe five times in TNE buffer to reach a final concentration of 0.2 ng/μl. The binding mix for each sample is the following: add 1.5 μl of binding buffer (10×) to 6.5 μl of distilled water and 1 μl of bovine serum albumin (BSA) (1 mg/ml). Then add 1 μl of poly(dI–dC) (1.3 μg/μl) and 1 μl of purified labelled probe (*see* **Note 5**). Then add 5 μg of nuclear proteins (max. volume of 4 μl), incubate the mixture for 30 min at room temperature and then place on ice. Just before use, add 4 μl of EMSA loading buffer to each sample. Load the gel and perform the migration for 3 h at 300 V and at 4°C (*see* **Note 6**). Once migration is complete, carefully remove the gel, place it between a Whatman and a plastic sheet and dry it for 40 min at 80°C in an automatic dryer (Bio-Rad GmbH, Germany). Put the gel in an X-ray cassette with an appropriate film (Fuji, X-Ray, Belgium) and place it at –80°C. The exposure time is usually between 1 and 4 days.
4. *Results.* In the experiment presented in **Fig. 6.3a**, we can clearly see that the binding of NF-κB to the labelled probe leads to an important uppershift [compare lane 1, TNF-α condition, with lane 2, the free probe (fp) alone]. Furthermore, we can also clearly notice that the 5-ALA-PDT treatment also induces a binding of NF-κB on its probe in a time-dependent way. There is indeed virtually no binding in untreated cells, while the binding increases with time to reach a maximum at around 2 h post-irradiation. In this experiment, 5-ALA (0.5 mM) was added 3 h before a 0.71 J/cm^2 irradiation and the samples were collected at different times post-irradiation.
5. *Supershift experiment*: The specificity of the NF-κB binding can be evaluated via two different ways: either by competition with a free probe (*see* **Note 7**) or by supershift of the complexes involved. For the supershift experiment, please refer to the general protocol given for the EMSA, except that the gel is a 4% acrylamide/bisacrylamide instead of a 6% as used for the EMSA experiment. This technique is based on the use of specific antibodies that can bind directly to the proteins that are part of the NF-κB–DNA probe complex, inducing a super-complex antibody–NF-κB–DNA probe that migrates at a lower rate in the non-denaturing gel. This technique not only ensures the specificity of the NF-κB binding but also allows identifying the subunits that are present in the complexes. For this, please incubate 1 μl of concentrated antibodies (**Section 2.4.2** or **2.4.3**) with the

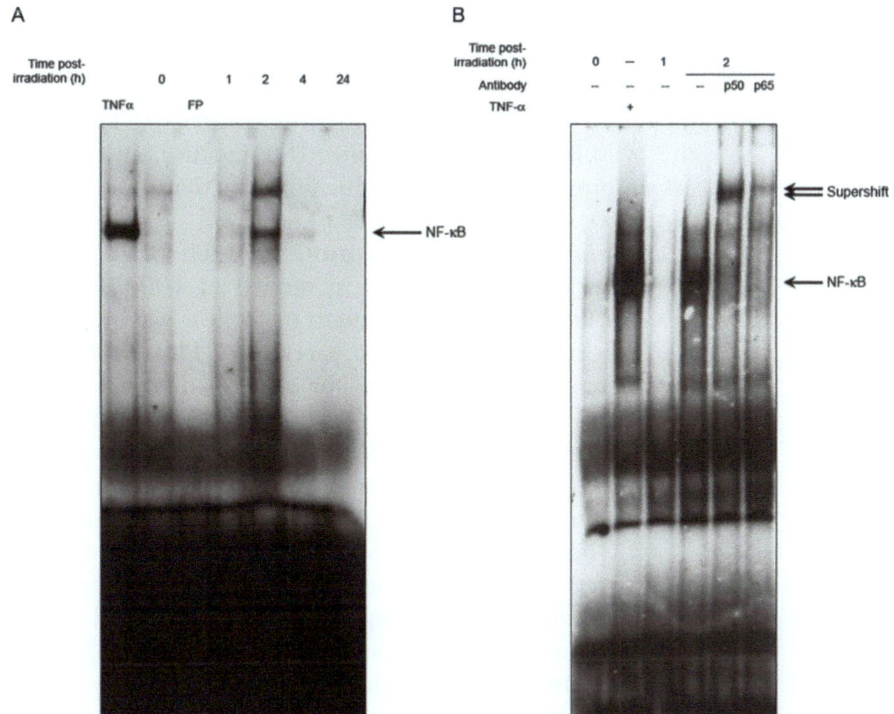

Fig. 6.3. (**a**) EMSA experiment to detect the binding of the NF-κB from nuclear extracts of 5-ALA treated and irradiated or non-irradiated HeLa cells to a specific radiolabelled probe. TNF-α is used as positive control. FP = free probe. (**b**) Supershift experiment to identify the NF-κB subunits involved in the complex bound to a specific radiolabelled probe. TNF-α is used as positive control.

nuclear proteins but without the DNA-binding mixture and the labelled probe for 15 min on ice. After this incubation period, add the DNA-binding mixture and labeled probe for 30 min at room temperature and then proceed as described for the EMSA experiment.

6. *Results*: It can be clearly seen in **Fig. 6.3b** that the incubation of the nuclear extracts from cells collected 2 h post-5-ALA treatment with specific antibodies directed against either p50 or p65, the main NF-κB subunits, induces a clear uppershift of the pre-formed complex. This clearly demonstrates that these NF-κB subunits are involved in the NF-κB complex whose translocation is induced by the PDT treatment (*see* **Notes 8** and **9**).

3.5. Nuclear NF-κB Activity Demonstrated Using a Luciferase Reporter Gene

After the demonstration that PDT treatment can induce a nuclear translocation of the NF-κB subunits and that p50 and p65 proteins are part of the NF-κB complex able to bind an NF-κB consensus probe, it still has to be proved that this complex is able to induce the expression of target genes. We have decided to address this question using a luciferase reporter gene

(LUC) under the control of an NF-κB promoter. For this, 24 h before 5-ALA-PDT treatment, HeLa cells were transiently transfected with a reporter plasmid (pNF-κB-Luc), where the luciferase reporter gene is under the control of a tandem repeat of the NF-κB consensus sequence (Stratagene), and then collected 18 h post-irradiation for luciferase activity measurement (*see* **Note 10**).

1. *HeLa cells transient transfection*: The day prior to transfection, HeLa cells were seeded at 100,000 cells/well in six-well plates. Transient transfection was performed using Fugene reagent (Roche, Germany). Please refer to the manufacturer's instructions for a detailed protocol. Briefly, for each sample, a mix of 100 ng of pNF-κB-Luc plasmid and 400 ng of pcDNA3.1 plasmid (Invitrogen) was prepared as carrier plasmid in a final volume of 50 μl of serum-free medium. A second mix composed of 1.25 μl of Fugene and 48.75 μl of serum-free medium was prepared and rested for 5 min at room temperature. The plasmids and the Fugene were then mixed together and left for 20 min at room temperature. Finally, the solution was dropped onto the cells and they were placed in the incubator.
2. Twenty-four hours post-transfection, the 5-ALA treatment was performed as previously described (**Section 3.1**). Eighteen hours post-irradiation, cells were rinsed with warm PBS, scrapped and collected as described above. The detection of the firefly luciferase activity was achieved using the Luciferase Reporter Gene Assay, High Sensibility (Roche, Germany). Please refer to the manufacturer's instructions for a detailed protocol. Briefly, 200 μl of the provided lysis buffer was added onto the cell pellets and they were left on ice for 20 min. The tubes were centrifuged at maximum speed for 5 min and then the supernatants collected. Next, the detection reaction was immediately started using a detection solution provided and by measuring the emitted light using a luminometer (Lumat LB 9507, EG&G Berthold). It is also important to measure protein concentration in each sample in order to relate this measure to the specific luciferase activity.
3. *Results*: As we can observe in **Fig. 6.4**, a 5-ALA-PDT treatment of HeLa cells induces an activation of the NF-κB promoter on the luciferase reporter gene as exemplified by the increased luciferase activity in a time-dependent way. Positive control for this experiment is a 16 h treatment of HeLa cells with TNF-α (200 U/sample).

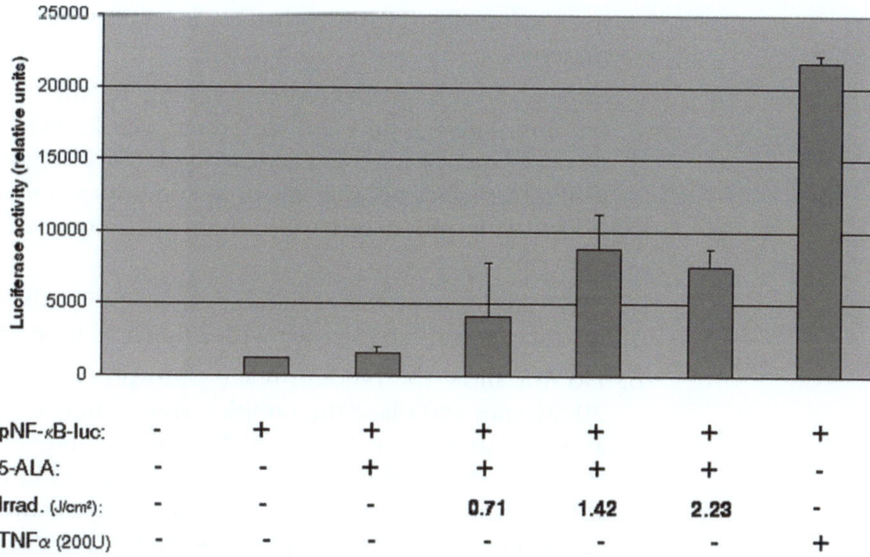

Fig. 6.4. Detection of the luciferase activity in cellular extracts of HeLa cells transiently transfected with a pNF-κB-Luc reporter plasmid with or without 5-ALA-PDT treatment. TNF-α is used as positive control.

4. Notes

1. For all the lysis buffers, it is very important to add the protease (PMSF, Complete, etc.) and the phosphatase inhibitors (Na_3VO_4, β-glycerophosphate, etc.) extemporaneously to ensure a maximum activity of these inhibitors, especially for monitoring protein phosphorylation and keeping the lysates on ice. One alternative protocol for the phosphoprotein detection is to perform a rapid cell lysis using a special buffer containing 62.5 mM Tris–HCl (pH 6.8), 2% SDS, 10% glycerol, 0.1% bromophenol blue and 50 mM DTT. Collect the cells from a 25-cm^2 flask, add 100 μl of this fast-lysing buffer, resuspend the pellet, place it on ice for 15 min and centrifuge at maximum speed for 20 min. It is also important to note that protein concentration cannot be measured via the technique described here but with the BCA method.
2. It is important to perform these experiments in the dark, at least from cell scraping to the end of the lysis. Indeed, NF-κB can be in some cases rapidly activated by light exposure (which is due to the illumination of the PS).
3. Be very cautious with the handling of radioactive [α-^{32}P]-dATP and [α-^{32}P]-dCTP and please refer to the correct

instructions from your institution for the use of this type of material.

4. Several NF-κB probes corresponding to the consensus-binding sites found in different well-known NF-κB-activated genes have been described. We suggest testing different probes because in some conditions, the different NF-κB subunits may have a slightly different affinity for each one.
5. After addition of the radiolabelled probe to the binding mixture, gently tap the tube with a finger to homogenize it.
6. Do not allow the binding reaction to proceed more than 20–30 min and place the samples immediately on ice right after and until the gel loading. This step is quite crucial for the experiment. Always use EMSA loading buffer prepared within the last 3 months because old solutions may impair the migration of the samples. Do not leave the wells of your gel dry and carefully clean them to remove acrylamide residues with a syringe filled with TNE (0.25×). For the loading, we strongly suggest using a Hamilton syringe and carefully drop the samples in the bottom of the well.
7. The specificity of the binding can be assessed by a competition experiment with a "cold" probe. For this, just perform the EMSA as described above but add increasing concentration of non-radiolabelled probe (from 10 to 50 ng in TNE) to the binding mixture and allow the reaction to take place 30 min as described. Be cautious that the volume of added cold probe should be as low as possible (1 μl) in order to keep a similar final volume of reaction.
8. As it is sometimes difficult to observe a clear supershift of the complex, it is often admitted that the supershift takes place either when the protein-DNA complex is upper-shifted by the antibodies or when its intensity is decreased when compared to the non-supershifted control band.
9. It is also possible to supershift other NF-κB subunits. Please find here some antibodies that work very well in our hands: mouse monoclonal anti-p52x antibody (ref SC-7286 X), rabbit polyclonal anti-RelBx antibody (ref SC-226 X), mouse monoclonal anti-C-relx (ref SC-6955 X) (Santa Cruz, USA).
10. We suggest to test different concentrations of transfected reporter plasmid and to use a positive control such as TNF-α to optimize the assay. However, you should keep in mind that the kinetics of NF-κB activation might be slower after a PDT treatment than with TNF-α.

Acknowledgments

IC is supported by a grant FRIA from the FNRS (Brussels, Belgium), JP is Research Director from the FNRS (Brussels, Belgium) and SB is supported by a grant from the Walloon Region (Belgium).

References

1. Luo, J. L., Kamata, H., and Karin, M. (2005) The anti-death machinery in IKK/NF-kappaB signaling. *J Clin Immunol*, **25**(6), 541–550.
2. Bonizzi, G. and Karin, M. (2004) The two NF-kappaB activation pathways and their role in innate and adaptive immunity. *Trends Immunol*, **25**(6), 280–288.
3. Ghosh, S. and Hayden, M. S. (2008) New regulators of NF-kappaB in inflammation. *Nat Rev Immunol*, **8**(11), 837–848.
4. Karin, M. and Greten, F. R. (2005) NF-kappaB linking inflammation and immunity to cancer development and progression. *Nat Rev Immunol*, **5**(10), 749–759.
5. Ryter, S. W. and Gomer, C. J. (1993) Nuclear factor kappa B binding activity in mouse L1210 cells following Photofrin II-mediated photosensitization. *Photochem Photobiol*, **58**(5), 753–756.
6. Volanti, C., Gloire, G., Vanderplasschen, A., Jacobs, N., Habraken, Y., and Piette, J. (2004) Downregulation of ICAM-1 and VCAM-1 expression in endothelial cells treated by photodynamic therapy. *Oncogene*, **23**(53), 8649–8658.
7. Matroule, J. Y., Hellin, A. C., Morliere, P. et al. (1999) Role of nuclear factor-kappa B in colon cancer cell apoptosis mediated by aminopyropheophorbide photosensitization. *Photochem Photobiol*, **70**(4), 540–548.
8. Granville, D. J., Carthy, C. M., Jiang, H. et al. (2000) Nuclear factor-kappaB activation by the photochemotherapeutic agent verteporfin. *Blood*, **95**(1), 256–262.
9. Volanti, C., Hendrickx, N., Van Lint, J., Matroule, J. Y., Agostinis, P., and Piette, J. (2005) Distinct transduction mechanisms of cyclooxygenase 2 gene activation in tumour cells after photodynamic therapy. *Oncogene*, **24**(18), 2981–2991.
10. Matroule, J. Y., Volanti, C., and Piette, J. (2006) NF-kappaB in photodynamic therapy: discrepancies of a master regulator. *Photochem Photobiol*, **82**(5), 1241–1246.
11. Volanti, C., Matroule, J. Y., and Piette, J. (2002) Involvement of oxidative stress in NF-kappaB activation in endothelial cells treated by photodynamic therapy. *Photochem Photobiol*, **75**(1), 36–45.
12. Matroule, J. Y., Bonizzi, G., Morliere, P. et al. (1999) Pyropheophorbide-a methyl ester-mediated photosensitization activates transcription factor NF-kappaB through the interleukin-1 receptor-dependent signaling pathway. *J Biol Chem*, **274**(5), 2988–3000.

Chapter 7

Application of 5-Aminolevulinic Acid and Its Derivatives for Photodynamic Therapy In Vitro and In Vivo

Asta Juzeniene, Petras Juzenas, and Johan Moan

Abstract

Photodynamic therapy (PDT) with 5-aminolevulinic acid (ALA) is the most widely used form of PDT in clinical practice. Topical application of ALA leads to overproduction of the endogenous photosensitizer protoporphyrin IX (PpIX). ALA-PDT is efficient treatment of superficial skin lesions, but not for thicker lesions. The main reason for this is suboptimal penetration of ALA molecules through cellular membranes and through stratum corneum of intact skin. Different approaches (formulations, mechanical and physical penetration enhancers, ALA derivatives) are currently used to increase the penetration. The content and distribution of ALA intracellularly and in tissues is difficult to measure, but PpIX content, on a relative scale, can be easily measured by fluorimetric assays.

Key words: Photodynamic therapy, 5-aminolevulinic acid, 5-aminolevulinic acid derivatives, protoporphyrin IX, fluorescence spectroscopy, extraction method.

1. Introduction

5-Aminolevulinic acid (ALA), a precursor in the haeme synthesis pathway, is currently used to induce endogenous synthesis of the protoporphyrin IX (PpIX) for photodynamic therapy (PDT) and for fluorescence diagnosis (FD) (1, 2). The ALA molecule is small enough to penetrate the stratum corneum, and, due to this, topical application of ALA is efficient and often used for treating different skin ailments. However, such application of ALA results in a shallow penetration depth (<2 mm) into tissue due to the hydrophilic nature of ALA. Several methods have been proposed in order to increase this penetration (3–5). Different formulations

C.J. Gomer (ed.), *Photodynamic Therapy*, Methods in Molecular Biology 635,
DOI 10.1007/978-1-60761-697-9_7, © Springer Science+Business Media, LLC 2010

(creams, lotions, gels, bioadhesive patches, liposomes, nanoparticles, bases with addition of penetration enhancers) are used to enhance the penetration through the stratum corneum and to increase the diffusion in tissue. Enhanced penetration can also be achieved by physical methods (curettage, ultrasound, iontophoresis, electroporation and electrophoresis) and by chemical derivatization of ALA. A number of new derivatives of ALA are continuously being synthesized and tested. Different derivatives may be optimal for different applications. It is necessary to determine the optimal ALA ester: one with good stability, deep penetration, high efficiency of PpIX generation, homogenous tissue distribution, allowing short application times and low drug dose (for reduction of costs), and, thus, overall possessing the best diagnostic and therapeutic properties. The ultimate criterion for choice should be the treatment outcome.

Haeme biosynthesis is normally so tightly regulated that the concentrations of intermediate products are far below the threshold of photosensitization. After addition of exogenous ALA or its derivatives, porphyrins accumulate, because both of the rate-limiting enzyme ALA synthase and the haeme feedback mechanism are bypassed. Analysis of different tissues by HPLC shows that the predominant porphyrin synthesized in different tissues is PpIX (6). Flow cytometry (7), HPLC (6), confocal fluorescence microscopy (8) and fluorescence spectroscopy (9) are used to measure PpIX synthesis in cells. Fluorescence spectroscopy is simple, useful, reliable and noninvasive technique in monitoring PpIX production in healthy skin and its lesions in vivo. Direct PpIX fluorescence measurements and chemical extraction of PpIX from cells and tissues are often used, and are described in this chapter.

2. Materials

2.1. Cell Culture

1. Dulbecco's Modified Eagle's medium (DMEM) (Lonza Group Ltd., Switzerland) supplemented with 100 U/ml penicillin, 100 g/ml streptomycin, 2 mM L-glutamine (Sigma-Aldrich, St. Louis, MO, USA) and foetal calf serum (FCS) (GIBCO BRL, Life Technologies, Roskilde, Denmark).
2. The stock solutions of 5-aminolevulinic acid hydrochloride (ALA), methyl 5-aminolevulinate hydrochloride (MAL) (Sigma-Aldrich, St. Louis, MO, USA), 5-aminolevulinic acid hexyl ester hydrochloride (HAL) (Biosynth AG, Staad, Switzerland) and other ALA esters are dissolved in DMEM

without FCS immediately before taken into the experiments. The stock solutions are sterilized by filtration (0.22 μm pore size) (*see* **Note 1**).

3. Costar cell scrapers (Corning, Corning, NY, USA) are used to bring cells into suspension.

2.2. Mice

1. Female NCR athymic nude mice may be used in the study. All procedures and experiments, involving animals, must be carried out according to the ethical guidelines and requirements approved by a local Animal Research Authority as well as according to the policy of the international Federation of European Laboratory Animal Science Associations (FELASA) and The European Convention for the protection of vertebrate animals used for experimental and other scientific purposes.
2. Creams containing different concentration of ALA and its derivatives: the drugs are dissolved directly in a cream (Unguentum, Merck, Darmstadt, Germany) (*see* **Note 2**).

2.3. Solvent for Porphyrin Extraction from the Cells and Tissues

1. 200 ml of the porphyrin extraction solvent supplemented with 1% sodium dodecyl sulphate (SDS) in 1 N perchloric acid and methanol (1:1 v/v). Store at room temperature (*see* **Note 3**).

2.4. Solutions Necessary for PpIX Calibration Curve

1. PpIX solvent, which is the same as the extraction solvent: 1% sodium dodecyl sulphate (SDS) in 1 N perchloric acid and methanol (1:1 v/v) (*see* **Note 3**).
2. A concentrated 0.125 mM PpIX stock solution: dissolve 3.52 mg PpIX (Sigma-Aldrich) in 50 ml solvent. Store at 0–4°C in the dark (*see* **Note 4**).
3. 5 μM PpIX stock solution.

2.5. Fluorescence Measurements

1. A spectrofluorometer (for instance Perkin-Elmer LS50B, Waltham, MA), connected to an external computer for data processing (*see* **Note 5**).
2. A fibre-optic probe coupled to a luminescence spectrometer (*see* **Section 2.5**, step 1) is needed (*see* **Note 6**).

3. Methods

Porphyrins in cells and tissues are often quantified by direct fluorescence measurements (10). This method is fast and sensitive, and it is reliable for comparison between two or more experimental group, for example, when comparing different ALA formulations, studying the presence of different physical methods or different ALA derivatives in order to find which of them is best. Relative intensity values are usually obtained by fluorescence measurements. However, if one needs to quantify PpIX production in different cells or tissues, this method is not reliable due to the following reasons. PpIX has a strong tendency to aggregate in aqueous solutions (11) and the aggregates have much lower fluorescence quantum yields than monomers (12). Different degrees of aggregation may take place in different cells or organs. In addition, different pigmentation of the tissues make direct fluorescence measurements of limited value in pharmacological studies where concentration levels in different organs are measured (10, 13). Direct PpIX fluorescence measurements in a cuvette and using an optical fibre probe as well as the chemical extraction of PpIX from the cells and tissues are described here.

3.1. Incubation of Cells with ALA and Its Derivatives

1. A431 human squamous carcinoma cells are grown in DMEM, supplemented with 100 U/ml penicillin, 100 g/ml streptomycin, 2 mM L-glutamine and 10% FCS, in plastic flasks (Nunclon^{TM}, Nunc, Roskilde, Denmark) at 37°C in a humidified atmosphere of 5% CO_2 and subcultured every 2–3 days using Trypsin–EDTA solution. All tests should be performed in the exponential growth phase of the cell cultures.
2. Calculate how many samples you need and prepare two sets of triplicates for each sample, which will be used for determination of PpIX amount, cell number and cellular protein content independently. A431 cells are seeded on six-well plates (5×10^5 cells, 3 ml medium per well) and incubated for 48 h. At this point the cultures are rinsed twice with DMEM without FCS and incubated for different periods of time in DMEM without FCS containing different concentrations of ALA and its derivatives. Exposure to ambient light must be avoided during incubation with ALA or ALA esters and during all procedures afterwards. Controls are the cells without ALA and its derivatives, which will be treated the same way as the cells with ALA or its esters.
3. After incubation for different periods of time (e.g. 0, 1, 3, 6, 9, 12, 24 h), the cells are washed twice with 0.5 ml ice-cold phosphate buffered saline (PBS) per well. Rinsing should be performed carefully to prevent damage to the cell monolayer: pipette avoiding strong flow and aspirate PBS by placing pipette tip in a corner of each well.
4. Further experimental procedures will depend on which method is chosen to measure formation of PpIX in cells.

If you choose direct fluorescence measurements *see* **Section 3.2.1**, if you choose cellular extraction *see* **Section 3.2.2**.

3.2. Quantification of the Endogenous PpIX Content

3.2.1. Direct Fluorescence Measurements In Vitro

1. The cells are detached with 0.3 ml trypsin per well and 2.5 ml PBS is added to each well.
2. Then each cell suspension is transferred into appropriately marked centrifuge tube.
3. The cells are pelleted by centrifugation for 5 min at 1,000×*g* (around 2,500–3,200 rpm, depending on the rotor radius of the centrifuge, being from 14.5 to 9 cm in this example).
4. The supernatant is carefully removed and discarded. To each pellet 1 ml of PBS is added. The cells are carefully suspended and counted using a haemocytometer or a Coulter counter.
5. Each cell suspension is transferred to a standard 10 mm semi-micro cuvette (1 ml volume; other cuvettes can also be used provided necessary volume of cell suspension is prepared) and fluorescence emission spectra are recorded as described in **Section 2.5**. Fluorescence emission intensities are read at around 636 nm.
6. Fluorescence intensities of cell samples incubated with ALA or its esters are corrected for autofluorescence by subtracting the intensity readings of control samples (blank).
7. The data are expressed as arbitrary fluorescence units per determined number of cells for each sample (for example, F value/10^6 cells).

3.2.2. Fluorescence Measurements of Cell Extracts In Vitro

1. Old medium is aspirated and 1 ml of the porphyrin extraction solvent is added to each well. The cells are brought into suspension with a cell scraper.
2. The plates are kept on a platform and rocked for 10 min at room temperature.
3. The cells are then transferred into centrifuge tubes and centrifuged for 5 min at 1,500×*g* (around 3,000–3,900 rpm, depending on the rotor radius of the centrifuge, being from 14.5 to 9 cm in this example) to remove the cell debris. New vials with transferred supernatants are put on ice, until measurements can be carried out.
4. The supernatant is transferred to a standard 10 mm cuvette and fluorescence emission spectra are measured as described in **Section 2.5**. Fluorescence intensities are recorded at around 606 nm, corresponding to the fluorescence emission

maximum of PpIX in the extraction solvent (*see* **Note 7** and **Section 3.4**).

5. Standard curves are prepared by gradually adding known amounts of PpIX (e.g. 2 + 5 + 10 + 20 + 40 + 60 + 80 + 100 μl of a 5 μM PpIX stock solution, in 1 ml of the extraction solvent) into the supernatant of extracted control cells (not treated with ALA or its esters) and measuring their fluorescence intensities. Peak fluorescence signals of the samples must be within the linear range of the standard curve (*see* **Note 8**).
6. Independent samples are used to determine cell number or cellular protein content. The cell number is determined using a haemocytometer or a Coulter counter. The protein content in the lysates is measured by DC BioRad assay as described by the manufacturer's protocol (BioRad Laboratories, Hercules, CA, USA), or using any other available protein reagent.
7. Fluorescence intensities of cell samples incubated with ALA and its esters are corrected for autofluorescence by subtracting the intensity readings of control samples (blank).
8. Using the calibration curve (obtained in step 5) the concentration of PpIX in each sample is determined. Finally, the data are expressed as ng PpIX per cell number or mg protein (ng PpIX/10^6 cells or ng PpIX/mg protein) (*see* **Note 9**).

3.3. Direct PpIX Fluorescence Measurements with an Optical Fibre Probe

1. After topical application of ALA and its derivatives for different times, the fluorescence of PpIX is measured noninvasively with a fibre-optic probe coupled to a luminescence spectrometer (*see* **Section 2.5**). At least three fluorescence spectra are recorded from the same area.
2. The autofluorescence background, the fluorescence of the skin/tumour measured before the application of the drugs, is subtracted from the fluorescence data.
3. Every fluorescence value is calculated as an average of at least three recordings and the final data are presented as means from all animals (or humans) within the group.

3.4. Preparation of Tissue Homogenates and Supernatants

1. Prepare necessary number of laboratory 10 ml tubes. Mark them in advance with sample names and weigh every empty tube.
2. Each tissue sample (skin, tumour, liver, etc.) excised from animals is put into the appropriate tube. Again weigh the tubes and calculate the weight of every excised tissue sample.
3. To each tube add 2 ml of the extraction solvent.

4. Each sample is then separately homogenized for approximately 1 min by immersing into each sample a homogenizer probe (model PRO200, PRO Scientific, Inc., Monroe, CT). Before immersion into next sample and when finished, thoroughly rinse the homogenizer probe with the extraction solvent or ethanol and then with distilled water. Do not operate the homogenizer without being immersed in a liquid or being wet. After rinsing, remove excess liquid using soak paper. The skin homogenates are then frozen and kept overnight in a freezer (–20°C).
5. The homogenates are thawed within approximately 15 min at room temperature.
6. Each sample is then sonicated for 30 s (longer sonication times will lead to vial heating and possibly to sonochemical destruction of the extracted photosensitizer) by immersing into the samples a thin 20 kHz ultrasound probe (set the amplitude of ultrasonic power at 20%; available ultrasound units: Sonics converter CV18 together with a proprietary 130 W generator VCX130, Sonics and Materials Inc., Meyrin/Satigny, Switzerland; Branson converter CL70028A (set the microtip position at 3–4, max 5) with a proprietary generator Sonifier B-12A, Branson Sonic Power Comp., Danbury, CT). Before next sample and when finished, thoroughly rinse the ultrasound probe with the extraction solvent or with ethanol and then with distilled water. After rinsing, remove excess liquid with soak paper.
7. Each suspension is then diluted 1:50 in the extraction solvent (80 μl original extract in 3.92 ml of the extraction solvent). Other dilutions can be prepared if necessary.
8. The rest of the original extracts can be stored frozen at –20°C for future reference.
9. The diluted samples are centrifuged for 10 min at 600×*g* (1,900–2,400 rpm, depending on the radius a centrifuge rotor, being from 14.5 to 9 cm in this example).
10. The supernatants are then separated from the pellets by careful aspiration and transferred into new appropriately marked tubes.
11. Resuspend each pellet in the extraction solvent (1 ml or other volume corresponding to a cuvette to be used). Both the supernatants and the pellets can be frozen if fluorescence measurements cannot be performed the same day.
12. The fluorescence (full spectra or peak readings) of the supernatant and pellet is measured in a cuvette as described above (*see* **Sections 2.5** and **3.2.2**, step 5).

13. Standard curves are prepared for each tissue type by gradually adding known amounts of PpIX (e.g. 2 + 5 + 10 + 20 + 40 + 60 + 80 + 100 μl of a 5 μM PpIX stock solution, in 1 ml of the extraction solvent) into the control samples of each tissue type. This is to account for any spectral differences occurring due to different chromophores present in different tissues.
14. Determine the PpIX amount in each sample form the standard curves (obtained in step 13).
15. Finally, calculate PpIX amount per sample of wet tissue (μg PpIX/1 g wet tissue) (*see* **Note 9**).

4. Notes

1. Working solutions are prepared by dilution in DMEM without serum. Serum-free medium is used in order to avoid porphyrin extraction from the cells (14, 15).
2. Approximately 75 mg/cm^2 of the freshly prepared cream is applied topically on the tumours or on the normal skin and covered with a occlusive transparent adhesive dressing (OpSite Flexigrid, Smith & Nephew Medical Ltd., Hull, UK). The creams are maintained continuously on the test spots for the duration of the experiment (maximally 24 h). The fluorescence measurements are carried out through the transparent occlusive dressing, which reduces the fluorescence signal by less than 10%.
3. First fill a vial with 91.4 ml of cold distilled water and then add 8.6 ml of 70% $HClO_4$. Add 100 ml of methanol to the solution. Dissolve 2 g of SDS and mix well. To check if the porphyrin extraction solution is of good quality, shake it and look at it. If it becomes transparent quickly, it is suitable for measurements. If not, make new solution. By the way, the porphyrin extraction solvent was first described by Gomer et al. (16).
4. Sonicate the solution for 1 min to completely dissolve PpIX. Prolonged sonication will lead to vial heating and sonochemical destruction of PpIX.
5. Fluorescence emission spectra of porphyrins in the supernatant of extracts should be measured in the range of 550–750 nm using a spectrofluorometer. Photomultiplier voltage is usually set at 800 V. A long pass cut-off filter (515 nm) is used on the emission side of the spectrometer to block scattered excitation light. The fluorescence, originating from PpIX, is excited at 407 nm.

6. The fibre-optic probe used for direct fluorescence measurements is commercially available accessory (Perkin-Elmer). It consists of two 1-m fused silica fibre bundles joined in parallel at the measuring tip fit with a cylinder-shaped aluminium spacer (6.5 mm diameter), which provides a constant fixed distance of 10 mm between the fibre ends and the sample surface. This assures a relatively uniform distribution of the excitation light over the area to be measured and provides the maximum fluorescence signal for a given setup.
7. In acidic solutions protonation of porphyrins occurs by forming cations or dications. Thus, spectral changes of porphyrins in the extraction solvent are observed in comparison with that in PBS or in tissues. Note that PpIX fluorescence peak is at 605 nm in the extracts while it is at 636 nm in direct PpIX fluorescence measurements.
8. Calibration curve should be a straight line for PpIX concentrations up to 200 ng/ml.
9. Around 90% of PpIX induced by ALA or its derivatives can be extracted from cancer cells, normal skin or tumour by this extraction method.

Acknowledgements

We appreciate financial support from the Norwegian Cancer Society (Kreftforeningen). As well P. Juzenas would like to acknowledge researcher grant received from the Research Council of Norway (Forskningsrådet). The authors also thank Vladimir Iani and Dr. Li-Wei Ma for technical assistance, reading the manuscript and giving valuable comments and suggestions.

References

1. Peng, Q., Warloe, T., Berg, K., Moan, J., Kongshaug, M., Giercksky, K. E., and Nesland, J. M. (1997) 5-Aminolevulinic acid-based photodynamic therapy. Clinical research and future challenges. *Cancer*, **79**, 2282–2308.
2. Morton, C. A., McKenna, K. E., and Rhodes, L. E. (2008) Guidelines for topical photodynamic therapy: update. *Br J Dermatol*, **159**, 1245–1266.
3. Donnelly, R. F., McCarron, P. A., and Woolfson, A. D. (2005) Drug delivery of aminolevulinic acid from topical formulations intended for photodynamic therapy. *Photochem Photobiol*, **81**, 750–767.
4. Morrow, D. I., Garland, M. J., McCarron, P. A., Woolfson, A. D., and Donnelly, R. F. (2007) Innovative drug delivery strategies for topical photodynamic therapy using porphyrin precursors. *J Environ Pathol Toxicol Oncol*, **26**, 105–116.
5. Donnelly, R. F., McCarron, P. A., Morrow, D. I., Sibani, S. A., and Woolfson, A. D. (2008) Photosensitiser delivery for photodynamic therapy. Part 1: topical carrier platforms. *Expert Opin Drug Deliv*, **5**, 757–766.

6. Hua, Z., Gibson, S. L., Foster, T. H., and Hilf, R. (1995) Effectiveness of delta-aminolevulinic acid-induced protoporphyrin as a photosensitizer for photodynamic therapy in vivo. *Cancer Res*, **55**, 1723–1731.
7. Luksiene, Z., Eggen, I., Moan, J., Nesland, J. M., and Peng, Q. (2001) Evaluation of protoporphyrin IX production, phototoxicity and cell death pathway induced by hexylester of 5-aminolevulinic acid in Reh and HPB-ALL cells. *Cancer Lett*, **169**, 33–39.
8. Sato, N., Moore, B. W., Keevey, S., Drazba, J. A., Hasan, T., and Maytin, E. V. (2007) Vitamin D enhances ALA-induced protoporphyrin IX production and photodynamic cell death in 3-D organotypic cultures of keratinocytes. *J Invest Dermatol*, **127**, 925–934.
9. Gaullier, J. M., Berg, K., Peng, Q., Anholt, H., Selbo, P. K., Ma, L. W., and Moan, J. (1997) Use of 5-aminolevulinic acid esters to improve photodynamic therapy on cells in culture. *Cancer Res*, **57**, 1481–1486.
10. Moan, J., Ma, L. W., Juzeniene, A., Iani, V., Juzenas, P., Apricena, F., and Peng, Q. (2003) Pharmacology of protoporphyrin IX in nude mice after application of ALA and ALA esters. *Int J Cancer*, **103**, 132–135.
11. Margalit, R., Shaklai, N., and Cohen, S. (1983) Fluorimetric studies on the dimerization equilibrium of protoporphyrin IX and its haemato derivative. *Biochem J*, **209**, 547–552.
12. Moan, J. (1984) The photochemical yield of singlet oxygen from porphyrins in different states of aggregation. *Photochem Photobiol*, **39**, 445–449.
13. Juzenas, P., Juzeniene, A., Stakland, S., Iani, V., and Moan, J. (2002) Photosensitizing effect of protoporphyrin IX in pigmented melanoma of mice. *Biochem Biophys Res Commun*, **297**, 468–472.
14. Hanania, J. and Malik, Z. (1992) The effect of EDTA and serum on endogenous porphyrin accumulation and photodynamic sensitization of human K562 leukemic cells. *Cancer Lett*, **65**, 127–131.
15. Iinuma, S., Farshi, S. S., Ortel, B., and Hasan, T. (1994) A mechanistic study of cellular photodestruction with 5-aminolaevulinic acid-induced porphyrin. *Br J Cancer*, **70**, 21–28.
16. Gomer, C. J., Jester, J. V., Razum, N. J., Szirth, B. C., and Murphree, A. L. (1985) Photodynamic therapy of intraocular tumors: examination of hematoporphyrin derivative distribution and long-term damage in rabbit ocular tissue. *Cancer Res*, **45**, 3718–3725.

Chapter 8

Hypoxia and Perfusion Labeling During Photodynamic Therapy

Theresa M. Busch

Abstract

The development of tumor hypoxia during illumination for photodynamic therapy (PDT) can negatively affect treatment outcome. Furthermore, the spatial distribution of this hypoxia may impact the balance between tumor cell damage and vascular damage as mechanisms of photodynamic effect. The hypoxia markers EF3 [(2-(2-nitroimidazol-1 [H]-yl)-*N*-(3,3,3-trifluoropropyl)acetamide)] or EF5 [(2-(2-nitroimidazol-1 [H]-yl)-*N*-(2,2,3,3,3-pentafluoropropyl)acetamide)] can provide a quantitative description of the intratumor distribution of hypoxia during PDT. In vivo perfusion labeling coupled with immunohistochemical staining for vascular structure can provide accompanying information on the status of tumor blood flow at treatment conclusion. Taken together these data can be used to access the relative spatial distributions of hypoxia and perfusion during PDT.

Key words: Photodynamic therapy, hypoxia, EF3, EF5, perfusion, immunohistochemistry.

1. Introduction

Photodynamic therapy (PDT) can have profound effects on tumor microenvironment, even during the period of light exposure. Oxygen consumption by the photochemical process can create hypoxia, as can PDT effects on blood flow in the treated field. Intra-treatment effects of PDT on oxygen concentration and blood flow can impact therapeutic outcome, and numerous studies have demonstrated that choice of treatment conditions to minimize photochemical oxygen consumption can significantly improve long-term tumor response (1, 2). To the interested investigator, a number of technologies are suitable for measuring PDT effects on tissue oxygenation and/or blood flow (3). The

C.J. Gomer (ed.), *Photodynamic Therapy*, Methods in Molecular Biology 635,
DOI 10.1007/978-1-60761-697-9_8,

analysis of hypoxia marker binding during PDT is one such technique that is particularly well suited for the quantitative microscopic analysis of the spatial distribution of hypoxia (4).

The hypoxia markers EF3 [(2-(2-nitroimidazol-1 [H]-yl)-*N*-(3,3,3-trifluoropropyl)acetamide)] and EF5 [(2-(2-nitroimidazol-1 [H]-yl)-*N*-(2,2,3,3,3-pentafluoropropyl)acetamide)] form long-lasting covalent bonds with hypoxic cells. Binding increases linearly as a function of incubation time and drug concentration, and inversely with oxygen concentration (5–7). The cell-bound hypoxia marker can then be detected by a fluorochrome-labeled antibody and visualized by fluorescence microscopy. Through methods developed by us and outlined below, EF3 labeling was used to assess the level and distribution of hypoxia during Photofrin-PDT of murine tumors (8, 9). With the addition of in vivo perfusion labeling, hypoxia can be visualized relative to the distribution of perfused blood vessels, and when both in vivo perfusion labeling and immunohistochemical staining for vascular structure are performed it is possible to determine the fraction of vascular structure with perfusion at the conclusion of illumination. Such data are valuable for the identification of PDT treatment protocols that are oxygen-sparing at the desired target of interest, e.g., tumor cells and/or the vasculature.

2. Materials

2.1. In Vivo *Labeling of Hypoxia and Perfusion*

1. EF3 (266 g/mole) at 20 mM in sterile saline or EF5 (302 g/mole) at 10 mM in sterile saline (Imaging Service Center, Department of Radiation Oncology, University of Pennsylvania, www.hypoxia-imaging.org). To aid dissolution the mixture can be heated and/or sonicated. Store final solution at room temperature, protected from light.
2. Hoechst 33342 (Sigma-Aldrich, St. Louis, MO): 3 mg/ml in sterile saline; store frozen, protected from light.
3. Tissue-Tek O.C.T. compound (Electron Microscopy Services, Hatfield, PA).

2.2. Sectioning and Fixation

1. Poly-L-lysine coated slides (LabScientific Inc., Livingston, NJ).
2. 4% paraformaldehyde (PF): 4% (w/v) paraformaldehyde (Sigma-Aldrich) in 1X PBS. Dissolve PF in nine parts of warm water then add 1 part 10X PBS (*see* **Section 2.4**, step 2). Filter solution (0.45 μm paper; Buchner funnel). Adjust pH to 7.3 by addition of sodium hydroxide (NaOH) as needed. Store at 4°C for use within 2 weeks (*see* **Note 1**).

2.3. Fluorescence Microscopy for Perfusion Label (see Note 2)

1. Filter cube appropriate for Hoechst 33342 (e.g., Nikon UV 2E/C DAPI with Ex 330-380, DM 400, BA 435-485).
2. Raised cover slip; place strips of laboratory tape (colored label tape; Fisher, Pittsburgh, PA) along two opposite edges of a hemacytometer cover slip (this is thicker than a standard cover slip).

2.4. Immunohisto-chemistry

1. PAP pen (Sigma-Aldrich) or other solubilized wax pen.
2. 10X PBS (Dulbecco's Phosphate Buffered Solution; Sigma-Aldrich); prepare in distilled, deionized water using the lot-specific manufacturer-indicated density. Thimerosal (Sigma-Aldrich) is added as a preservative to final concentration of 100 μM. Store at room temperature.
3. 1X PBS; dilute from the 10X PBS stock in distilled, deionized water. Store at 4°C; good for a minimum of 3 weeks (*see* **Note 3**).
4. PBS with Tween 20 (PBStt); dissolve Tween 20 (Bio Rad, Hercules, CA) to 0.3% (w/v) in 1X PBS and stir thoroughly to dissolve. Add thimerosal to 100 μM and sodium azide (Sigma-Aldrich) to 2 mM. Store at 4°C.
5. Antibody carrier: PBStt with 1.5% (w/v) lipid-free albumin (albumin from bovine serum; Sigma-Aldrich). Store at 4°C.
6. Block: antibody carrier with 5% (v/v) normal mouse serum (Jackson Immunoresearch, West Grove, PA) and 20% (v/v) nonfat milk. Nonfat milk, e.g., nonfat carnation powder, is dissolved at 10% (w/w) in 1X PBS. Store block at 4°C for use within 3 weeks.
7. 1% PF: 4% PF diluted in 1X PBS.
8. A8-Cy3 (for EF3) or ELK3-51-Cy3 (for EF5) antibody (Imaging Service Center, Department of Radiation Oncology, University of Pennsylvania, www.hypoxia-imaging.org): 0.075 mg/ml in antibody carrier; stored at 4°C, protected from light.
9. Competed A8-Cy3 (for EF3) or competed ELK3-51-Cy3 (for EF5) antibody: A8-Cy3 or ELK3-51-Cy3 antibody-containing 1 mM EF3 or 0.05 mM EF5, respectively.
10. CD31 antibody: rat anti-mouse CD31 antibody (BD Pharmingen, San Diego, CA); dilute 1:100 in antibody carrier immediately before use.
11. CD31 secondary antibody: Cy5 AffiniPure mouse anti-rat IgG (H+L) min X Hu, Bov, Hrs, Ms, Gt, Rb, Sr Prot (Jackson Immunoresearch); dilute 1:100 in antibody carrier immediately before use.

2.5. Fluorescence Photography for Hypoxia, Blood Vessels, and Tissue Area

1. Calibration dye composed of a standard concentration of Cy3 dye in 1% PF. Standard concentration is determined as that required to result in a mean absorption of 1.25 at 549 nm. Store at 4°C, protected from light.
2. Filter cubes appropriate for Hoechst 33342 (*see* **Section 2.3**, step 1), Cy 5 (e.g., Nikon Cy5, ex 590-650, DM 660, BA 663-735), and Cy 3 (e.g., Nikon TRITC, ex 530-560, DM 570, BA 590-650).

2.6. Image Analysis

1. Adobe® Photoshop® Creative Suite (CS) (Adobe Systems Incorporated, San Jose, CA).

3. Methods

In order to quantify the severity and distribution of PDT-created hypoxia, tumor-bearing animals are injected with hypoxia marker immediately prior to the start of illumination, and tumor is excised from the anesthetized animals and frozen within minutes of the conclusion of illumination. The presence of vascular perfusion is labeled by animal injection with a fluorescent dye at 90 s before tumor excision and freezing. After sectioning, staining, and photography of the tumors, PDT effects on hypoxia and perfusion are determined by comparing these features to those found in control animals exposed to the hypoxia and perfusion labels for the same exposure time, but in the absence of PDT.

EF3 is specified as the hypoxia marker in **Section 3**. However, EF5 can be used alternately in conjunction with its antibody, as listed in **Section 2**.

3.1. In Vivo Labeling of Hypoxia and Perfusion During PDT

1. This protocol assumes that tumors are used at a size free of pre-existing necrosis and that PDT is performed through surface illumination, i.e., not using interstitial fibers that will cause tissue damage. EF3 will be reduced in and thus bind to only viable tissue so tissue anoxia/hypoxia secondary to necrosis will not be labeled.
2. The setup for PDT should be pre-arranged to ensure that treatment begins as soon as possible after hypoxia marker injection. For example, laser output should be measured and adjusted as needed and all treatment fibers should be properly positioned for light delivery to the tumor (*see* **Note 4**).
3. EF3 at 52 mg/kg is injected iv (tail vein) in the awake mouse (*see* **Note 5**). Immediately after EF3 injection the animal is anesthetized and PDT is begun (*see* **Note 6**).

4. At 90 s before the end of PDT, Hoechst 33342 at 30 mg/kg is injected (retro-orbital) without disturbing the laser treatment.
5. At the conclusion of PDT the tumor is excised from the anesthetized animal and frozen (*see* **Note 7**). Use of bright lights should be avoided to minimize photobleaching of Hoechst-labeled perfusion. The tumor is frozen to a slip of labeled filter paper moistened with saline and placed on a pre-cooled aluminum plate that lies on a layer of dry ice. After placement on the filter paper the tumor is covered in O.C.T. compound. The filter paper with attached frozen tumor is stored at –80°C in a cryovial that also contains a chip of wet ice to help prevent tissue desiccation.

3.2. Tissue Sectioning and Fixation

1. The frozen tumor is moved from the –80°C freezer to the –25°C cryostat at ~60 min prior to sectioning to allow it to equilibrate to the higher temperature.
2. Groups of five sections (14 μm thick) are cut from two to three different levels spaced to be representative of the tumor. Care must be taken to protect the sections from light to avoid photobleaching of Hoechst-labeled perfusion.
3. Immediately after a section is collected onto a labeled slide (*see* **Note 8**), fixation is performed by placing the slide in a Coplin jar containing a pre-cooled solution of 4% PF (1 h ± 10 min; on ice).
4. After fixation, slides are rinsed three times for 5 min each in Coplin jars containing 1X PBS (on ice).

3.3. Fluorescence Photography for Perfusion Label

1. Photography for the perfused-Hoechst label, which is called endogenous Hoechst (EH) from this point forward, is performed immediately following section fixation and rinses. In order to keep the section moist during photography it is covered with several drops of room temperature 1X PBS and a raised cover slip (*see* **Note 9**).
2. Photographs are generally taken with a 4× or 10× lens. Because Hoechst is photolabile, an approximate exposure time is estimated from a section to subsequently be used for control EF3 or CD31 staining (described below). Exposure time is selected to provide images that utilize the maximal range in signal intensity, e.g., 0–4,095 on a 12 bit system or 0–255 on an 8 bit system. However, to avoid overexposure care should be taken to ensure that only a few pixels demonstrate maximal intensity. Furthermore, the exposure time should not be longer than a value that results in background signal (on nontissue-containing areas) greater than ~5% of the maximum range in signal intensity (*see* **Note 10**).

3. The stage coordinates of the location of the image should be recorded to allow the user to return to the same location for subsequent photography of hypoxia, etc. Multiple adjacent frames can be photographed as desired to provide an image of EH labeling in a larger area of interest (*see previous* **Note 2**).

3.4. Immunohistochemistry

3.4.1. Blocking

1. After photography for EH, sections are circled with a PAP pen to confine the subsequent reagents. Add mouse block drop-by-drop, enough to cover the section but remaining within the boundaries of the PAP pen. Slides are laid on a water-moistened Kimwipe placed inside the lid to a 96-well plate (four slides fit per lid) and covered by another lid to ensure that moisture is maintained in the slide environment. Lids can be stacked to accommodate more than four slides. The stack of slide-containing lids is placed in a refrigerator for blocking overnight at 4°C (*see* **Note 11**).
2. After blocking, slides are rinsed for 1 min (*see* **Note 12**) in a Coplin jar containing PBStt (room temperature) and then divided into staining groups as summarized in **Table 8.1**.

Table 8.1
Example of slide assignments[a]

Level	Section #	Photography for EH	Stain
1	1	Yes	EF3
	2	Yes	CD31
	3	Optional	CS[b]-EF3
	4	Optional	NS[c]-EF3
	5	Optional	Second antibody control for CD31
2	1	Yes	EF3
	2	Yes	CD31
	3	Optional	CS-EF3
	4	Optional	NS-EF3
	5	Optional	Second antibody control for CD31

[a]Depending on the size of the tumor it may be desirable to collect sections from more than two levels. Typically, a group of tissue sections from one plane of a tumor (level 1) is separated by an intervening space of at least 500 μm from the next group (level 2). Also, within each level, duplicate sections are sometimes collected for each stain in order to provide an alternative if one is inadvertently damaged

[b]Competed stain (CS) control

[c]No stain (NS) control

3.4.2. EF3 Staining

1. A8-Cy3 antibody is added drop-by-drop to sections to be stained for EF3 until the section is covered. Controls for competed stain (CS) are covered in competed A8-Cy 3 antibody and controls for no stain (NS) are covered in antibody carrier. Slides are laid on a water-moistened Kimwipe placed inside the lid to a 96-well plate and covered by another lid for 5 h of staining at 4°C.
2. Rinse EF3-stained slides and NS slides twice for 45 min each in Coplin jars containing PBStt (4°C). EF3-stained and NS slides, as well as those stained with CS (below), must be kept separate from each other to avoid antibody transfer until 1 h after final storage in 1% PF.
3. Rinse CS slides by the drop-by-drop addition of PBStt with 500 μM EF3 until the section is covered (*see* **Note 13**). Let the section rinse for 2 min, remove the rinse solution by gently tapping the slide on its edge or wicking away with a Kimwipe, and then repeat this process for a total of four times over ~10 min. The fifth rinse takes place over 35 min with the slide laying on a water-moistened Kimwipe inside a stack of 96-well-plate lids (4°C). Repeat this process in conjunction with the second 45 min rinse of the EF3-stained and NS slides.
4. All slides, EF3-stained, NS, and CS, are rinsed for about 45 min in Coplin jars of 1X PBS (4°C).
5. Slides are stored in Coplin jars containing 1% PF (4°C) until photography.

3.4.3. CD31 Staining

1. Sections to be stained for CD31 receive the drop-by-drop addition of diluted CD31 antibody until the section is covered. Secondary antibody controls for CD31 are instead exposed to antibody carrier. Slides are laid on a water-moistened Kimwipe placed inside the lid to a 96-well plate and covered by another lid for 1 h of staining at room temperature.
2. Slides are rinsed three times for 15 min each in Coplin jars containing PBStt (room temperature).
3. After rinses, diluted secondary antibody is added drop-by-drop to all sections for a staining time of 45 min (room temperature). Slides are laid on a water-moistened Kimwipe placed inside the lid to a 96-well plate and covered by another lid during staining.
4. Slides are rinsed three times for 7 min each in Coplin jars containing PBStt (room temperature).
5. Slides are stored in a Coplin jar containing 1% PF (4°C) until photography.

3.5. Fluorescence Photography for Hypoxia, Blood Vessels, and Tissue Area

3.5.1. Setup for Photography

1. Photography should be performed within ~3 weeks of the conclusion of staining.
2. Rinse 1% PF from slides in a Coplin jar of 1X PBS.
3. Flood each slide to be photographed with Hoechst 33342 in order to label all cell nuclei. This is accomplished by placing the slides in a Coplin jar that contains 20 μM of Hoechst 33342 in 1X PBS for 5 min (room temperature). This is followed by a rinse in 1X PBS for a minimum of 5 min (room temperature).
4. Load the calibration dye in a hemacytometer and photograph (10×) the center square with a filter cube for Cy3.

3.5.2. Photography for EF3

1. Photograph the EF3-stained slides with a filter cube for Cy3. If merged images of hypoxia vs. perfusion are desired, images should be collected using the same objective and at the same coordinates as were used for the EH photograph. As with the EH photos, exposure time should be set to utilize the maximal range in signal intensity. In order to keep the section moist during photography it is covered with several drops of room temperature 1X PBS and a raised cover slip.
2. After photography for EF3, re-photograph at the same coordinates with the filter cube for Hoechst to obtain an image of tissue-containing areas within the photographed field. This is called a flooded Hoechst (FH) image. The FH image is taken only after photography for EF3 in order to prevent photobleaching of Cy3 with the UV excitation for Hoechst.
3. Control sections (CS and NS) are photographed using the same exposure time as was used for the section stained for EF3; however, a smaller area of the section is typically photographed for controls.
4. After photography of each CS and NS section in turn, re-photograph at the same coordinates with the Hoechst filter to obtain an image of tissue-containing areas within the photographed field.

3.5.3. Photography for CD31

1. Photograph the CD31-stained slides with a filter for Cy5. Images should be collected with the same objective and at the same coordinates as were used for the EH photo. As with the EH photos, exposure time should be set to utilize the maximal range in signal intensity. In order to keep the section moist during photography it is covered with several drops of room temperature 1X PBS and a raised cover slip.

2. After photography for CD31, re-photograph at the same coordinates with the filter cube for Hoechst to obtain an image of tissue-containing areas within the photographed field.
3. CD31 secondary antibody control sections are photographed using the same exposure time as was used for the section stained for CD31.
4. After photography for CD31 control, re-photograph at the same coordinates with the filter cube for Hoechst to obtain an image of tissue-containing areas within the photographed field.

3.6. Image Analysis

3.6.1. Masking of Images

1. Creation of bitmap masks and subsequent image analysis can be performed in Adobe Photoshop.
2. Confirm that images are *grayscale* (under *mode* subheading of *image*).
3. EH and CD31 masks are created using the *auto levels* and then *threshold* functions (under *adjustments* subheading of *image*); on each image a threshold value is selected that suitably identifies the positive-stained regions of interest.
4. FH masks are created after applying a series of filters. Apply the *equalize* function (under *adjustments* subheading of *image*), followed by a *maximum filter* (radius 1; *other* subheading of *filter*) and *median filter* (radius 5; *noise* subheading of *filter*), then select a *threshold* value that suitably identifies the positive-stained regions of interest.

3.6.2. Analysis of EF3 Binding

1. Open FH mask and corresponding EF3 image for that section.
2. Change EF3 image to *grayscale* if needed.
3. Copy the FH mask and paste it onto the EF3 image to create a layer.
4. On the FH mask under *select*, choose *color range*, and select *highlights* to outline the cells.
5. Throw the FH mask layer into the layers window trash (the outlined area should remain on the EF3 image).
6. Create a *histogram* (under *windows*) and record mean, median, and 95% levels (confirm cache level 1).
7. To measure background, outline an area that does not contain any tissue, create *histogram* and record the mean, median, and 95% levels (confirm cache level 1).

8. Open image of hemacytometer-loaded calibration dye standard, create *histogram*, and record mean fluorescence level.
9. For the purpose of inter-tissue comparisons, EF3 binding values are corrected not only for their exposure time but also for day-to-day variation in the intensity of the lamp used for fluorescence microscopy (determined from the standard). A calibrated EF3 tissue value (e.g., median) is calculated as the median tissue fluorescence intensity multiplied by the exposure time (ms) of the standard dye photograph and then divided by the product of the mean fluorescence intensity of the standard dye photograph and the exposure time (ms) for the tissue image.
10. If desired, background correction can be performed by first repeating the above step using values obtained from the background measurement. The resulting calibrated background value is subtracted from the calibrated tissue value on the same image in order to produce a background-corrected, calibrated EF3 tissue level.

3.6.3. Analysis of Perfused Vascular Structure

1. Open FH, EH, and CD31 masks for a given section.
2. Convert images to *grayscale*, if needed.
3. Open *layers* (under *Window*).
4. Select *channels* – within this window select *merge channels.*
5. Choose RGB color (red, green, blue) and designate three channels.
6. In the *merge RGB channels* window designate red as the EH mask, green as the CD31 mask, and blue as the FH mask. Click Ok.
7. Under *select* choose *color range* and select *magenta* or use the *sampled colors* pen to identify magenta on the image.
8. Create a *histogram* of magenta-selected area and record the number of pixels (confirm cache level 1).
9. Clear the magenta-selected area with *deselect* under *select.*
10. Repeat above steps to identify the number of *cyan, blue,* and white pixels in the image (white requires using the *sampled colors* pen).
11. The number of EH-stained pixels in tissue identified by FH is the sum of the magenta and white pixels. The number of CD31-stained pixels in tissue identified by FH is the sum of the cyan and white pixels. The number of CD31-stained pixels that also demonstrate EH-labeled perfusion is the number of white pixels. The number of FH-stained pixels is the sum of the blue, cyan, magenta, and white pixels.

3.6.4. Visualization of Hypoxia Versus Perfusion

1. Open the EH and FH masks and EF3 image for a given section (*see* **Fig. 8.1**).
2. Convert images to *grayscale*, if needed.
3. Create an inverse of the FH mask by selecting *invert* under the *adjustments* subheading in the *image* menu.
4. Open *layers*.
5. Select *channels* within this window select *merge channels*.
6. Choose RGB color (red, green, blue) and designate three channels.
7. In the *merge RGB channels* window designate red as the EF3 image, green as the EH mask, and blue as the inverse of the FH mask. Click Ok.
8. On the merged image adjust the input and output of the blue (non-tissue containing areas), green (perfusion), and red (EF3 binding) colors after selecting each color under the *levels* menu of the *adjustments* subheading in the *image* menu (*see* **Note 14**).

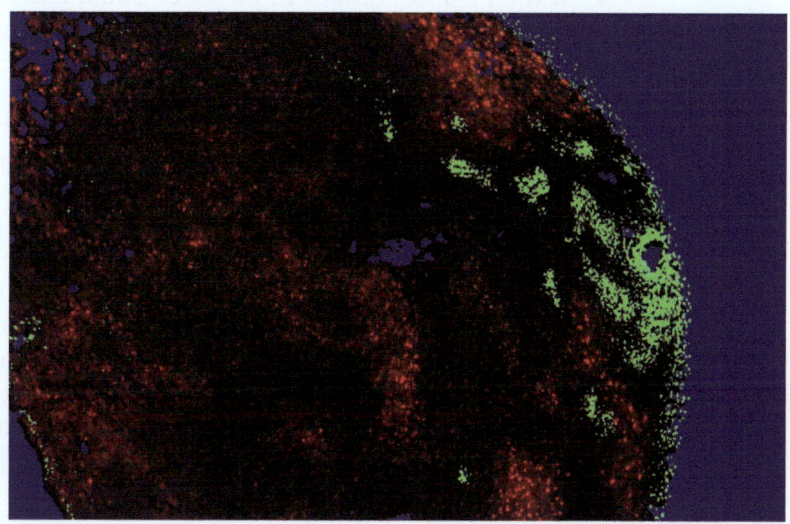

Fig. 8.1. Representative image of hypoxia (EF3 binding; *red*), perfusion (injected Hoechst label; *green*), and nontissue areas (inverse of flooded Hoechst label; *blue*) created through the merge channels feature in Adode Photoshop. Section (14 μm) is from a RIF (radiation-induced fibrosarcoma) tumor treated with Photofrin (5 mg/kg, 24 h) PDT at 75 mW/cm^2, 135 J/cm^2, 630 nm. EF3 labeling took place during the 30 min of PDT and injected Hoechst labeling took place during the last 90 s of PDT, as per the protocol described in **Section 3**. Image depicts a 2.2 × 1.4 mm area.

4. Notes

1. Proper chemical hygiene should be exercised when performing these studies, especially when working with fixatives (paraformaldehyde) and preservatives (thimerosal and sodium azide). It is recommended that paraformaldehyde be purchased in prills (Sigma-Aldrich), which make it less dusty to handle.
2. It is sometimes desirable to photograph multiple adjacent fields to provide an image of a larger area. This is most accurately performed on a microscopy system that consists of an automated stage and controlling software (e.g., IP Lab) because this ensures that the imaging frames are contiguous and electronic stage control enables the user to return to precisely the same location on the section for photography with a different filter for another feature of interest.
3. The reagents of steps 3–6 (**Section 2.4**) may need to be made without sodium azide for peroxidase-based immunohistochemistry.
4. If the PDT conditions to be tested could create perfusion-limited delivery of EF3 then "euthanized animal" studies should be performed to establish sufficient EF3 access to the tumor volume. This involves injecting EF3 at a chosen fluence(s) during PDT, allowing circulation for 5 min, and then euthanizing the animal to create a uniformly hypoxic tumor. The euthanized animal is kept warm for 1 h to allow the creation of tissue hypoxia, caused by respiration, followed by hypoxia marker binding. The process of drug metabolism typically takes place over the first 30–45 min of the 1 h incubation. Sections cut from this tumor are examined for uniform, albeit low levels of, hypoxia marker binding. The presence of FH-stained tissue without EF3 labeling suggests perfusion-related limitations in drug delivery.
5. If EF5 is used instead of EF3 an injected dose of 30 mg/kg is recommended (10).
6. The specified protocol has been used for PDT treatment times of $\geq$30 min. Control animals (not receiving PDT) should be exposed to EF3 for the same length of time as the EF3 incubation that took place during PDT.
7. After in vivo hypoxia labeling, tumors are surgically removed from anesthetized animals rather than harvested from euthanized animals because (1) during euthanasia additional hypoxia marker binding will occur as the animal becomes hypoxic and (2) tumor removal from the

already-anesthetized animal ensures that as little time passes as possible between the end of PDT and tumor freezing.

8. Sections should not be allowed to dry out during any step of these studies.
9. Using cold PBS to keep the section moist during photography will lead to the formation of air bubbles as the solution warms to room temperature and these air bubbles will become trapped under the cover slip causing artifacts in the fluoromicrographs.
10. To reduce photobleaching on the section of interest, a neutral density filter can be used to lower-light levels while viewing the section or taking "test" photographs.
11. If it is desirable to perform CD31 staining on the same day as sectioning, blocking of these sections can be performed for 1 h at room temperature instead of at 4°C overnight.
12. Rinsing in PBStt for more than several minutes could lead to disintegration of the PAP marking, which would then need to be reapplied as needed for subsequent steps.
13. If EF5 is used instead of EF3 the PBStt rinse for CS sections should contain 250 μM EF5.
14. When adjusting input and output levels on the red (EF3 stain) color, care must be taken not to misrepresent the EF3 staining levels. The best approach is to adjust the input levels on two comparative images only to account for any differences in the exposure time and lamp intensity between these images.

Acknowledgments

This work was supported by RO1 CA853831, PO1 CA87971, and CA87645.

References

1. Henderson, B. W., Busch, T. M., and Snyder, J. W. (2006) Fluence rate as a modulator of PDT mechanisms. *Lasers Surg Med*, **38**, 489–493.
2. Busch, T. M. (2006) Local physiological changes during photodynamic therapy. *Lasers Surg Med*, **38**, 494–499.
3. Woodhams, J. H., Macrobert, A. J., and Bown, S. G. (2007) The role of oxygen monitoring during photodynamic therapy and its potential for treatment dosimetry. *Photochem Photobiol Sci*, **6**, 1246–1256.
4. Evans, S. M. and Koch, C. J. (2003) Prognostic significance of tumor oxygenation in humans. *Cancer Lett*, **195**, 1–16.
5. Busch, T. M., Hahn, S. M., Evans, S. M., and Koch, C. J. (2000) Depletion of tumor oxygenation during photodynamic therapy: detection by the hypoxia marker EF3 [2-(2-nitroimidazol-1

[*H*]-yl)-*N*-(3,3,3,-trifluoropropyl)acetamide]. *Cancer Res*, **60**, 2636–2642.

6. Koch, C. J. (2008) Importance of antibody concentration in the assessment of cellular hypoxia by flow cytometry: EF5 and pimonidazole. *Radiat Res*, **169**, 677–688.
7. Koch, C. J. (2002) Measurement of absolute oxygen levels in cells and tissues using oxygen sensors and 2-nitroimidazole EF5. *Methods Enzymol*, **352**, 3–31.
8. Busch, T. M., Wileyto, E. P., Emanuele, M. J., Del Piero, F., Marconato, L., Glatstein, E., and Koch, C. J. (2002) Photodynamic therapy creates fluence rate-dependent gradients in the intratumoral spatial distribution of oxygen. *Cancer Res*, **62**, 7273–7279.
9. Busch, T. M., Wileyto, E. P., Evans, S. M., and Koch, C. J. (2003) Quantitative spatial analysis of hypoxia and vascular perfusion in tumor sections. *Adv Exp Med Biol*, **510**, 37–43.
10. Chen, B., Pogue, B. W., Hoopes, P. J., and Hasan, T. (2005) Combining vascular and cellular targeting regimens enhances the efficacy of photodynamic therapy. *Int J Radiat Oncol Biol Phys*, **61**, 1216–1226.

Chapter 9

Targeting the Tumor Microenvironment Using Photodynamic Therapy Combined with Inhibitors of Cyclooxygenase-2 or Vascular Endothelial Growth Factor

Angela Ferrario and Charles J. Gomer

Abstract

Photodynamic therapy (PDT) involves the administration of a photosensitizer (PS) followed by localized exposure of a targeted tissue to PS adsorbing light. PDT induces cytotoxicity to exposed malignant cells and also effects non-malignant components of the tumor microenvironment. This indirect action of PDT leads to inflammatory and proangiogenic responses and modulates treatment effectiveness. Preclinical studies designed to determine how PDT modulates the tumor microenvironment use murine tumor models to investigate the expression and/or the activation of growth factors, proteinases, and inflammatory molecules following treatment. These studies demonstrate that improvements in treatment responsiveness following PDT are achieved using inhibitors targeting angiogenic and/or inflammatory pathways.

Key words: Photodynamic therapy, angiogenesis, inflammation, tumor microenvironment.

1. Introduction

Many tumors have an active microenvironment rich in growth factors, chemokines, and photolytic enzymes promoting angiogenesis, tissue breakdown, and tissue remodeling. Inflammation-dependent angiogenesis is an important determinant of tumor viability and has lead to direct targeting of the inflammatory angiogenic process as a method to treat and/or prevent cancer (1–3). Cellular responses associated with PDT such as oxidative stress and hypoxia can lead to the transcriptional activation of VEGF (4, 5). Likewise several laboratories have shown that

C.J. Gomer (ed.), *Photodynamic Therapy*, Methods in Molecular Biology 635,
DOI 10.1007/978-1-60761-697-9_9, © Springer Science+Business Media, LLC 2010

PDT-mediated inflammation induces expression and/or activation of additional proangiogenic molecules including COX-2 and prostaglandins (6–8). Procedures designed to suppress angiogenesis and inflammation improves tumor responsiveness following PDT (9–11). This chapter describes tumor models and combined treatment protocols designed to improve the tumoricidal action of PDT. Celecoxib and NS-398 are used to target COX-2 enzymatic activity in a mouse mammary carcinoma tumor model and Avastin (bevacizumab) is used to target human VEGF in a human Kaposi's sarcoma xenograft model. The efficacy of the inhibitors was monitored through quantitative analysis of VEGF and PGE_2 levels in treated and untreated tumors. The effectiveness of the combined treatment regimens targeting VEGF or COX-2 was documented by measuring the tumoricidal response and normal skin phototoxicity.

2. Materials

2.1. Animal and Tumor Models

1. The mouse BA mammary carcinoma cell line was obtained from the NIH (National Institutes of Health), Bethesda, MD, tumor bank and the human Kaposi's sarcoma cell line KS-Imm was obtained from Dr. Albini, National Institute for Cancer Research, Genoa, Italy (12).
2. Female C3H/HeJ mice were purchased from The Jackson Laboratory, Bar Harbor, ME, at 8–12 weeks of age. Female Balb/c nude mice were purchased from Harlan Sprague–Dawley, Indianapolis, IN, at 8–12 weeks of age. Animals were housed in autoclaved mouse cages (four mice per cage) in compliance with the vivarium facility guidelines, the Animal Welfare Act and the NIH Guide for Care and Use of Laboratory Animals.
3. Hair clipper equipped with a size 40 blade set from Oster Professional Products, McMinnville, TN.
4. Euthanasia equipment from Euthanex Corp., Palmer, PA, delivering a CO_2 mixture (increasing from 30 to 70%) at a flow rate of 70 standard ft^3/min.
5. Sterile sharp-pointed scissors, straight microscissors, and straight jewelers microforceps from Fisher Scientific, Pittsburg, PA.
6. Sterile stainless steel Cancer Implant Needles 16 × 3–1/4" (82.6 mm) from Popper & Sons Inc., New Hyde Park, NY.
7. Isoflurane from Phoenix Pharmaceutical Inc., St. Joseph, MO, and Isoflurane Anesthetic Vaporizer from Universal Vaporizer Support, Menlo Park, CA.

2.2. PDT Treatment

1. Photofrin [porfimer sodium (PH)] is a gift from Axcan Scandipharm Inc., Birmingham, AL. PH is stored at 4°C in the dark and dissolved in 5% dextrose in water to make a 2.5 mg/ml stock solution. Stock solutions are aliquoted into glass tubes wrapped in aluminum foil and kept at –20°C. A working solution of 0.5 mg/ml is obtained by diluting the thawed stock solution with saline immediately before use. All procedures are performed in dim light.
2. Mouse scale from Taconic Farms, Germantown, NY.
3. Disposable 1-ml tuberculin syringes and PrecisionGlide 19-, 25-, and 27-gauge needles from BD Biosciences, San Jose, CA.
4. Sylvania infrared heating lamp and an autoclavable polycarbonate cage from Fisher Scientific with custom-made vertical slit for tail vein injection.
5. Ear punch from Fisher Scientific to make identification holes in the distil portion of mouse ears.
6. 630 PDT diode laser, Model T2USA, from Diomed Limited, Cambridge Research Park, Cambridge, UK, emitting monochromatic light at a wavelength of 630 nm.
7. Quartz light delivery fibers with a 400 μm core diameter and a distil microlens tip, Model ML2-0400-DC, from PDT Systems Inc., Santa Barbara, CA.
8. Light beam splitter (630 nm) from Laser Therapeutics, Buellton, CA.
9. Power Meter, Model 210, from Coherent Radiation, Palo Alto, CA.
10. Precision Caliper from Fisher Scientific to measure tumor size and laser beam spot size.

2.3. PDT-Mediated Normal Skin Response: Animal and Quantitative Scoring System

1. Female albino Swiss Webster mice at 8–12 weeks of age were purchased from Harlan Sprague–Dawley, Indianapolis, IN.
2. Hair clipper equipped with a size 40 blade set.
3. Quantitative scoring chart (described in **Table 9.1**) to document the degree of normal tissue damage induced by each treatment.

2.4. Cyclooxygenase-2 (COX-2) and Vascular Endothelial Growth Factor (VEGF) Inhibitors

1. The COX-2 inhibitors NS-398 [*N*-(2-cyclohexyloxy-4-nitrophenyl)-methane sulfonamide], purchased from Cayman Chemical Co., Ann Arbor, MI, and celecoxib, purchased from Pfizer Inc., New York, NY, are dissolved in dimethyl sulfoxide (DMSO) (Sigma-Aldrich, St. Louis, MO) to make 4.0 mg/ml stock solutions and then stored in

Table 9.1
Grading Scores for Acute Skin Photosensitization Reactions

Score	Observation
A. *Reaction appearing*	
0	Normal
1	Slight edema
2	Severe edema
3	Erythema
4	Skin desquamation
5	Areas of necrosis
B. *Reaction subsiding*	
4	Extensive scab formation
3	Decreased scab and epilation
2	Extensive papery skin
1	Slight abnormal appearance
	Slight scab formation
	Reduction of papery skin
	Sparse regrowth of hair
0	Normal

single-use aliquots at –80°C (*see* **Note 1**). Working solutions at 2.0 mg/ml are obtained by diluting stock solutions with saline prior to use.

2. The human VEGF inhibitor Avastin (bevacizumab) obtained from Genentech Inc., South San Francisco, CA, is stable for 1 year when stored at 4°C (Genentech Communication). Working solutions at 2.0 mg/ml are obtained by diluting stock solutions with saline prior to use.

_2.5._ Quantitative Analysis of Prostaglandin E_2 (PGE_2) and VEGF in Tumor Lysates

1. Reporter lysis buffer (5×) from Promega, Madison, WI, stored at room temperature and diluted to 1× in ddH_2O prior to use.
2. Sterile 14-ml polypropylene round-bottom tubes from BD Biosciences and sterile 1.5-ml microcentrifuge tubes from USA Scientific Inc., Ocala, FL.
3. Polytron Virtishear, catalog # 225326, from Virtis Co. Inc., Gardiner, NY, set at 1,500–2,000 rpm to obtain tumor homogenates.
4. Bio-Rad Protein Assay Dye Reagent, catalog # 500-0006, from Bio-Rad Laboratories, Inc., Hercules, CA.

5. Protein Standard, 2 mg BSA (Sigma), reconstituted with 5 ml of ddH_2O and stored at 4°C.
6. Polystyrene–acrylic cuvettes from Sarstedt, Newton, NC.
7. DU-65 Spectrophotometer from Beckman, Fullerton, CA.
8. Prostaglandin E_2 EIA Kit, catalog # 514010, from Cayman Chemical Co., Ann Arbor, MI, and Quantikine human and mouse VEGF immunoassays, catalog # DVE00 and MMV00, from R&D Systems, Minneapolis, MN.
9. Microplate spectrophotometer.

3. Methods

3.1. Tumor Transplantation

1. Mouse BA mammary carcinomas grow in syngeneic female C3H/HeJ mice and human KS-Imm tumors grow in immunodeficient Balb/c nude mice.
2. Hair is removed, using the Oster clipper, from the right hind limb of the C3H/HeJ mice. This step is not needed for the nude mice. *See* **Notes 2** and **3**.
3. Euthanize a tumor-bearing mouse to obtain fresh tumor tissue for transplantation. The tumor used to propagate the line should not exceed 10 mm in the largest diameter.
4. Sterile surgical instruments are used to remove the tumor; place the dissected tumor in a Petri dish and obtain small 1.0- to 1.5-mm pieces (*see* **Note 4**).
5. While anesthetizing four mice at the time, introduce a small 1-mm^3 piece of tumor into the distal slit of the trochar (cancer implant needle). Remove one mouse at a time from the anesthesia chamber and place face down. Stretch the shaved hind limb, wipe the area with an alcohol swab, introduce the tip of the trochar subcutaneously, and push the tumor piece in place (*see* **Note 5**).
6. Return the tumor-transplanted mice to labeled cages. It normally takes 10–14 days for tumors to reach the desirable size for PDT treatment; 5.5–6.5 mm is the largest diameter.

3.2. PDT Treatment: I.V. Injection of Photofrin Followed by Light Exposure

1. Mice with a single tumor measuring 5.5–6.5 mm in the largest diameter are placed in a cage and exposed to an infrared lamp for 5 min to promote dilation of tail veins.
2. In a dim light environment, dilute the aliquoted and thawed stock solution of PH (2.5 mg/ml) to a working solution of 0.5 mg/ml with 0.9% saline using a sterile glass tube.

3. In a darkened environment (the light generated by the heating lamp is sufficient to perform this procedure), remove a mouse from the heated cage and place it into the injection cage while sliding the tail outside through the slit. Wipe the tail with an alcohol swab. Use a 1-ml tuberculin syringe and a 27-gauge needle to inject PH into one of the two lateral veins of the tail (*see* **Note 6**).
4. Cages containing PH-injected mice are left in a darkened environment for the 24-h preceding light treatment. Immediately prior to light treatment, mice (three at a time) are restrained face down on small plastic boards by immobilizing the four limbs and tail with surgical tape (*see* **Note 7**).
5. The light doses used in these studies range from 0 to 200 J/cm^2 and the light dose rate is kept constant at 75 mW/cm^2 to minimize thermal effects (*see* **Note 8**). The treated tumor area is set at 1 cm in diameter (0.785 cm^2).
6. **Figure 9.1** illustrates the light source and the delivery system used for PDT treatments of tumor-bearing mice. Three tumor-bearing mice are treated simultaneously.

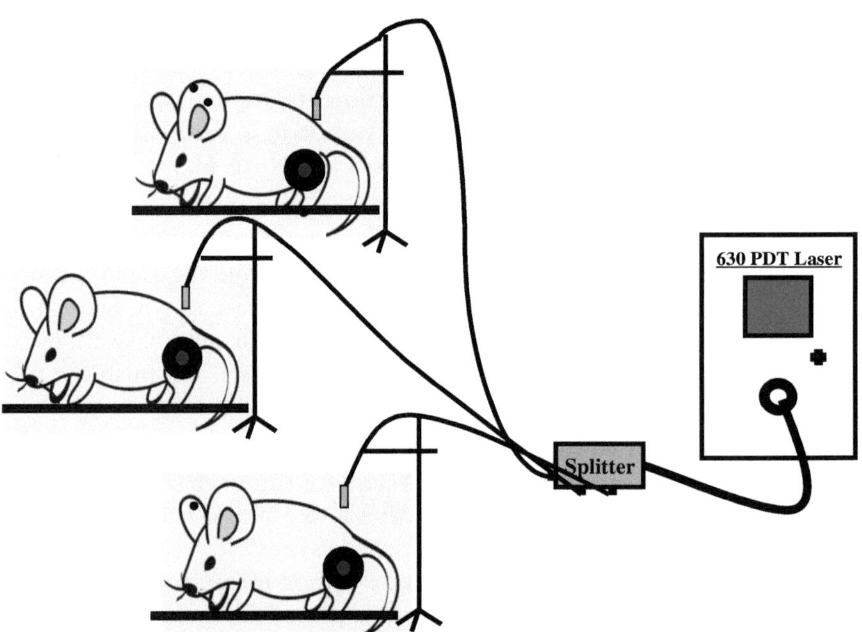

Fig. 9.1. Light treatment of tumor-bearing mice: source and delivery system. The light source (diode laser emitting 630 nm light) is coupled, via a single quartz fiber, to a three-output-beam splitter that permits the simultaneous treatment of three tumor-bearing mice. The light emitted from each fiber is delivered via a 400-μm quartz distal microlens system. The ends of the three fibers are secured on metal tripods, while the distal microlens is positioned above the tumor (supported by a sliding movable clamp) to generate a 1-cm-diameter treatment spot size.

7. Select the treatment parameters (length of the treatment and power of the emitted light) on the screen of the Diomed Laser by following the steps of the operator manual (*see* **Note 9**).
8. The low-power laser-aiming beam is used to position the laser light to the tumor area of the restrained mice. The clamp supporting the light delivery fiber is moved vertically to produce a uniform 1-cm-diameter light spot over the tumor.
9. When all the parameters (power, time, and spot size) have been set, start the light treatment.
10. Mice are returned to labeled cages following treatment. Mice are monitored thrice weekly for detection of tumor recurrence. In case of tumor recurrence, lesion size is recorded and volume is calculated as: $L \times W^2 \times \pi/6$. Tumor cures are defined as treated mice being disease-free for at least 90 days following PDT.

3.3. Treatment Protocol for PDT Combined with COX-2 or VEGF Inhibitors

1. Each inhibitor (NS-398, celecoxib or Avastin) is administered by an i.p. injection (10 mg/kg) starting immediately after light exposure (time 0) and then repeated at 4, 24, 48 h after treatment and then once every other day up to 20 days post-PDT.
2. Mice are monitored for tumor recurrence up to 90 days after single and combined treatments. **Figure 9.2a,b** shows examples of Kaplan–Meier curves generated by plotting the percentages of mice without tumor recurrences as a function of time following treatments.
3. Direct comparisons of the percentage of tumor cures at the end of the 90-day observation period, as well as differences in tumor regrowth rates, are used to determine the effectiveness of each treatment protocol (*see* **Note 10**).

3.4. PDT-Mediated Normal Skin Response

1. Remove the hair (using the Oster clipper) from the right hind limb of Swiss Webster mice.
2. Treat the mice with either a single PDT treatment (following the steps in **Section 3.2**, steps 2–10) or PDT plus inhibitor (**Section 3.3**, step 1).
3. Place the treated mice into labeled cages and monitor thrice weekly for skin reactions according to the skin scoring system (**Table 9.1**). Evaluations continue until the exposed skin returns to normal. The skin response is calculated as an average for each treatment group and plotted as a function of time (**Fig. 9.3**).

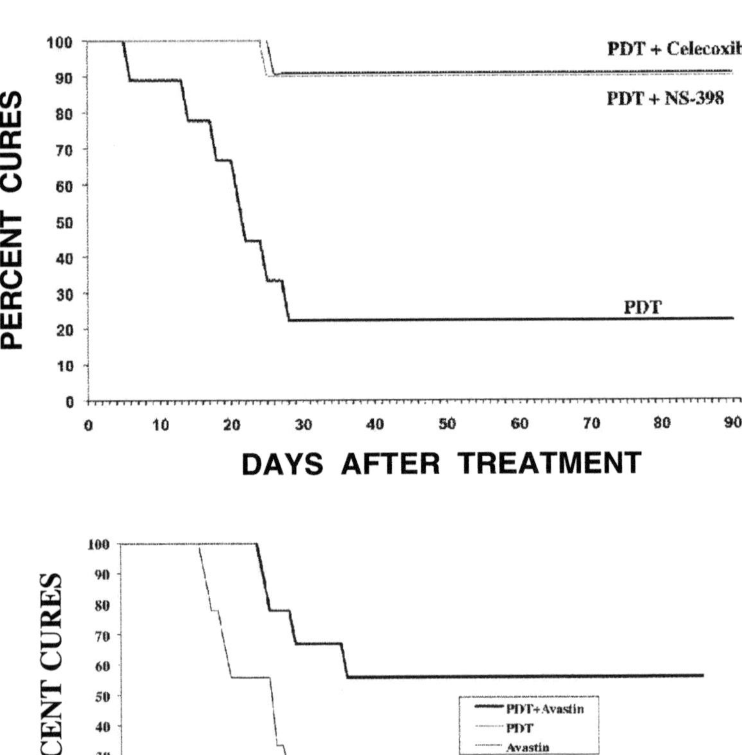

Fig. 9.2. Selective COX-2 inhibitors (**a**) and a VEGF inhibitor (**b**) enhance tumoricidal action of PDT. Percentage of tumor-free mice as a function of time after PDT alone, PDT combined with NS-398 or celecoxib (**a**), and PDT combined with Avastin (**b**). Mice were treated with PDT when BA carcinoma (**a**) or KS-Imm tumors (**b**) were 5.5–6.5 mm in diameter. Photofrin (5 mg/kg) was administered via i.v. injection and 24 h later, tumors were treated with 200 J/cm^2 (**a**) or 100 J/cm^2 (**b**) of 630 nm light. After PDT, randomly selected mice received multiple 10 mg/kg i.p. injections of NS-398, celecoxib (**a**), or Avastin (**b**). Injections started immediately after PDT and then followed at 4, 24, 48 h and then every other day up to day 20. Mice were monitored for tumor recurrences thrice weekly for up to 90 days.

4. The plotted curves are compared to determine the effect of the inhibitors on PDT-induced normal skin phototoxicity.

3.5. Quantitative Analysis of PGE_2 and VEGF Levels in Tumor Lysates

1. Tumor-bearing mice are treated with PDT as described above (*see* **Note 11**). Tumor samples are collected 24 h after PDT.
2. Mice exposed to combined treatment regimens receive celecoxib, NS-398, or Avastin i.p. at 20 mg/kg (twice the dose utilized for the tumor response analysis) starting

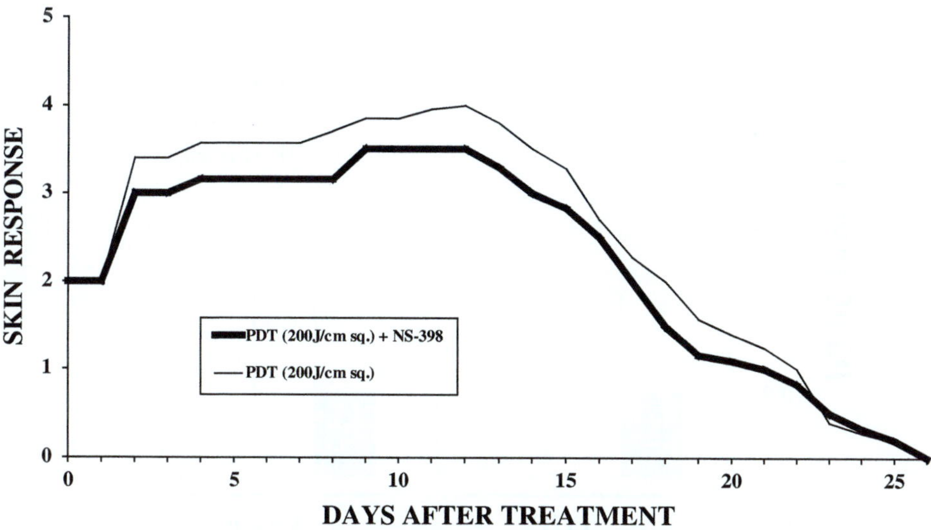

Fig. 9.3. NS-398 does not affect PDT-mediated normal skin photosensitization. Skin photosensitization in albino Swiss Webster mice treated with PDT (200 J/cm^2) or PDT plus NS-398 (10 mg/kg) administered immediately after PDT, 4, 24 and 48 h after PDT, and then every other day up to day 20. A 1-cm-diameter treatment area of a hind limb was treated and then evaluated for the appearance/disappearance of skin phototoxicity according to the scoring system described in **Table 9.1**. Mice were monitored and scored until skin appearance returned to pretreatment conditions.

immediately after irradiation and then at 4 and 23 h (*see* **Note 12**).

3. Tumor samples are collected 24 h after PDT from euthanized mice and placed in an individual 14-ml polypropylene round-bottom tube containing 0.5–0.7 ml of 1× reporter lysis buffer (obtained by diluting the 5× stock in ddH_2O).
4. Tumor samples are also collected from control mice to document constitutive expression of PGE_2 or VEGF.
5. Tumor samples are homogenized in 1× reporter lysis buffer on ice using the Virtis Polytron set at 1,500–2,000 rpm for 20–30 s (*see* **Note 13**).
6. Homogenized samples are left on ice for 15–20 min.
7. Transfer the homogenized samples into 1.5-ml microcentrifuge tubes and spin at 10,000 rpm for 10 min at 4°C.
8. Transfer aliquoted supernatants to new microcentrifuge tubes for storage at –80°C.
9. Thaw the samples and determine protein concentrations by following the Bio-Rad protein protocol for "low concentration assay in test tubes." Dilute 2 μl of each supernatant in 798 μl of ddH_2O; add 200 μl of dye reagent concentrate. Transfer to a clear cuvette and read adsorption with the spectrophotometer set at 595 nm. Protein

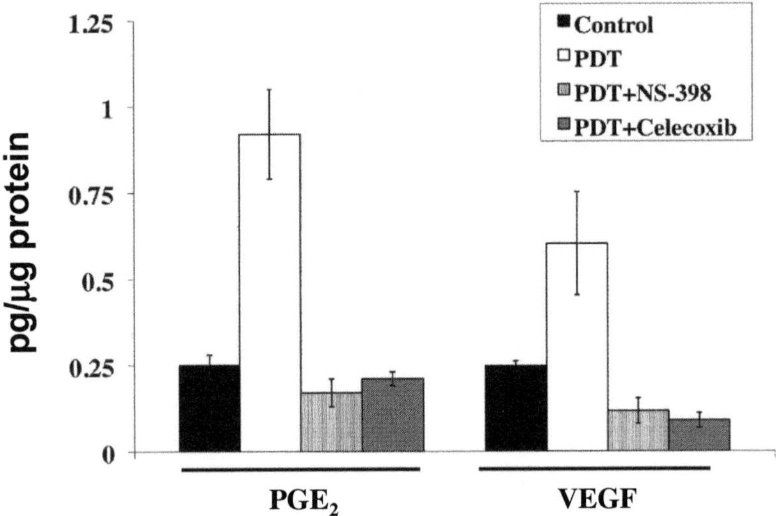

Fig. 9.4. COX-2 inhibitors modulate in vivo expression pattern of PGE_2 and VEGF in BA tumors treated with PDT. Mice were treated with PDT at a dose of 200/cm^2. NS-398 or celecoxib were given i.p. at a dose of 20 mg/kg immediately after light treatment and again 4 and 23 h later. Tumor lysates were collected 24 h after PDT and assayed for levels of PGE_2 and VEGF using a prostaglandin E_2 EIA kit and a Quantikine mouse VEGF immunoassay kit.

concentrations of the samples are then read off a standard curve generated with known concentrations of BSA.

10. Perform immunoassays for VEGF or PGE_2 following manufacturer's instructions.
    For the PGE_2 EIA kit, dilute the homogenates, if needed, in EIA buffer (provided in the kit) to reach a protein concentration of 2.5 μg/50 μl. For the Quantikine human or mouse VEGF immunoassay, dilute samples, if needed, with 1× reporter lysis buffer to reach a concentration of 20 μg/100 μl volume (*see* Note **14**). Each sample should be assayed in duplicate.
11. Calculate levels of VEGF or PGE_2 for each sample by referring to internal standard curves. This analysis is designed to document constitutive, inducible, and suppressed levels of PGE_2 and VEGF in untreated tumors and tumors treated with single or combined treatments (**Fig. 9.4**).

3.6. Data Interpretation

1. Calculate tumor enhancement ratios by using PDT dose alone versus PDT dose plus inhibitor required to produce a specific biological effect such as an increased tumor delay of a certain number of days or a specific percentage of long-term cures.
2. Calculate normal skin enhancement ratios by using PDT dose alone versus PDT dose plus inhibitor required to produce a specific skin response such as erythema.

3. Calculate therapeutics gain for combined therapy (PDT plus inhibitor) using both the tumor and the skin enhancement values. A positive therapeutic response requires that the tumor enhancement is greater than the normal skin enhancement (13).

4. Notes

1. Celecoxib (100 or 200 mg) capsules are open and the powder containing celecoxib is dissolved in DMSO to a concentration of 4 mg/ml. Aliquots are stored at –80°C.
2. Techniques for handling the mice for this procedure can vary. For instance, mice can rest on top of the cage and simply be held by their tails while shaving the hind limb. Alternatively, the limb can be shaved while restraining the mouse with one hand.
3. The hind limbs of mice are chosen as tumor sites for local PDT treatment to avoid potential damages to internal organs.
4. Dissected tumor pieces are maintained in 0.9% saline.
5. It is important not to invade the underlying muscle with the tip of the trochar in order to avoid diffusely growing tumors. Lesions growing subcutaneously and suitable for PDT treatment can be gently pulled (with index and thumb) away from the muscle underneath.
6. Mice not injected properly should be withdrawn from the study.
7. General anesthesia is not used in order to minimize interference with metabolism and blood flow of the treated mouse.
8. Higher light dose rates can lead to local hyperthermia. This could affect and/or mask some of PDT-mediated responses.
9. Most of the power coming out of the diode laser is lost throughout the beam splitter; therefore the power has to be set higher than the actual sum of the three single final outputs.
10. Alternatively, data can be plotted as tumor growth (volume) as a function of time following individual or combined treatments.
11. Use slightly larger tumors of about 6.5–7.0 mm in the largest diameter in order to collect enough tissue for analysis.

12. The dose of inhibitor is increased to 20 mg/kg to compensate for the decreased number of injections delivered in this short-term analysis.
13. The 1× reporter lysis buffer can get very foamy with the Polytron. Let the foamy sample sit for a few minutes before processing. If the tumor is not completely homogenized following the first attempt, re-homogenize with the Polytron.
14. Change dilution factors if samples need to be re-assayed due to either very low readings or plateau values.

References

1. Coussens, L. M. and Werb, Z. (2002) Inflammation and cancer. *Nature*, **420**, 860–867.
2. Hussain, S. P. and Harris, C. C. (2007) Inflammation and cancer: an ancient link with novel potentials. *Int J Cancer*, **121**, 2373–2380.
3. Macarthur, M., Hold, G. L., and El-Omar, E. M. (2004) Inflammation and cancer II. Role of chronic inflammation and cytokine gene polymorphisms in the pathogenesis of gastrointestinal malignancy. *Am J Physiol Gastrointest Liver Physiol*, **286**, G515–G520.
4. Ferrario, A., von Tiehl, K. F., Rucker, N., Schwarz, M. A., Gill, P. S., and Gomer, C. J. (2000) Anti-angiogenic treatment enhances photodynamic therapy responsiveness in a mouse mammary carcinoma. *Cancer Res*, **60**, 4066–4069.
5. Ferrario, A. and Gomer, C. J. (2006) Avastin enhances photodynamic therapy treatment of Kaposi's sarcoma in a mouse tumor model. *J Environ Path Tox Oncol*, **25**, 251–259.
6. Ferrario, A., von Tiehl, K. F., Wong, S., Luna, M., and Gomer, C. J. (2002) Cyclooxygenase-2 inhibitor treatment enhances photodynamic therapy-mediated tumor responsiveness. *Cancer Res*, **62**, 3956–3961.
7. Ferrario, A., Fisher, A. M., Rucker, N., and Gomer, C. J. (2005) Celecoxib and NS-398 enhance photodynamic therapy by increasing in-vitro apoptosis and decreasing in-vivo inflammatory and angiogenic factors. *Cancer Res*, **65**, 9473–9479.
8. Gollink, S. O., Evans, S. S., Baumamann, H., Owczarczak, B., Maier, P., Vaughan, L., Wang, W. C., Unger, E., and Henderson, B. W. (2003) Role of cytokines in photodynamic therapy-induced local and systemic inflammation. *Br Cancer*, **88**, 1772–1779.
9. Makowski, M., Grzela, T., Niderla, J., Azarczyk, M., Mroz, P., Kopee, M., Legat, M., Strusinska, K., Koziak, K., Nowis, D., Mrowka, P., Wasik, M., Jakobisiak, M., and Golab, J. (2003) Inhibition of cyclooxygenase-2 indirectly potentiates antitumor effects of photodynamic therapy in mice. *Clin Cancer Res*, **9**, 5417–5422.
10. Akita, Y., Kozaki, K., Nakagawa, A., Saito, T., Ito, S., Tamada, Y., Fujiwara, S., Nishikawa, N., Uchida, K., Yoshikawa, K., Noguchi, T., Miyaishi, O., Shimozato, K., Saga, S., and Matsumoto, Y. (2004) Cyclooxygenase-2 is a possible target of treatment approach in conjunction with photodynamic therapy for various disorders in skin and oral cavity. *Br J Dermatol*, **151**, 472–480.
11. Gomer, C. J., Ferrario, A., Luna, M., Rucker, N., and Wong, S. (2006) Photodynamic therapy: combined modality approaches targeting the tumor microenvironment. *Lasers Surg Med*, **38**, 516–521.
12. Marchio, S., Primo, L., Pagano, M., Palestro, G., Albini, A., Veikkola, T., Cascone, I., Alitalo, K., and Bussolino, F. (1999) Vascular endothelial growth factor-C stimulates the migration and proliferation of Kaposi's sarcoma cells. *J Biol Chem*, **274**, 27617–27622.
13. Hall, E. (2000) Radiobiology for the Radiologist. Philadelphia, PA: J.B. Lippincott.

Chapter 10

Photochemical Internalization (PCI): A Technology for Drug Delivery

Kristian Berg, Anette Weyergang, Lina Prasmickaite, Anette Bonsted, Anders Høgset, Marie-Therese R. Strand, Ernst Wagner, and Pål K. Selbo

Abstract

The utilization of macromolecules in therapy of cancer and other diseases is becoming increasingly relevant. Recent advances in molecular biology and biotechnology have made it possible to improve targeting and design of cytotoxic agents, DNA complexes, and other macromolecules for clinical applications. To achieve the expected biological effect of these macromolecules, in many cases, internalization to the cell cytosol is crucial. At an intracellular level, the most fundamental obstruction for cytosolic release of the therapeutic molecule is the membrane-barrier of the endocytic vesicles. Photochemical internalization (PCI) is a novel technology for release of endocytosed macromolecules into the cytosol. The technology is based on the use of photosensitizers located in endocytic vesicles that upon activation by light induces a release of macromolecules from their compartmentalization in endocytic vesicles. PCI has been shown to potentiate the biological activity of a large variety of macromolecules and other molecules that do not readily penetrate the plasma membrane, including type I ribosome-inactivating proteins (RIPs), gene-encoding plasmids, adenovirus, oligonucleotides, and the chemotherapeutic bleomycin. PCI has also been shown to enhance the treatment effect of targeted therapeutic macromolecules. The present protocol describes PCI of an epidermal growth factor receptor (EGFR)-targeted protein toxin (Cetuximab–saporin) linked via streptavidin–biotin for screening of targeted toxins as well as PCI of non-viral polyplex-based gene therapy. Although describing in detail PCI of targeted protein toxins and DNA polyplexes, the methodology presented in these protocols are also applicable for PCI of other gene therapy vectors (e.g., viral vectors), peptide nucleic acids (PNA), small interfering RNA (siRNA), polymers, nanoparticles, and some chemotherapeutic agents.

Key words: Photochemical internalization, photodynamic, photosensitizer, drug delivery, gene therapy, immunotoxin, siRNA, PNA.

C.J. Gomer (ed.), *Photodynamic Therapy*, Methods in Molecular Biology 635,
DOI 10.1007/978-1-60761-697-9_10, © Springer Science+Business Media, LLC 2010

1. Introduction

A major goal in the development of cancer therapy protocols is to achieve efficient, site-specific delivery of the therapeutic agent. Thus, the utilization of macromolecules in therapy of cancer and other diseases is becoming increasingly relevant. Recent advances in molecular biology and biotechnology have made it possible to improve targeting and design of cytotoxic agents, DNA complexes, and other macromolecules for clinical applications. To achieve the expected biological effect of these macromolecules, in many cases, internalization to the cell cytosol is crucial. At an intracellular level, the most fundamental obstruction for cytosolic release of these therapeutic molecules is the membrane-barrier of the endocytic vesicles. As an example, the poor escape of nucleic acids from endosomes and their consequent degradation in lysosomes is a barrier for obtaining efficient gene delivery. Consequently, many of the delivery methods developed are based on improved endocytic uptake and release of the therapeutic molecule from the endocytic vesicles into the cytosol. Photochemical internalization (PCI) is a method for light-inducible permeabilization of endocytic vesicles (**Fig. 10.1**) (1). The technology is based on photosensitizers localizing in the endocytic membranes. Light activation of the photosensitizers initiates photochemical reactions, which cause rupture of the vesicles. This leads to the release of endocytosed compounds (e.g., macromolecules) from the endocytic vesicles into the cytosol where they may act on their target directly or further translocate in the cytoplasm or to the nucleus. The PCI technology may be viewed not only as a method for intracellular delivery of molecules that do not readily penetrate the cellular membranes but also as a technology to enhance therapeutic efficacy and specificity.

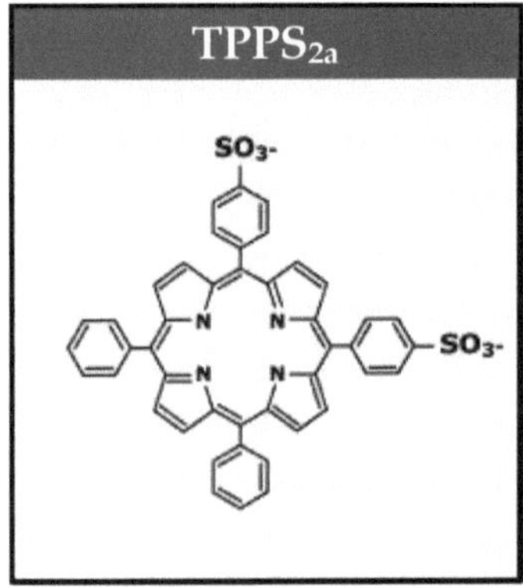

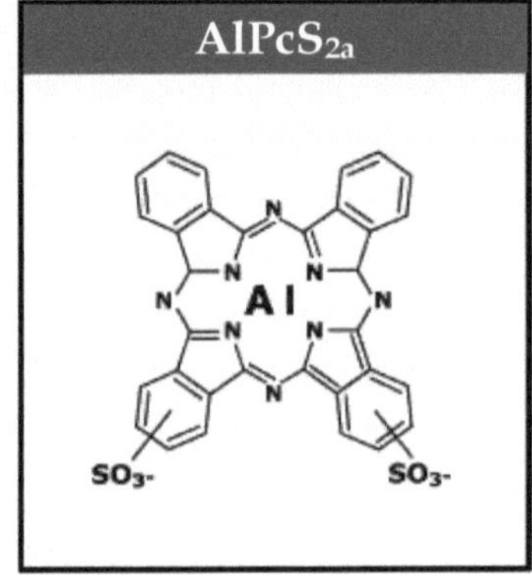

Fig. 10.1. Structure of the amphiphilic photosensitizers $AlPcS_{2a}$ and $TPPS_{2a}$.

PCI derives from the field of photodynamic therapy (2), taking advantage of the photochemical effects induced by a photosensitizer, light, and oxygen. Photosensitizers are compounds that upon absorption of light at specific wavelengths induce chemical or physical alterations in other chemical entities. The most applied photosensitizers for PCI are aluminum phthalocyanine with two sulfonate groups on adjacent phthalate rings ($AlPcS_{2a}$) and *meso*-tetraphenylporphine with two sulfonate groups on adjacent phenyl rings ($TPPS_{2a}$) (**Fig. 10.2**). These photosensitizers are amphiphilic compounds and localize in the membranes of endocytic vesicles. Photosensitizers that localize to other cellular structures are not efficient for inducing the PCI effect (1, 3). It is also of major importance that the photosensitizer is located in or close to the membranes of the endocytic vesicles. Photosensitizers, such as $TPPS_4$ and $TPPS_{2a}$ with the sulfonate groups on opposite pyrroles, located in the matrix of these vesicles may inactivate the macromolecules upon light exposure (3). The photochemical reactions induced following excitation of the photosensitizer proceed mainly via formation of singlet oxygen ($^1O_2$) (2). Singlet oxygen is highly reactive and is generated after interaction between the excited photosensitizer in its triplet state and ground state molecular oxygen (O_2). Singlet oxygen has a short lifetime and a short range of action (10–100 nm) in cells (4). Accordingly, only structures very close to the photosensitizer will be affected following light exposure, whereas distant molecules will be left unaffected.

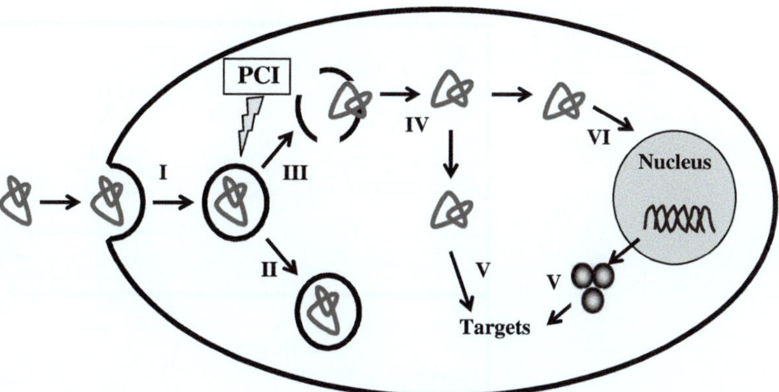

Fig. 10.2. Photochemical internalization (PCI) of a macromolecule. The macromolecule is endocytosed (I). Amphiphilic photosensitizers localize to the membranes of the endocytic vesicles. Upon light exposure of the cells, the photosensitizer generates reactive oxygen species of which singlet oxygen ($^1O_2$) dominates. The oxidative damage of endocytic membranes by singlet oxygen promotes rupture of the vesicular membranes (III) and the release of the macromolecule into the cytosol (IV). In the cytosol, the macromolecule may reach its target in the cytoplasma (V) or in the nucleus (VI) where transgene synthesis can be activated (V). Alternatively, the macromolecules may be degraded by hydrolytic enzymes in late endosomes and lysosomes (II).

The use of the PCI technology has been documented for proteins (1, 5), genes carried by nonviral and viral vectors (6–8), peptide nucleic acids (PNA) (9, 10), nanoparticles (11–13), siRNA (14), and some chemotherapeutic agents. In vivo, PCI has been shown to enhance the therapeutic efficacy of the plant toxin gelonin (15), genes delivered by a nonviral vector (11, 16), siRNA (17), polymer-bound chemotherapeutic agents, and bleomycin (18). Biologically targeted gene vectors may also be applied in combination with PCI (19, 20).

The PCI treatment procedures are illustrated in **Fig. 10.3**. The in vitro standard procedure we use is to incubate the cells overnight with the photosensitizer and change to a photosensitizer-free medium 4 h prior to light exposure. This procedure ensures that a low level of photosensitizer is located on the plasma membrane at the time of light exposure and a high level is located in the endocytic vesicles. The molecule to be delivered to the cytosol by PCI can be administered at different time points in the treatment sequence depending on the molecule of interest. It may even be possible to administer this molecule after the photochemical treatment. The procedure is principally the same for in vivo treatment, although a somewhat longer drug-light interval (48 h) is needed to reduce plasma membrane damage of the target cells than for the in vitro procedure. As pointed out above, PCI can be utilized to deliver a large variety of molecules to the cytosol, both targeted and nontargeted molecules. The present protocols will describe the photochemical delivery of genes by

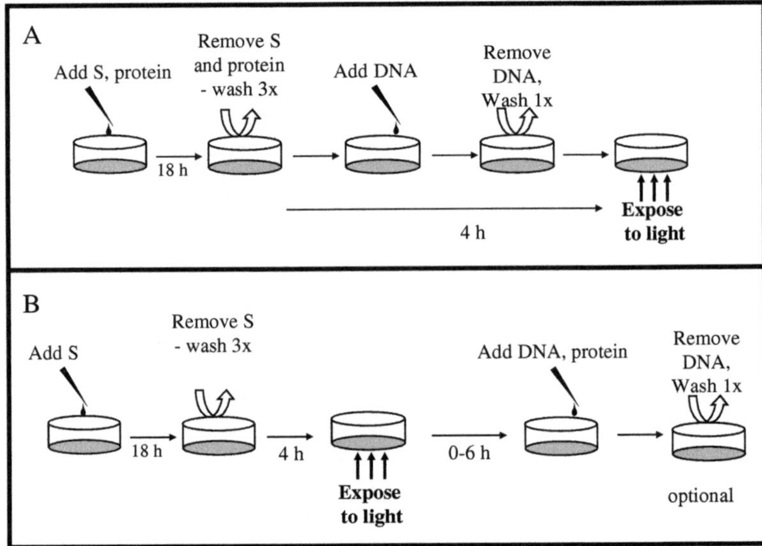

Fig. 10.3. Experimental scheme of PCI of DNA polyplexes on cultured cells. Two different treatment regimens are described and protein and DNA are used as examples of drugs to be delivered by PCI. S: photosensitizer.

nonviral nontargeted polyplex vectors and a method to screen targeted delivery of a protein toxin as illustrations of the utilization of PCI. In the latter case, the strong binding between biotin and streptavidin is utilized to link a targeting ligand such as a mAb or a growth factor to the protein toxin saporin.

2. Materials

1. Photosensitizers: Al(III) phthalocyanine disulfonate chloride (adjacent isomer) ($AlPcS_{2a}$) and *meso*-tetraphenylporphine disulfonic acid dihydrochloride (adjacent isomer) ($TPPS_{2a}$): dissolve 5 mg of $AlPcS_{2a}$ or 2 mg $TPPS_{2a}$ (Frontier Scientific, Logan UT) in a small volume (approx. 0.1–0.2 ml) of 0.1 M NaOH, dilute with phosphate-buffered saline (PBS) to a final volume of 1 ml (*see* **Note 1**), sterilize by filtration through a 0.22 mm filter, and store at –20°C in small aliquots up to 6 months (*see* **Note 2**).
2. Light source: LumiSource™ (PCI Biotech AS, Oslo, Norway) or other light sources that emit light absorbed by the photosensitizers (*see* **Note 9**).
3. Anti-EGFR antibody: Cetuximab (Merck, marketed under the name Erbitux®).
4. Biotinylation agent: 10 mM NHS-biotin (Pierce Biotechnology, Inc., Rockford, IL) in anhydrous dimethyl sulfoxide (DMSO, 99.9%) was freshly made before the conjugation (*see* **Note 3**).
5. Desalting column: Sephadex 25 (Amersham Biosciences, Amersham Place, UK).
6. Storage buffer (for desalting column): 10 mM Tris, 150 mM NaCl, pHix, pH 8.2 (*see* **Note 4**).
7. Plasmid DNA: Stock solution at 5 mg/ml in TE buffer (10 mM Tris, pH 7.5; 1 mM EDTA). Sterilize by filtration and store at –20°C (*see* **Note 5**).
8. Poly-L-lysine: Poly-L-lysine hydrobromide (MW 20700) (Sigma, St. Louis, MO). To make stock solution (1 mg/ml), dissolve 1 mg poly-L-lysine in 1 ml distilled water. Sterilize by filtration and store at 4°C.
9. Polyethylenimine: Linear polyethylenimine with an average molecular weight of 22 kDa (PEI22) (21). PEI22 can be synthesized by acid-catalyzed deprotection of poly(2-ethyl-2-oxazoline) (50 kDa, Sigma Aldrich, St. Louis, MO, USA)

(22). Complete deprotection of nitrogen is important and can be monitored by proton NMR analysis (23). For polyplex preparation, PEI22 was used at a 1 mg/ml working solution, neutralized with hydrochloric acid. Linear PEI is also available from Polyplus-transfection (Illkirch, France).

3. Methods

3.1. Determination of the Light Dose

The optimal photochemical dose has to be determined individually for every cell line, photosensitizer, and light source prior to photochemical transfection of the cells. For this purpose, survival of cells preloaded with the photosensitizer should be determined as a function of the light dose. Light doses causing a 30–50% reduction of cell viability are recommended for photochemical transfections (*see* **Note 6**).

1. Seed the cells in cell culture dishes at a density of typically 2×10^4 cells/cm^2 in the cell culture medium recommended for the cell line in use (*see* **Note 7**). Allow the cells to attach to the substratum for at least 6 h at 37°C in a CO_2 incubator.
2. Working solution of the photosensitizer should be freshly made before application to the cells. Add 1 μl of $AlPcS_{2a}$ or 0.1 μl $TPPS_{2a}$ stock solutions (5 or 2 mg/ml, respectively) to 1 ml of complete cell culture medium to the final concentrations 5 and 0.2 μg/ml. Other concentrations may also be used, depending on the cell line. Typical range: 5–20 μg/ml $AlPcS_{2a}$ and 0.1–0.6 μg/ml $TPPS_{2a}$.
3. In subdued light, add ,e.g., 5 μg/ml $AlPcS_{2a}$ or 0.2 μg/ml $TPPS_{2a}$ to the cells and incubate for 16–18 h at 37°C in a CO_2 incubator (*see* **Note 8**).
4. Wash the samples three times with photosensitizer-free cell culture medium. Chase for 4 h at 37°C in photosensitizer-free cell culture medium.
5. Expose the samples to different light doses with a suitable light source (*see* **Note 9**).
6. Measure cytotoxicity 24–48 h after illumination by one of the common cell viability or survival tests such as the MTS/MTT-test, protein synthesis, or clonogenic analysis.

3.2. Preparation of Cetuximab–Saporin

3.2.1. Biotinylation of a Targeting Ligand

A standard procedure for biotinylation of proteins as provided by the supplier (e.g., Pierce Biotechnology, Inc., Rockford, IL, http://www.piercenet.com/) is used with some minor modifications, exemplified by conjugation to the clinically used mAb to epidermal growth factor receptor (EGFR), Cetuximab (5).

1. One hundred microliter 1 M $NaHCO_3$ was added to 2 ml of 2 mg/ml Cetuximab to increase the pH of the solution to about 8.
2. Fifty-four microliter of the 10 mM NHS-biotin solution was added to 2 ml of the Erbitux solution.
3. The mixture was gently shaken for 30 min at room temperature.
4. The biotinylated Cetuximab is purified by a prepacked Sephadex G25 desalting column.
5. The column is washed with 25 ml of a storage buffer and biotinylated Cetuximab added on top of the column.
6. After the solution has passed into the column, stop the chromatography, add a small volume (e.g., 2–300 μl) of storage buffer, and let the solution elute into the column; repeat this procedure 2–3 times and then add 3.5 ml of storage buffer.
7. The effluent is collected in small tubes, about 14 droplets (≈0.56 ml) per tube.
8. Each fraction is monitored at 280 nm by a spectrophotometer, and the fractions with the highest content of protein are mixed.
9. Protein concentration is measured by a standard protein assay kit (e.g., DC protein assay kit 2 (BioRad, Laboratories, Philadelphia, PA) or by measuring absorbance at 280 nm and correlate to a standard curve based on Cetuximab.

3.2.2. Complexation of Cetuximab–Saporin

1. Streptavidin is a 60 kDa nonglycosylated tetramer with identical subunits, each with a binding site for biotin. Streptavidin has a high affinity for biotin (binding constant 10^{15}/M). The binding is practically irreversible, not sensitive to pH and is rapidly formed (24). Streptavidin–saporin (MW 113 kDa) is commercially available (Advanced Targeting Systems, CA, USA) or may be conjugated by standard procedures (e.g., disulfide link, www.piercenet.com).
2. Biotinylated Cetuximab (10 μM, see above) was mixed with streptavidin–saporin at a molar ratio of 4:1 and incubated for 15 min. This ratio is based on the assumption that all the antibody molecules were biotinylated and that four Cetuximab bind to each streptavidin. Quantification of the biotinylation may be performed by commercially available kits (www.piercenet.com).
3. The solution is diluted to 300 nM with sterile PBS (pH 7.0)
4. The immunotoxin is aliquoted and stored at –80°C.

3.3. Preparation of the Plasmid DNA/Poly-L-lysine Complex

The complex should be freshly prepared before application to the cells. We routinely make the complex with a charge ratio 1.7 (*see* **Note 10**); therefore, the amounts presented below correspond to the complex having the charge ratio 1.7.

1. Prepare plasmid DNA solution in a separate sterile microcentrifuge tube: 5 μg of plasmid DNA (we use 1 μl of DNA stock solution, 5 mg/ml) diluted to 75 μl in sterile water. Gently mix by pipetting the solution several times. Do not vortex.
2. Prepare poly-L-lysine solution in a separate sterile microcentrifuge tube: 5.3 μg of poly-L-lysine (i.e., 5.3 μl of stock solution, 1 mg/ml) diluted to 75 μl in sterile water. Gently mix by pipetting the solution several times. Do not vortex.
3. Slowly transfer the poly-L-lysine solution (*see* Step 2) into the microcentrifuge tube containing DNA solution (*see* Step 1). The final volume of the mixture is 150 μl. Gently mix by pipetting the mixture several times. Do not vortex.
4. Leave the mixture on the bench at room temperature for 30 min to allow formation of the DNA/poly-L-lysine complex.
5. Transfer the whole DNA/poly-L-lysine mixture into another sterile tube containing growth medium to bring the final volume to 1 ml. Mix carefully by pipetting several times. The solution is now ready for application to the cells.

3.4. Preparation of the Plasmid DNA/PEI Complex

1. Dilute the DNA and the PEI polymer conjugates separately in HBG (HEPES buffered glucose (HBG): 5% (w/vol) glucose, 20 mM HEPES, pH 7.1) in equal volumes to 40 μg/ml (DNA) and 31 μg/ml (PEI conjugates), respectively, in the case of a molar PEI nitrogen/DNA phosphate (N/P) ratio of 6. For other N/P ratios, the concentration of conjugates has to be adjusted, for example 21 μg/ml PEI conjugates for N/P 4 (*see* **Note 11**).
2. Add the DNA to an equal volume of PEI polymer buffer solution and mix carefully with a pipette. This results in a 20 μg/ml DNA polyplex solution. More concentrated polyplexes (up to 200 μg/ml DNA) can be generated by applying more concentrated DNA and polymer solutions. Allow the polyplexes to form for 20 min at room temperature before use. Shortly before transfection, dilute the polyplexes in cell culture medium to the appropriate DNA concentrations (0.2–5 μg/ml) (*see* **Note 12**)

3.5. The PCI Treatment

1. Seed the cells in cell culture dishes at a density of 2×10^4 cells/cm^2 in the cell culture medium recommended for the

cell line in use. Allow the cells to attach to the substratum for at least 6 h at 37°C in a CO_2 incubator.

2. In subdued light, add 5 μg/ml $AlPcS_{2a}$ or 0.2 μg/ml $TPPS_{2a}$ to the cells, incubate for 16–18 h at 37°C in a CO_2 incubator (*see* **Note 8**), and wash the cells three times with photosensitizer-free cell culture medium.
3. Treatment with the drug to be delivered by PCI
   (a) *Immunotoxin.* Co-incubate with Cetuximab–saporin or any other immuno- or affinity-complex in the pico-nanomolar range with the photosensitizer in the ordinary cell culture medium (16–18 h).
   (b) *DNA polyplex.* Add the DNA polyplexes to the cells and incubate for up to 4 h at 37°C (*see* **Notes 13–15**).
4. Aspirate off the medium and wash the cells once with cell culture medium. Expose the cells to light from an appropriate light source; use the light dose(s) empirically determined as described in **Section 3.1** (*see* **Note 9**).
5. Grow the cells further in the dark for 24–48 h and analyze for cell survival, transgene expression, or transgene effect (*see* **Note 16**).

4. Notes

1. The photosensitizers usually dissolve well in this way, but if complete solubilization of the photosensitizer is difficult we recommend treating the solution in a sonicator bath.
2. Long-term storage or repeated freezing and thawing may cause aggregation and hence reduce the efficacy of the photosensitizer. The photosensitizer solution should also be protected from light to avoid photoinduced damage to the photosensitizer.
3. It is important that DMSO is kept anhydrous.
4. Storage buffer (per liter): 1.43 g Trizma 8.0, 8.77 g NaCl, 3–4 droplets pHix (5 mg/ml pentachlorophenol in 95% ethanol, pH 8.2).
5. PCI has no restriction on the size of DNA to be delivered to the cell. Thus, any required plasmid may be applied. We have used the plasmid pCMVLuc (*Photinus pyralis luciferase* gene under the control of the CMV enhancer/promoter) (25) and the plasmid pEGFP-N1 (encoding enhanced green fluorescent protein (eGFP) under the control of CMV promoter), purchased from Clontech Laboratories, Inc. (Palo Alto, CA).

6. Ours and others experience is that oligonucleotides (e.g., peptide–nucleic acids and siRNA) may be photochemically translocated to cytosol even at nontoxic doses (9, 26). For delivery of cytotoxic drugs, the whole range of doses may be utilized.
7. Our experience is that PCI efficiently stimulate intracellular drug delivery in all monolayer cells tested, i.e., >30 cell lines. We have much less experience with cells not attached to a substratum. The rate of endocytosis is obviously a limiting factor.
8. In order to avoid uncontrollable activation of the photosensitizer and to protect the cells from undesirable photochemical damage, all the procedures starting from point 2 in **Sections 3.1** and **3.3** should be carried out in subdued light. For in vitro studies, it may be sufficient to turn off the light in the sterile bench. To test if the light in the laboratory is sufficiently subdued, the toxicity of the photosensitizer without irradiating the cells with light from the light source could be analyzed. With the photosensitizer concentrations recommended here, we have not experienced any significant toxicity from the photosensitizer in the cell lines tested thus far.
9. In principle, all light sources that emit light absorbed by the photosensitizer may be used for PCI. The LumiSource^{TM} red lamp consists of 4 × 18 W Philips Fluotone 18/950 light tubes and a PMMA PSC-S110 filter, and it delivers light with an irradiance of 1.5 mW/cm^2. For cells that have been incubated with 5 μg/ml of $AlPcS_{2a}$ for 18 h, a typical range of light doses would be 0.9–1.4 J/cm^2 (i.e., 10–16 min). The LumiSource^{TM} blue lamp consists of 4 × 18 W Osram L 18/67 standard light tubes and delivers blue light with an irradiance of 13.5 mW/cm^2. For cells that have been incubated with 0.2 μg/ml of $TPPS_{2a}$ for 18 h, a typical range of light doses would be 0.5–1.0 J/cm^2 (i.e., 40–75 s). Both lamps are air-cooled during light exposure, which prevents cells from being exposed to hyperthermia and keeps the irradiance stable over time.
10. We routinely use DNA/poly-L-lysine complexes with the charge ratio 1.7 (*see* **Section 3.4**). However, charge ratios in the range 1.0–2.5 gave similar efficiency of photochemical transfection (6); therefore, readers might try other charge ratios as well (the charge ratio is the number of positive charges provided by the amino groups of poly-L-lysine divided by the negative charges provided by the phosphate groups of DNA. 1 μg of DNA has 3.03 nmol of phosphate groups which are neutralized by the addition of 0.63 μg poly-L-lysine carrying 3.03 nmol of amino groups, so that charge ratio 1.0 is obtained).

11. Our experience is that PCI is more efficient when the N/P is relatively low, e.g., N/P 2. We assume that this is due to the relatively low efficacy of PEI in releasing the plasmid into the cytosol under such conditions. The transfection effect of PEI is caused by the proton-sponge effect, which requires accumulation of large quantities of cations (with pK around physiologic pH) into the endocytic vesicles (27). In case of poly-L-lysine, the pK of the amino group is above physiological pH and the transfection efficacy is less sensitive to the N/P ratio.
12. Other polymer vectors and other targeting ligands than those described here may be applied in photochemical transfection. Readers are encouraged to test their transfection vector of choice while applying the same main principles of photochemical transfection as described in the current protocol. The size and charge of the polyplexes should be verified prior to transfection, for example using a Malvern Zetasizer instrument (Malvern Instruments Ltd, Worcestershire, UK). Charge shielded complexes with diameters $\leq$ 200 nm are preferred for in vitro and in vivo applications where target specificity is required.
13. Photosensitizer located on the plasma membrane will cause a cytotoxic effect upon light exposure without resulting in intracellular delivery of drugs. The photosensitizer is therefore removed from the medium 4 h prior to the light exposure. The amount of photosensitizer on the plasma membrane is in this way reduced by diffusion into the serum-containing medium and by adsorptive endocytosis. The kinetics of these processes is however somewhat cell-line dependent.
14. The cells may be treated with the photosensitizer for 18 h, washed three times, chased 4 h in photosensitizer-free medium, and exposed to light before the drug to be delivered by PCI is added. In the latter case, the polyplexes should be added within 6 h after the light exposure (28) while little is know about this for other drugs of interest. However, the photochemical treatment may damage the cell surface receptors and cause a reduced effect of PCI-induced drug delivery.
15. For drug delivery by PCI, the cells may be incubated with the photosensitizer and the macromolecule at the same time (e.g., for 18 h prior to removal of the photosensitizer). In the case of delivery of proteins, PNA, or siRNA to cells, molecules have been added to the cells at the same time as the photosensitizer and incubated for 18 h prior to 4 h chase and light exposure (1, 9). However, for gene delivery, incubation with the photosensitizer prior to the gene is recommended to enhance the photochemical

effect on transfection (i.e., this protocol would maximize the amount of photosensitizer in the endocytic vesicles and minimize the degradation of the transgenes). Shorter incubation times than 4 h with the DNA complex (e.g., 0.5–1 h pulse) are also possible. Then the cells should be chased in photosensitizer-free medium before incubation with the DNA complex, so that the total incubation time in photosensitizer-free medium before irradiation is 4 h. We have also observed improved specificity of PCI of EGF–saporin by reducing the incubation time with the affinity toxin to 1–3 h (29).

16. When a ribosome-inactivating protein toxin is applied, the treatment effect may be evaluated by incorporation of ^{3}H-leucine by the cells (1) instead of a cell survival assay. If a plasmid encoding luciferase is applied, transgene expression may be analyzed by a commercial luciferase assay (e.g., Promega). If a plasmid encoding eGFP is applied, transgene expression may be analyzed by fluorescence microscopy or flow cytometry. Expression of the transgene is somewhat delayed by the transient inhibition of protein synthesis caused by the photochemical treatment.

References

1. Berg, K., Selbo, P. K., Prasmickaite, L., Tjelle, T. E., Sandvig, K., Moan, J. et al. (1999) Photochemical internalization: a novel technology for delivery of macromolecules into cytosol. *Cancer Res*, **59**, 1180–1183.
2. Dolmans, D. E., Fukumura, D., and Jain, R. K. (2003) Photodynamic therapy for cancer. *Nat Rev Cancer*, **3**, 380–387.
3. Prasmickaite, L., Høgset, A., and Berg, K. (2001) Evaluation of different photosensitizers for use in photochemical gene transfection. *Photochem Photobiol*, **73**, 388–395.
4. Moan, J. and Berg, K. (1991) The photodegradation of porphyrins in cells can be used to estimate the lifetime of singlet oxygen. *Photochem Photobiol*, **53**, 549–553.
5. Yip, W. L., Weyergang, A., Berg, K., Tønnesen, H. H., and Selbo, P. K. (2007) Targeted delivery and enhanced cytotoxicity of Cetuximab–saporin by photochemical internalization in epidermal growth factor-positive cancer cells. *Mol Pharm*, **4**, 241–251.
6. Høgset, A., Prasmickaite, L., Tjelle, T. E., and Berg, K. (2000) Photochemical transfection: a new technology for light-induced, site-directed gene delivery. *Hum Gene Ther*, **11**, 869–880.
7. Høgset, A., Engesæter, B. Ø., Prasmickaite, L., Berg, K., Fodstad, O., and Mælandsmo, G. M. (2002) Light-induced adenovirus gene transfer, an efficient and specific gene delivery technology for cancer gene therapy. *Cancer Gene Ther*, **9**, 365–371.
8. Bonsted, A., Høgset, A., Hoover, F., and Berg, K. (2005) Photochemical enhancement of gene delivery to glioblastoma cells is dependent on the vector applied. *Anticancer Res*, **25**, 291–298.
9. Folini, M., Berg, K., Millo, E., Villa, R., Prasmickaite, L., Daidone, M. G., Benatti, U., and Zaffaroni, N. (2003) Photochemical internalization of a peptide nucleic acid targeting the catalytic subunit of human telomerase. *Cancer Res*, **63**, 3490–3494.
10. Shiraishi, T. and Nielsen, P. E. (2006) Photochemically enhanced cellular delivery of cell penetrating peptide-PNA conjugates. *FEBS Lett*, **580**, 1451–1456.
11. Nishiyama, N., Iriyama, A., Jang, W. D., Miyata, K., Itaka, K., Inoue, Y., Takahashi, H., Yanagi, Y., Tamaki, Y., Koyama, H., and Kataoka, K. (2005) Light-induced gene transfer from packaged DNA enveloped in a dendrimeric photosensitizer. *Nat Mater*, **12**, 934–941.

12. Cabral, H., Nakanishi, M., Kumagai, M., Jang, W. D., Nishiyama, N., and Kataoka, K. (2008) A photo-activated targeting chemotherapy using glutathione sensitive camptothecin-loaded polymeric micelles. *Pharm Res.* E-pub.
13. Lai, P. S., Lou, P. J., Peng, C. L., Pai, C. L., Yen, W. N., Huang, M. Y., Young, T. H., and Shieh, M. J. (2007) Doxorubicin delivery by polyamidoamine dendrimer conjugation and photochemical internalization for cancer therapy. *J Control Release*, **122**, 39–46.
14. Oliveira, S., Fretz, M. M., Høgset, A., Storm, G., and Schiffelers, R. M. (2007) Photochemical internalization enhances silencing of epidermal growth factor receptor through improved endosomal escape of siRNA. *Biochim Biophys Acta*, **1768**, 1211–1217.
15. Selbo, P. K., Sivam, G., Fodstad, O., Sandvig, K., and Berg, K. (2001) In vivo documentation of photochemical internalization, a novel approach to site specific cancer therapy. *Int J Cancer*, **92**, 761–766.
16. Ndoye, A., Dolivet, G., Hogset, A., Leroux, A., Fifre, A., Erbacher, P. et al. (2006) Eradication of p53-mutated head and neck squamous cell carcinoma xenografts using nonviral p53 gene therapy and photochemical internalization. *Mol Ther*, **13**, 1156–1162.
17. Oliveira, S., Høgset, A., Storm, G., and Schiffelers, R. M. (2008) Delivery of siRNA to the target cell cytoplasm: photochemical internalization facilitates endosomal escape and improves silencing efficiency, in vitro and in vivo. *Curr Pharm Des*, **14**, 3686–3697.
18. Berg, K., Dietze, A., Kaalhus, O., and Høgset, A. (2005) Site-specific drug delivery by photochemical internalization enhances the antitumor effect of bleomycin. *Clin Cancer Res*, **11**, 8476–8485.
19. Prasmickaite, L., Høgset, A., Tjelle, T. E., Olsen, V. M., and Berg, K. (2000) Role of endosomes in gene transfection mediated by photochemical internalisation (PCI). *J Gene Med*, **2**, 477–488.
20. Kloeckner, J., Prasmickaite, L., Høgset, A., Berg, K., and Wagner, E. (2004) Photochemically enhanced gene delivery of EGF receptor-targeted DNA polyplexes. *J Drug Target*, **12**, 205–213.
21. Zou, S. M., Erbacher, P., Remy, J. S., and Behr, J. P. (2000) Systemic linear polyethylenimine (L-PEI)-mediated gene delivery in the mouse. *J Gene Med*, **2**, 128–134.
22. Brissault, B., Kichler, A., Guis, C., Leborgne, C., Danos, O., and Cheradame, H. (2003) Synthesis of linear polyethylenimine derivatives for DNA transfection. *Bioconjug Chem*, **14**, 581–587.
23. Thomas, M., Lu, J. J., Ge, Q., Zhang, C., Chen, J., and Klibanov, A. M. (2005) Full deacylation of polyethylenimine dramatically boosts its gene delivery efficiency and specificity to mouse lung. *Proc Natl Acad Sci USA*, **102**, 5679–5684.
24. Green, M. (1990) Avidin and streptavidin. *Methods Enzymol*, **184**, 51–67.
25. Plank, C., Zatloukal, K., Cotton, M., Mechtler, K., and Wagner, E. (1992) Gene transfer into hepatocytes using asialoglycoprotein receptor mediated endocytosis of DNA complexed with an artificial tetra-antennary galactose ligand. *Bioconjug Chem*, **3**, 533–539.
26. Boe, S., Longva, A. Sa. nd, and Hovig, E. (2008) Evaluation of various polyethylenimine formulations for light-controlled gene silencing using small interfering RNA molecules. *Oligonucleotides*, **18**, 123–132.
27. Berg, K., Folini, M., Prasmickaite, L., Selbo, P. K., Bonsted, A., Engesaeter, B. Ø., Zaffaroni, N., Weyergang, A., Dietze, A., Maelandsmo, G. M., Wagner, E., Norum, O. J., and Høgset, A. (2007) Photochemical internalization: a new tool for drug delivery. *Curr Pharm Biotechnol*, **8**, 362–372.
28. Prasmickaite, L., Høgset, A., Selbo, P. K., Engesæter, B. Ø., Hellum, M., and Berg, K. (2002) Photochemical disruption of endocytic vesicles before delivery of drugs: a new strategy for cancer therapy. *Br J Cancer*, **86**, 652–657.
29. Weyergang, A., Selbo, P. K., and Berg, K. (2006) Photochemically stimulated drug delivery increases the cytotoxicity and specificity of EGF–saporin. *J Control Release*, **111**, 165–173.

Chapter 11

Photodynamic Therapy-Generated Cancer Vaccines

Mladen Korbelik

Abstract

Eradication of cancer by an intervention producing a potent immune response capable of rejecting both primary and metastatic deposits remains the most pragmatic approach in cancer therapy. Cancer vaccine generated by photodynamic therapy (PDT) is therefore of considerable interest, particularly as it is becoming increasingly clear that it holds unique prospects for optimally presenting tumor antigens and because of emerging indications that its efficacy can be further potentiated by continued development. The present report dissects the preparation of PDT vaccine in a mouse model of squamous cell carcinoma.

Key words: Photodynamic therapy, cancer vaccine, autologous whole-cell vaccine, anti-tumor immune response, tumor cell death.

1. Introduction

Photodynamic therapy (PDT), a regulatory approved modality for treatment of various malignant and non-oncological lesions (1–3), continues to be developed and expanded for different novel applications. Among such novel applications, one of the most exciting is the development of PDT-generated cancer vaccines (4, 5). In standard PDT, cytotoxic reactive oxidative species are produced directly in targeted lesions. This is achieved by tumor localized illumination with light of the wavelength matching absorption characteristics of the photosensitizing drug that has accumulated at that site after its (usually systemic) administration (1). In contrast with PDT vaccine application the photosensitizer is not administered to the host nor is the tumor exposed to light. Instead, the host is injected a vaccine consisting of autologous tumor cells or their lysates treated by PDT in

C.J. Gomer (ed.), *Photodynamic Therapy*, Methods in Molecular Biology 635,
DOI 10.1007/978-1-60761-697-9_11, © Springer Science+Business Media, LLC 2010

vitro (3–6). The first publication on pre-clinical development of PDT vaccines was by Gollnick and co-workers, who used lysates of PDT-treated mouse tumor cells as a prophylactic vaccine that protected against the challenge with the same tumor (4). In our laboratory, we have established therapeutic cancer vaccines based on PDT-treated tumor cells or ex vivo tumor tissue (3, 5, 6). In this work we used mouse tumor models SCCVII (squamous cell carcinoma) and LLC (Lewis lung carcinoma). Vaccination of mice bearing established SCCVII tumors with in vitro expanded and PDT-treated SCCVII cells results reproducibly with cures or growth retardation of these poorly immunogenic lesions (5, 6).

The PDT vaccine we developed belongs to the class of autologous whole-cell vaccines. There are clear advantages of whole-cell/polypeptide vaccination over targeting specific epitopes (7, 8). Such polyvalent vaccines secure greater coverage of potential/diverse tumor antigens (even if most of them are unknown), including the necessary determinants for helper T cells, and are thus less likely to encounter "tumor escape" by downregulation of antigen expression (8–10). Autologous whole-cell vaccines are optimally conditioned to express relevant (and even unique) antigens in individualized patient-specific manner and provide patient-matched MHC through which tumor peptides can be recognized. The distinct advantage of using PDT for the generation of such vaccines is evidenced by the fact their efficacy cannot be rivaled by vaccines prepared by exposing cells to other treatments, such as X-rays, UV, hyperthermia, or lysis (4, 5). In comparison to other polyvalent vaccination strategies like whole-cell RNA-mediated transfection (11), the PDT vaccine advantage is in photooxidative changes-modified antigenic fingerprint and neoantigens characterized by greater immunogenicity (12) that are presented it in the context of complex immunostimulating environment including unique molecular changes unfolding in cells dying from PDT-mediated oxidative stress (13).

The accumulated evidence establishes unequivocally that the PDT vaccine effect is based on tumor-specific immune response executed by cytotoxic T-cell response. This evidence includes the ineffectiveness against mismatched tumor types, acquisition of resistance against re-challenge with the cured tumor, effectiveness against tumors growing distantly from the vaccination site, elicited accumulation of dendritic cells and their functional maturation, induction (among host splenocytes) of vaccinated tumor-specific interferon-γ-secreting T cells with increased specific tumoricidal activity, detection of high numbers of degranulating CD8 T cells in lesions regressing after vaccination but not in poorly responding lesions, and absence of the vaccine effect in $CD8^+$-depleted hosts (4–6).

A key factor contributing to PDT vaccine activity is the expression of PDT-induced molecular/biological changes on vaccine cells such as those associated with cell death. Consequently, the therapeutic results are more pronounced if the vaccine cells are not administered immediately after in vitro PDT treatment but left, before vaccination, overnight (16 h) in culture to allow the expression of these changes (6). Another critical event that we predict to play a role in the potency of this vaccine is the release of lysoalkylphospolipids and alkylphospholipids from PDT-damaged cells (14). These degradation products of alkylphospholipids (major constituents of cancerous but not non-cancerous cells) are principal activators of macrophages, the immune effector cells that are both directly tumoricidal and act as professional antigen-presenting cells.

Importantly, effective vaccines can be prepared not only from cultured single cells but also from freshly excised or previously frozen tumor tissue exposed ex vivo to PDT (6). The implication that surgically removed tumor tissue can be directly used for PDT vaccine (avoiding delays/restrictions with establishing cancer cell culture) has significant clinical ramifications, as it opens attractive prospects for employing cancer vaccines tailored for individual patients targeting specific antigens of the patient's tumor.

Increasing number of investigators is joining the research on developing various PDT vaccines (15–17). This topic has attracted popular press coverage and inspired the development of current ongoing clinical trials testing PDT vaccines in cancer patients.

2. Materials

2.1. Treatment of Cells for PDT Vaccine

1. Cultures of mouse squamous cell carcinoma SCCVII cells (18, 19).
2. Alpha modification of Minimal Essential Medium Eagle (alpha MEM) obtained from Sigma Chemical Co. (St. Louis, MO); for routine cell cultivation and expansion supplemented with 10% fetal bovine serum (HyClone Laboratories Inc., Logan, UT).
3. Ex-cell serum and protein-free medium (S8284, Sigma).
4. Phosphate-buffered saline (PBS): 8 g NaCl, 0.2 g KCl, 1.44 g $Na_2HPO_4 \times 12H_2O$, and 0.24 g KH_2PO_4 in 1 l of double distilled water (pH adjusted to 7.4).
5. Chlorin e6 (ce6, Frontier Scientific Inc., Logan, UT) dissolved at 0.2 mg/ml in 7.5% sodium bicarbonate aqueous solution.

6. PDT light source, FB-QTH-3 high throughput illuminator (Sciencetech Inc., London, Ontario, Canada) equipped with a 150 W QTH lamp and suitable interference filter; the light was delivered through an 8-mm core diameter liquid light guide (model 77638, Oriel Instruments, Stratford, CT).
7. Tissue culture 175 mm^2 T-flasks, cat. no. 83.1812 (Sarstedt Inc., Newton, NC).
8. Cell scrapers, cat. no. 3086 (Falcon, Becton Dickinson, Lincoln Park, NJ).

2.2. Tumor Implantation, Treatment, and Response Monitoring

1. C3H/HeN female mice, 7–9 week old (Simonsen Laboratories Inc., Gilroy, CA).
2. In-house constructed plexiglass holder for immobilizing mice during tumor inoculation.
3. Precision glide needles (20G1) and 1 ml tuberculin slip tip syringes, both from Becton Dickinson.
4. Micrometer steel calliper (metric) from Fisher Scientific, Pittsburgh, PA.

3. Methods

The standard PDT vaccine protocol that emerged after detailed optimization studies (5, 6) calls for injecting 2×10^7 PDT-treated cells per mouse. Usually, six mice are included in each experimental treatment group. Hence, an experiment with five experimental groups involves 24 mice receiving PDT vaccine and thus requires in total 4.8×10^8 cells. Since it is impractical to have such large cell numbers freshly available in culture, adequate numbers of SCCVII cells (obtained by expansion of cultures in vitro) are stored frozen in liquid nitrogen. At least one among the following control groups is included: the untreated tumors, sham vaccine injection group (saline in the same volume the real vaccine), group receiving cells treated with X-rays only (no PDT), and group receiving vaccine prepared by PDT treatment of a mismatched tumor cell line. All these control mice are with tumors implanted in the same cohort as other experimental groups.

An additional optimization step critical for boosting the vaccine potency is the post-PDT incubation with the cells returned to culture growth conditions where they are kept overnight (16 h) in especially enriched serum- and protein-free medium before being collected and used for vaccination without further delay.

3.1. Preparation of PDT Vaccine

1. Sufficient number of SCCVII cells are retrieved from liquid nitrogen, thawed, and cryoprotectant (DMSO) removed by centrifugation. For an experimental group consisting of six mice and requiring 20 million vaccine cells per mouse, the number of needed SCCVII cells is 1.2×10^8 cells. The cells for one experimental group are re-suspended in 39.9 ml of serum-free alpha MEM medium and then 0.1 ml of the photosensitizer stock (0.2 mg/ml) is added to have a final ce6 concentration of 0.5 μg/ml in 40 ml of cell suspension that is kept in 37°C incubator for 30 min.
2. After this exposure to ce6, the cells are washed with ice-cold PBS by centrifugation and pelleting, and then exposed (while re-suspended in PBS) to 1 J/cm^2 of 665 ±10 nm light (15 mW/cm^2).
3. Immediately after PDT light exposure, the cells are re-suspended in serum- and protein-free medium and distributed at 4×10^7 per 175 mm^2 T-flask and incubated for 16 h at 37°C.
4. The cells are then collected (detached if necessary using a cell scraper), concentrated by centrifugation, and transferred into 5-ml tubes in the volume required for injecting all mice of the particular treatment group (0.2 ml per mouse) (*see* **Note 1**). Immediately before injecting into mice, the tubes with cells are exposed to X-rays (60 Gy) using a Philips RT 250 (250 kV, 0.5 mm Cu, dose rate 3.26 Gy/min) (*see* **Note 2**).

3.2. Vaccination and Monitoring Tumor Response

1. The size of subcutaneous SCCVII tumors growing in syngeneic immunocompetent hosts (C3H/HeN mice) at the time of PDT vaccine treatment should not exceed 5 mm in largest diameter, unless used in a combined treatment with another modality such as radiotherapy. The vaccine is routinely administered peritumorally (2×10^7 vaccine cells per mouse in 0.2 ml) although it is also effective when injected at a distant site (6) (*see* **Note 3**).
2. The therapeutic effect of PDT vaccine is determined by monitoring changes in tumor size. This is done by measuring tumors every second day using a calliper. Tumor volume is calculated using a formula: $a \times b \times c \times \pi/6$, where a, b, and c are orthogonal diameters of the tumor (length, width, and height). With the tumors that continue to grow, the point will be reached when their hosts need to be sacrificed to prevent them starting suffering from tumor burden (tumor size exceeding 15 mm in the largest diameter,

volumes above 1,000 mm^3). In case when tumor shrinks and becomes impalpable, the host monitoring is continued until the absence of tumor growth persists for 90 days, which qualifies as tumor cure.

4. Notes

1. Injecting relatively large volumes such as 0.2 ml (of vaccine suspension) subcutaneously/peritumorally into mice requires particular care for preventing the loss of some of the injected contents by oozing out back through the needle track. Therefore, the bolus should be injected very slowly and the needle should be left in place for 20–30 s before withdrawing. An additional option is to inject smaller volumes at different positions around the tumor.
2. Immediately before injection, all vaccine cells are exposed to a lethal dose of X-rays (60 Gy). This simulates clinically acceptable safety restriction protocols for excluding the risk of secondary tumor generation (by vaccine cells themselves).
3. Effective PDT vaccines can be also generated using tumor tissue instead of tumor cells expanded in vitro (6). When using the same experimental model, tissue (brei) of growing SCCVII tumors (finely minced with scalpels and stored frozen in liquid nitrogen) is thawed and incubated ex vivo with ce6 (0.5 μg/ml in serum-free medium) and further processed following the protocols with SCCVII cells. For injection, 0.17 ml of wet brei together with 0.03 ml of PBS is injected per mouse (higher brei concentration becomes too viscous to pass through the needle).

Acknowledgments

Technical assistance in various phases of PDT vaccine development was provided by Jinghai Sun, Denise McDougal, Brandon Stott, and Soroush Merchant. Financial support was provided by the Canadian Institutes for Health Research (grant MPO-12165).

References

1. Dougherty, T. J., Gomer, C. J., Henderson, B. W., Jori, G., Kessel, D., Korbelik, M., Moan, J., and Peng, Q. (1998) Photodynamic therapy. *J Natl Cancer Inst*, **90**, 889–905.
2. Huang, Z. (2005) A review of progress in clinical photodynamic therapy. *Technol Cancer Res Treat*, **4**, 283–294.
3. Korbelik, M. and Cecic, I. (2003) Mechanisms of tumor destruction by photodynamic therapy. In: Nalwa, H. S. (ed.) Handbook of Photochemistry and Photobiology, Vol. 4. Stevenson Ranch, CA: American Scientific Publishers, pp. 39–77.
4. Gollnick, S. O., Vaughan, L., and Henderson., B. W. (2002) Generation of antitumor vaccines using photodynamic therapy. *Cancer Res*, **62**, 1604–1608.
5. Korbelik, M. and Sun, J. (2006) Photodynamic therapy-generated vaccine for cancer therapy. *Cancer Immunol Immunother*, **55**, 900–909.
6. Korbelik, M., Stott, B., and Sun, J. (2007) Photodynamic therapy-generated vaccines: relevance of tumor cell death expression. *Br J Cancer*, **97**, 1381–1387.
7. Copier, J. and Dalgleish, A. (2006) Overview of tumor cell-based vaccines. *Int Rev Immunol* , **25**, 297–319.
8. Emens, L. A. (2006) Cancer vaccines: toward the next revolution in cancer therapy. *Int Rev Immunol*, **25**, 415–443.
9. Khong, H. and Restifo, N. (2002) Natural selection of tumor variants in the generation of "tumor escape" phenotypes. *Nat Immunol*, **3**, 990–1005.
10. Thompson, P. L. and Dessureault, S. (2007) Tumor cell vaccines. *Adv Exp Med Biol*, **601**, 345–355.
11. Heisler, A., Maurice, M. A., Yancey, D. R., Coleman, D. M., Dahm, P., and Vieweg, J. (2001) Human dendritic cells transfected with renal tumor RNA stimulate polyclonal T-cell response against antigens expressed by primary and metastatic tumors. *Cancer Res*, **61**, 3388–3393.
12. Gollnick, S. O., Mazzacua, A., Vaughan, L., Owczarczak, B., Maier, P., and Henderson, B. W. (2001) Photodynamic therapy (PDT) treatment enhances tumor cell antigenicity. *Proc SPIE*, **4257**, 25–28.
13. Korbelik, M. (2006) PDT-associated host response and its role in the therapy outcome. *Lasers Surg Med*, **38**, 500–508.
14. Korbelik, M., Naraparaju, V. R., and Yamamoto, N. (1997) Macrophage directed immunotherapy as adjuvant to photodynamic therapy of cancer. *Br J Cancer*, **75**, 202–207.
15. Bau, S.-M., Kim, Y.-W., Kwak, S.-Y., Kim, Y. -W., Ro, D.-Y., Shin, J.-C., Park, C. -H., Han, S.-J., Oh, C. -H., Kim, C. -K., and Ahn, W.-S. (2007) Photodynamic therapy-generated tumor cell lysates with CpG-oligodeoxynucleotide enhance immunotherapy efficacy in human papillomavirus 16 (E6/E7) immortalized tumor cells. *Cancer Sci*, **98**, 747–752.
16. Friedberg, J. (2007) Photodynamic therapy-generated mesothelioma vaccine. *Wipo Patent WO2007133728*, www.freepatentsonline.com, 2007.
17. Zhang, H., Ma, W., and Li, Y. (2008) Generation of effective vaccines against liver cancer using photodynamic therapy. *Lasers Med Sci* (in press).
18. Suit, H. D., Sedlacek, R. D., Silver, G., and Dosoretz, D. (1985) Pentobarbital anesthesia and the response of tumor and normal tissue in the C3Hf/Sed mouse to radiation. *Radiat Res*, **104**, 47–65.
19. Khurana, D., Martin, E. A., Kasperbauer, J. L., O'Malley, B. W., Jr., Salomao, D. R., Chen, L., and Strome, S. E. (2001) Characterization of a spontaneously arising murine squamous cell carcinoma (SCC VII) as a prerequisite for head and neck cancer immunotherapy. *Head Neck*, **23**, 899–906.

Chapter 12

Antimicrobial Photodynamic Inactivation and Photodynamic Therapy for Infections

Liyi Huang, Tianhong Dai, and Michael R. Hamblin

Abstract

Photodynamic therapy (PDT) was initially discovered over 100 years ago by its ability to kill microorganisms, but its use to treat infections clinically has not been much developed. However, the present relentless increase in antibiotic resistance worldwide and the emergence of strains that are resistant to all known antibiotics has stimulated research into novel antimicrobial strategies such as PDT that are thought to be unlikely to lead to the development of resistance. In this chapter we will cover the use of PDT to kill pathogenic microbial cells in vitro and describe a mouse model of localized infection and its treatment by PDT without causing excessive damage to the host tissue.

Key words: Bacteria, fungus, microbiology, colony-forming units, *Photorhabdus luminescens* luciferase, bioluminescence imaging, mouse model of localized infection, antibiotic, wound healing.

1. Introduction

It has been known since the first days of PDT early in the last century that certain microorganisms can be killed by the combination of non-toxic dyes, known as photosensitizers (PSs), and harmless visible light in vitro (1, 2). Throughout the years since those times there have been additional reports of bacteria, yeasts, fungi, and viruses being killed or inactivated by various combinations of PSs and light (3, 4). In the 1990s it was observed that there was a fundamental difference in susceptibility to PDT between Gram-positive and Gram-negative bacteria. It was found that in general neutral or anionic PS molecules

C.J. Gomer (ed.), *Photodynamic Therapy*, Methods in Molecular Biology 635,
DOI 10.1007/978-1-60761-697-9_12,

are efficiently bound to and photodynamically inactivate Gram-positive bacterial and fungal cells, whereas Gram-negative bacterial cells are relatively resistant to these compounds (5). The high susceptibility of Gram-positive bacteria and fungi was explained by their physiology as their cytoplasmic membrane is surrounded by a relatively porous layer of peptidoglycan and lipoteichoic acid, or beta-glucan and chitin, respectively, and both these structures allow non-cationic PSs to cross (6). Then several groups of workers devised approaches that would allow PDI of Gram-negative species (5). These methods included using the polycationic peptide polymyxin B nonapeptide (5) and EDTA (7), which both increased the permeability of the Gram-negative outer membrane and allowed PSs that are normally excluded from the cell to penetrate to a location where the reactive oxygen species (ROS) generated on illumination to execute fatal damage. A second approach adopted by several groups is to use a PS molecule with an intrinsic positive charge. Wilson, Wainwright, and other groups have used the phenothiazinium salts such as toluidine blue O to carry out PDI of a large range of both Gram-positive and Gram-negative bacteria (8). The group in Italy led by Jori has used cationic porphyrins to photoinactivate Gram-negative species such as *Vibrio anguillarum* and *E. coli* (9). They found that washing the loosely bound PS from the cells before illumination decreased the killing and explained this finding by supposing that the first dose of light on PS bound to the outside of the outer membrane causes an initial limited photodamage that then allows further penetration of the PS (10). The group in Leeds, UK, led by Brown has used cationic phthalocyanines for PDI of Gram-negative bacteria (11). They investigated *E. coli* DH5a and in particular the mechanism of uptake. They found that incubation with PPC in the dark led to increased sensitivity of the bacteria to hydrophobic but not hydrophilic antibiotics. Incubation with PPC also led to increased uptake of radiolabeled protoporphyrin that was reversed in the presence of up to 50 mM Mg^{++} ions. These observations were consistent with the uptake of PPC proceeding through the self-promoted uptake pathway (12).

Our laboratory has introduced an approach to antimicrobial PDT in which an anionic PS (chlorin e6) is covalently conjugated to polymers with basic amino groups that can bear a cationic charge at biological pH values (13). These molecular constructs can be formed between poly-L-lysine chains (pL-ce6) or polyethylenimine polymers (either linear or branched; PEI-ce6). We have previously shown that these pL-ce6 and PEI-ce6 conjugates are highly effective in mediating the PDI of both Gram-positive and Gram-negative bacteria. Their positive charges help them to bind to the negatively charged bacteria and their polycationic nature enables them to penetrate the outer membrane of Gram-negative cells by disturbing the structure of the lipopolysaccharide layers. The macromolecular nature of these conjugates gives a temporal selectivity for bacteria over mammalian cells as the latter take them up by the time-dependent process of endocytosis, while they bind rapidly to bacteria.

Although PDI of bacteria has been known for over a 100 years (14), its use to treat infections has not been much developed (8). This may be partly due to the difficulty of monitoring the effectiveness of PDT in animal models of infection. The standard method of quantifying bacterial burdens in animal models of infection involves sacrificing the animal, removing tissue and homogenizing it, and carrying out serial dilutions to provide the number of CFU/g tissue. In order to improve this process of monitoring infection after PDT, we have developed a procedure that uses bioluminescent genetically engineered bacteria and a light-sensitive imaging system to allow real-time visualization of infections (15). The use of microbial cells that have been engineered to express luciferase and the imaging of their location and cell number has streamlined and refined studies involving PDT in animal infection models as the necessity to sacrifice the animals to acquire data on the progress of the infection has essentially been eliminated. Bacterial pathogenesis appeared to be unaffected by the presence of the luciferase genes, and bioluminescence can be detected throughout the study period in animals. Furthermore, the intensity of the bioluminescence measured from the living animal correlated well with the bacterial burden subsequently determined by standard protocols. When these bacteria are treated with PDT in vitro, the loss of luminescence parallels the loss of colony-forming ability.

We have developed several models of infections in wounds and soft-tissue abscesses in mice that can be followed by bioluminescence imaging. The size and intensity of the infection can be sequentially monitored in a non-invasive fashion in individual mice in real time. When photosensitizers are introduced into the infected tissue followed by illumination with red light, a light dose-dependent loss of luminescence is seen. If the bacterium is invasive, the loss of luminescence correlates with increased survival of the mice, while animals in control groups die of sepsis within 5 days. Healing of the PDT-treated wounds is not impaired and may actually be improved.

One problem that is evident when applying PDT for microbial infection is the fact that soon after cessation of illumination, the generation of antimicrobial ROS ceases and the lifetime of these ROS in tissue is very short. Therefore there is likely to be no reason why any microbial cell remaining alive cannot regrow without hindrance after illumination has finished. Bioluminescence imaging in fact demonstrates that in some circumstances this bacterial regrowth does occur. The hope for clinical application is that there exists some lower limit of infectious burden, so that if PDT is able to reduce the number of microbial cells beneath this limit, the host immune defense system will be able to "mop-up" the remaining microorganisms and cure will ensue. It may also be possible to repeat PDT for localized infections at defined time intervals.

The use of various animals as models for microbiological infections has been a fundamental part of infectious disease research for more than a century (16). Now, techniques of genetic alteration and manipulation have made possible the design of animals so as to be specifically applicable to the study of a myriad of diseases.

The intent for the use of animals as models of disease is to establish an infection that mimics that seen in humans. Ultimately, the goal is to seek means by which the infection can be thwarted. A key to developing an animal model is the selection of an animal whose physiology, reaction to an infection, and the nature of the infection itself all mirror as closely as possible the situation in humans. The data from animal models provide a means of indicating the potential of a treatment. Further study, involving humans, is always necessary before something such as a drug can be introduced for general use. Such human studies are subject to rigorous control.

2. Materials

The organisms described in this chapter are all classified as biosafety level two (BL2). This means that although these species are capable of causing disease in humans, they present no health hazard to laboratory personnel when standard universal precautions are taken in handling. These precautions include the use of personal protective equipment (gloves, laboratory coat, eye protection against splashes, and mask if aerosols are likely to be generated) and use of a Class 2 biosafety cabinet. All materials containing live microorganisms should be sterilized by autoclaving before disposal. Disinfectant sprays should be used to clean benches and hoods. UV light should be regularly used in biosafety cabinets to avoid contamination.

2.1. Microorganisms

1. Gram-positive bacterium *Staphylococcus aureus* strain 8325-4.
2. Gram-negative bacterium *Pseudomonas aeruginosa* strain 180.

In this report we will describe the use of *S. aureus* and *P. aeruginosa* in vitro and infections caused by *P. aeruginosa* in vivo (*see* **Note 1**).

2.2. Equipment

1. Shaking incubator
2. Stationary incubator
3. Class 2 biological safety cabinet
4. Centrifuge
5. Autoclave
6. Light source
7. Power meter
8. Vortex mixer
9. Spectrophotometer (not essential but useful)

2.3. Buffers, Reagents, Solutions

1. Brain-heart infusion broth (BHI) (Fisher Scientific, Waltham, MA).
2. Phosphate-buffered saline (PBS) (Fisher Scientific, Waltham, MA). PBS is used to wash microbial cells and for serial dilutions.
3. Liquid growth media: 200 ml of distilled water and 6 g of BHI powder. All liquid media are autoclaved at 120°C for 15 min before use.
4. Solid growth media: Liquid growth media with the addition of 1.5% microbiological agar. Microbiological agar is mixed with liquid growth media before autoclaving. Solid growth media is poured into petri dishes while warm and allowed to solidify on cooling.
5. Methylene blue (MB; 3,7-bis(dimethylamino)-phenothiazinium chloride) (Sigma-Aldrich, St. Louis, MO).

   Many photosensitizers (PSs) can be used to carry out PDI experiments of microorganisms (*see* **Note 2**). In this chapter we will describe the use of MB that can be purchased from chemical suppliers in a degree of purity suitable for antimicrobial PDI. It is soluble in distilled water and a stock solution of 5 mM can be prepared and stored in the dark at 4°C for a limited time (only a few days). PSs such as MB are of course light sensitive and unnecessary exposure to ambient light should be avoided (*see* **Note 3**) (*see* **Fig. 12.1**).

2.4. Light Source

A convenient light source consists of a non-coherent incandescent lamp capable of delivering light into a fiber-optic probe (FOP) fitted with a band-pass filter (LumaCare, Newport Beach, CA). For MB we use a 660 ± 15 nm band-pass filter that provides approximately 1 W of light that can be focused into a spot of

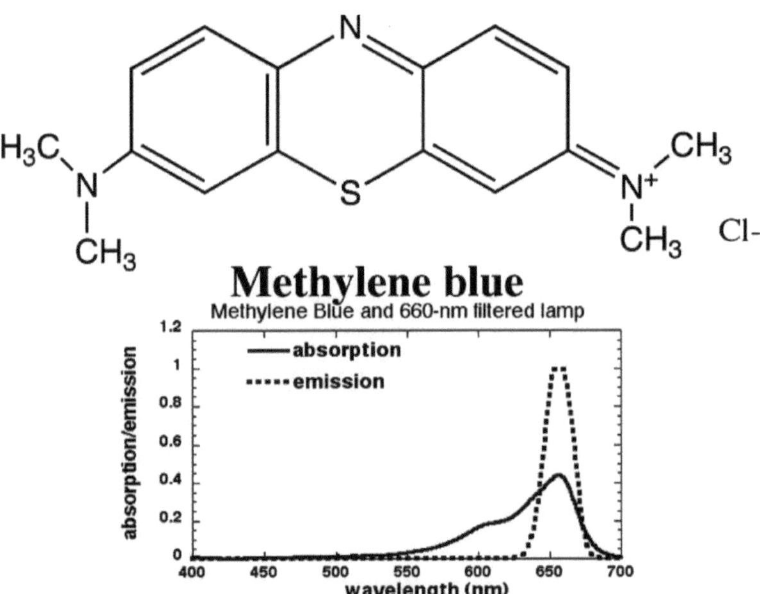

Fig. 12.1. Chemical structure of methylene blue, MB, absorption spectrum and lamp emission spectrum with 660 ± 15 nm filter showing overlap.

diameter between 1.5 and 5 cm depending on the distance from the end of the FOP.

2.5. Power Meter

The intensity of the light spot was measured as follows. A power meter (model DMM 199 with 201 standard head, Coherent, Santa Clara, CA) is used to measure the irradiance (power density in mW/cm^2).

2.6. Disposable Plasticware

Serial dilutions use a considerable amount of disposable plasticware.

1. Microcentrifuge tubes of 1.5 ml capacity (Fisher Scientific, Waltham, MA) are ideal for carrying out serial dilutions using 200 μL yellow pipette tips.
2. Square 10 × 10 cm plastic petri dishes (Fisher Scientific, Waltham, MA) are used for incubating the serial dilutions on agar medium in order to count colonies.

2.7. In Vivo PDT of Infections

Mice are used as an animal model. Female BALB/c mice (Charles River Lab, Wilmington, MA) are obtained at 6 weeks of age when they weigh on average 20 g. Anesthesia is conveniently obtained by intraperitoneal injection of a mixture of ketamine/xylazine (100 mg/kg; 10:1 ratio). Mice are shaved on the back and the next day burns are created using brass blocks obtained from Small Parts, Inc. (Miami, FL).

3. Methods

3.1. In Vitro PDI of Microorganisms

1. Preparation of suspension of microbial cells. Prepare liquid media (brain-heart infusion broth, BHI, for bacteria) and autoclave. Prepare solid media by addition of 1.5% microbiological agar to above broth and pour into 10 × 10 cm square petri dishes. Use a sterile loop to pick a single colony from the agar plate and put into a 15-ml centrifuge tube containing 3 ml of BHI. Leave it in the shaking incubator at 37°C overnight to allow adequate aeration. In the case of fast growing species (doubling times the order of 15–30 min) a small initial inoculum will give stationary cultures overnight that generally have cell densities of the order of 10^9 CFU/ml. It is possible to measure the approximate cell density by a simple visible absorption measurement in a spectrophotometer at 600 or 650 nm and this can be correlated to a one-off CFU determination. This will give a number such as an OD of 0.6 corresponding to a cell density of 10^8 CFU/ml. Stationary cultures should be refreshed after a dilution of 100:1 into fresh medium for about 1 h. Cell pellets are isolated by centrifugation (13,690 × g for 5 min) and resuspended in sterile PBS to the desired density (usually 10^8 CFU/ml) (*see* **Note 4**).
2. Incubation with PSs. The concentration of dye that is used and the amount of light that is delivered to some extent have a reciprocal relationship to each other. The PS that is used in this chapter, MB, has traditionally been used in higher concentrations compared to other reported antimicrobial PS. We recommend concentrations of 10 μM for *S. aureus* and 1 mM for *P. aeruginosa* (*see* **Note 5**). The incubation time can be short, and it has been found that 15 min is a reasonable time. One of the most important variables is whether the cell–PS suspensions are "washed" before illumination or not (*see* **Section 3.1**, Step 5). It is usual to protect the PS–microbial cell suspensions from ambient light by covering in aluminum foil.
3. Light delivery. The best way to carry out the actual illumination is in a 24- or 48-well plate. Place 1 ml of PS-loaded bacterial suspension into a well and remove an aliquot for CFU determination at $t = 0$. The light spot can be set up to illuminate four wells equally by adjusting its diameter to 3–4 cm. At an irradiance of 100 mW/cm^2 a fluence (energy density) of 6 J/cm^2 is delivered every minute.
4. In vitro PDI experiments. We will describe several variations of how these in vitro PDI experiments are carried out because we believe that they make an important and

interesting scientific point. First the suspensions of bacterial cells and dissolved MB can be washed (or not) by centrifugation and subsequent resuspension of the pellet in PBS. Centrifuge at 13,690 × *g* for 5 min and resuspend the bacterial pellet along with tightly bound MB in the same volume of PBS. Second the variable in the PDI experiments can be the MB concentration in the incubation mixture (from 0.3 to 30 μM as shown for *S. aureus* in **Fig. 12.3a, b**), and the light fluence (10 J/cm^2 of 660-nm light) can be kept constant. However, another way of conducting the in vitro PDI experiments is to keep the concentration of MB in the incubation mixture constant (1 mM MB in the case of *P. aeruginosa* as shown in **Fig. 12.4a, b**). In this case the variable is the delivered fluence that is increased up to 320 J/cm^2 for the difficult-to-kill *P. aeruginosa* (*see* **Fig. 12.2**).

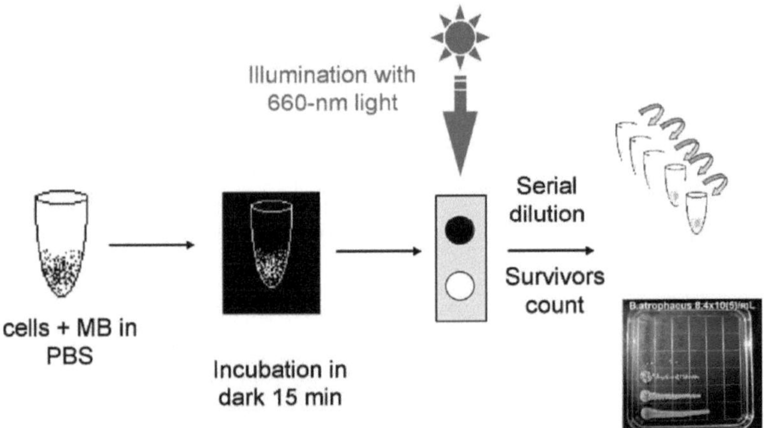

Fig. 12.2. Schematic cartoon illustrating an in vitro antibacterial PDT experiment with MB.

5. Serial dilutions. In order to construct a light dose–response curve with survival fraction the following aliquots of microbial cell suspension are obtained. First the original cell suspension, second the suspension after incubation for 15 min with MB solution (to quantify dark toxicity of the PS), then successive aliquots of suspension removed after successive fluences of light have been delivered (for instance, 5, 10, 20, and 40 J/cm^2). Each aliquot of microbial cell suspension is individually subjected to five ten-fold serial dilutions in sterile PBS. This will provide tubes with dilutions of 1×, 10×, 100×, 1,000×, 10,000×, and 100,000×. Ten μL of each dilution is horizontally streaked on square agar plates according to the method of Jett et al. (17) (*see* **Note 6**).

   After 24-h incubation the plates are counted. Ideally two or three rows can be counted on each plate, the results multiplied by the appropriate power of ten and averaged to give the number of CFU/ml in each aliquot of cell suspension. Survival fractions can be obtained by dividing the treatment CFU/ml by the CFU/ml in the original cell suspension (absolute control). It is possible to also perform a series of light-alone controls, but in our experience these do not show any appreciable difference from absolute control.

6. Results of in vitro PDI. **Figure 12.3a, b** shows PDI of the Gram-positive bacterium, *S. aureus*, with MB and red light. It is known that Gram-positive species are much easier to kill with PDI than Gram-negative species (5). When the bacterial suspension is illuminated without a wash then the bacteria are effectively eliminated (greater than six logs of killing) with MB concentrations higher than 10 μM, combined with 10 J/cm^2 of 660-nm light. In sharp contrast, when the bacterial suspensions are centrifuged before illumination to remove the MB solution, the killing obtained is dramatically reduced with barely one log of bacterial reduction even at 30 μM MB. The reason for this difference is probably that the extracellular reactive oxygen species produced also damage the bacteria and allow better penetration of MB into the bacterial cells and increase killing by intracellular reactive oxygen species (9). Similar findings to these have been previously reported (18).

   The Gram-negative bacterial species, *P. aeruginosa*, is very much harder to kill by PDI than Gram-positive *S. aureus*. Even though all Gram-negative species are more resistant to PDI than Gram-positive species, *P. aeruginosa* in particular is one of the most resistant of the Gram-negatives. This can

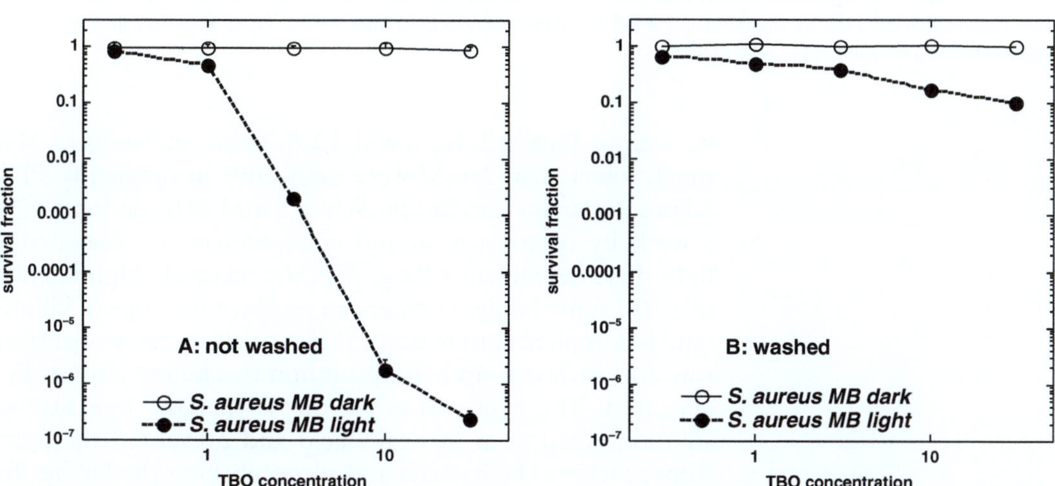

Fig. 12.3. Killing curves of MB concentration in the incubation media versus survival fraction obtained with MB-PDT (10 J/cm^2 of 660-nm light) of *S. aureus*. (**a**) The bacteria were illuminated without a wash; (**b**) the bacteria were washed before illumination.

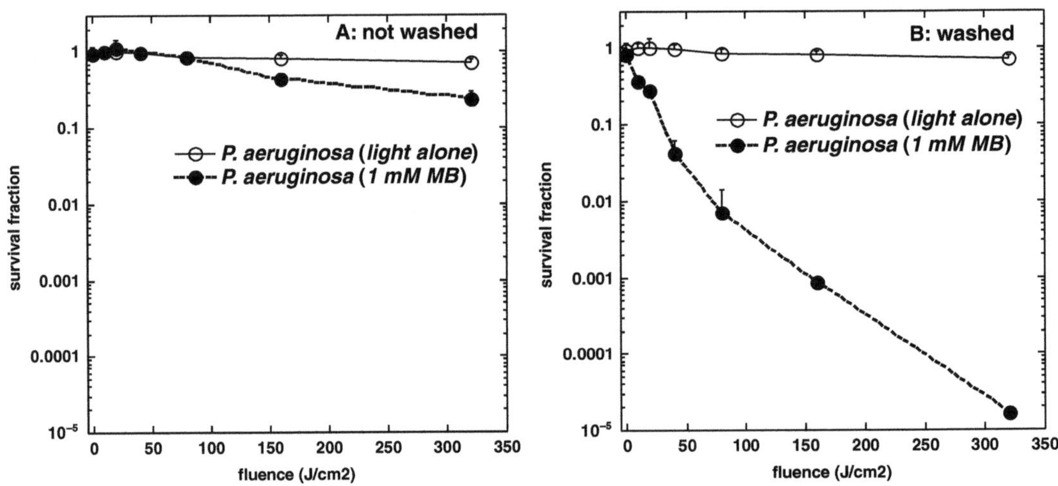

Fig. 12.4. Killing curves of delivered fluence versus survival fraction obtained with MB-PDT (incubated at 1 mM) of *P. aeruginosa*. (**a**) The bacteria were illuminated without a wash; (**b**) the bacteria were washed before illumination.

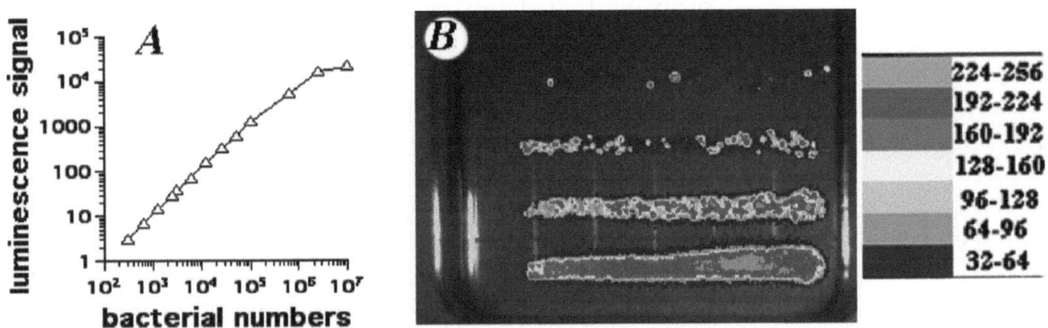

Fig. 12.5. Bioluminescent bacteria. *Panel* **a** shows the relationship between luminescence and bacterial number obtained with luminescent *P. aeruginosa* 180 over four logs of bacterial numbers as measured by a luminometer. Bacterial CFU were routinely determined by streaking out a set of serial dilutions onto agar plates. *Panel* **b** shows an example of bioluminescence imaging of the agar plates.

be seen in **Figs. 12.4a, b** and **12.5**. Concentrations of MB much lower than 1 mM were ineffective in mediating PDI killing under any conditions. When 1 mM MB was used with a wash by centrifugation and resuspension, we obtained a light dose-dependent killing, with the relatively high fluence of 320 J/cm^2 being necessary to produce five logs of killing (still incomplete elimination). When the bacterial suspension was not washed from MB in solution this killing almost disappeared. The explanation for this is that the free MB in solution acted as an optical shield and prevented the light from reaching the bacteria and accomplishing the killing. In other words the better killing effect of leaving the MB in solution only applies at fairly low MB concentrations, while at higher concentrations the MB in solution quenches PDI.

3.2. In Vivo PDT of Infections in Mouse Models

All animal procedures must be approved by the Institutional Animal Care and Use Committee (IACUC) and must meet the guidelines of National Institutes of Health. The animals are housed one per cage (to prevent mice interfering with each other's wounds) and maintained on a 12-h light/dark cycle with access to food and water ad libitum. Mice receive buprenorphine (0.03 mg/kg SC BID) for 3 days after wounding for pain relief. Mice are euthanized according to protocol when their condition is assessed to be moribund.

1. Preparation of mice. The day before the creation of the burn female BALB/c mice weighing 20–25 g are shaved on the back and depilated with Nair cream (Carter-Wallace Inc, New York, NY) (**Fig. 12.6a**).
2. Creation of a mouse burn infection (*see* **Note 8**). Mice are anesthetized with an i.p. injection of ketamine/xylazine cocktail. Burn wounds are created by applying two

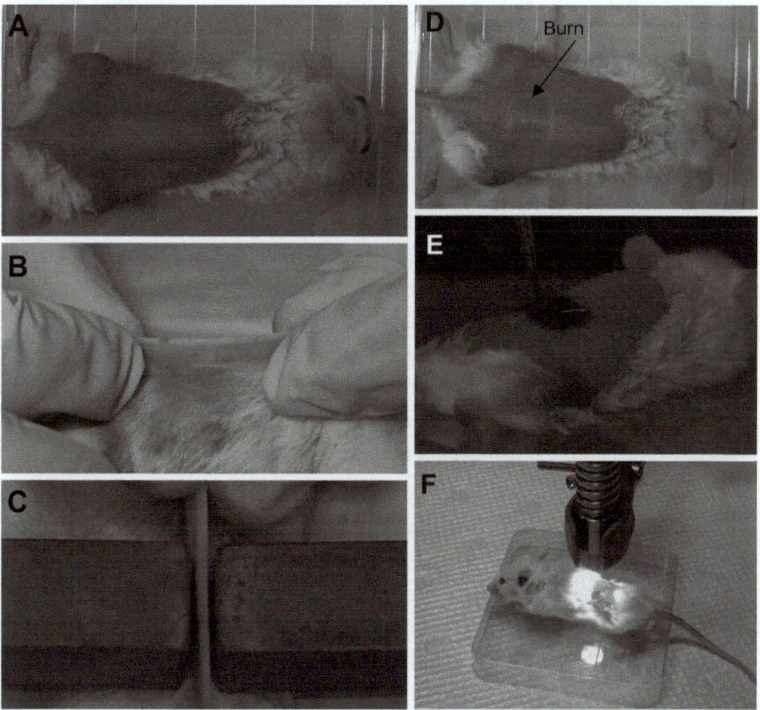

Fig. 12.6. Procedure of PDT for mouse burn infection. (**a**) Mouse is shaved and depilated on the back the day before experiment. (**b**) A skinfold is raised on the back of anesthetized mouse. (**c**) Two brass blocks that have been pre-heated to 95°C in boiling water are applied to either side of the skinfold for 10 s. (**d**) The resulting full-thickness burn on the mouse back measures 2 × 1 cm. (**e**) Fifteen minutes after application of the bacterial suspension to the mouse burn (not shown), MB solution is applied with a pipette tip. (**f**) Delivery of 660 ± 15 nm light from a non-coherent light source to the MB-treated infected burn.

pre-heated brass blocks (≈95°C, 1 × 1 cm^2 each in area; Small Parts, Inc., Miami, FL) to the opposing sides of an elevated skinfold on the back of each mouse (**Fig. 12.6b**) for 10 s (**Fig. 12.6c**) to make a full-thickness, non-lethal, third-degree burn measuring 2 × 1 cm (**Fig. 12.6d**) (19).

A PBS suspension (50 μL) containing 10^8 CFUs of mid-log-phase bioluminescent *P. aeruginosa* strain 180 (*see* **Note 7**) in sterile PBS (OD_{600} = 0.6–0.8) is inoculated onto each burn from a 200 μL yellow tip pipette and evenly spread over the surface (20). The mice are imaged with the luminescence camera immediately after adding bacteria to ensure even spread of bacteria across the burn and equal bacterial loading into each burn on different mice (21) (*see* **Note 9**).

3. Imaging of infections using bioluminescence. Mice are anesthetized with ketamine/xylazine and placed in a petri dish in a prone position with their backs uppermost on a laboratory stand inside the light-tight chamber 30 cm below the lens. The bioluminescence imaging setup (Hamamatsu Photonics KK, Bridgewater, NJ) consists of an intensified CCD camera mounted in a light-tight specimen chamber, fitted with a light-emitting diode, a setup that allows for a background gray-scale image of the entire mouse to be captured. In the photon-counting mode, an image of the emitted light from the bacteria is captured using an integration time of 2 min at a setting of 10 on the image intensifier control module. By use of ARGUS software (Hamamatsu), the luminescence image is presented as a false-color image superimposed on top of the gray-scale reference image. The image-processing component of the software calculated the total pixel values from the luminescence images of the infected area. The same analysis area of 1,200 pixels was used for all the wounds at all time points.

4. Addition of MB. MB is added 20–30 min after the inoculation of bacteria. MB is added as 50 μL of a solution in PBS (1 mM MB equivalent) (**Fig. 12.6e**), which is added to burns that will be PDT treated or dark controls. After a further 15–30 min to allow the MB to bind to and penetrate the bacteria the mice are again imaged to quantify any dark toxicity of the MB to the bacteria.

5. Light delivery. Mice are illuminated with 660 ± 15 nm light delivered by a non-coherent light source (LumaCare, Newport Beach, CA) (**Fig. 12.6f**) that provides a spot on the mouse with a diameter of 3 cm and an irradiance of 100 mW/cm^2. The power of light is routinely measured using a power meter. Mice are given total light doses of up to 240 J/cm^2 in aliquots (12, 24, 48, 96, and 60 J/cm^2),

with bioluminescence imaging taking place after each aliquot of light (*see* **Note 10**). At the conclusion of the experiment, mice are allowed to recover from anesthesia in an animal warmer and resume their normal activity. There are no visible differences between any of the burns at the completion of illumination or indeed at any time during the healing process.

6. Mouse follow-up. Burns are not dressed as the bacteria tend to grow on the moist undersurface of the dressing. On each of the next 2–5 days the mice are anesthetized with a small dose of ketamine/xylazine and imaged under the same conditions (*see* **Note 11**). The burns are measured in two dimensions each day and the areas calculated. The strain of *P aeruginosa* we have employed is invasive and bacterial inocula as low as 10^5 will reliably lead to development of bacteremia and death from sepsis. Depending on the bacterial load death occurs anywhere from 2 to 10 days after infection and is preceded by a significant weight loss (10–20% of body weight). Therefore, when mice are infected with *P aeruginosa* they are weighed each day and followed for survival in addition to their wounds being measured.

   Blood samples are withdrawn from the orbital plexus and cultured on BHI plates for determining the presence of bacteria in the bloodstream. That can be correctly identified as the colonies are bioluminescent.

   Mice are also followed for survival, body weight, and wound healing (wound area). When mice die they are dissected and organ samples (spleen, liver, and kidneys) taken for dissociation and determination of bacterial numbers and sectioned for hematoxylin–eosin staining for tissue damage.

7. Results of MB-PDT of mouse burn infection. **Figure 12.7** shows the bioluminescent images obtained during the PDT treatment of a *P. aeruginosa*-infected burn in a mouse model. In order to be able to visually compare the set of images they were all collected using the most sensitive bit range on the luminescent camera. This consideration means that

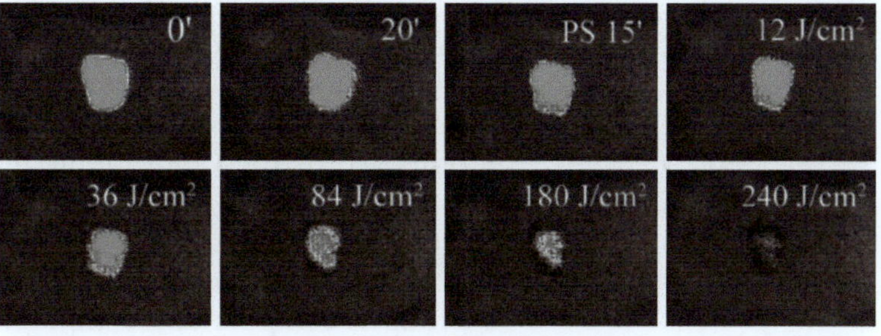

Fig. 12.7. Representative successive bioluminescence images of a 10-s mouse burn infected with 10^8 *P. aeruginosa* and treated with MB-PDT.

the images of the heaviest bacterial density contain saturated pixels. It can be seen that the bacterial bioluminescence remains fairly stable for the 20 min that the bacteria are given to adhere to the tissue of the burn and form an infection. Moreover when the MB is applied to the burn surface the loss of luminescence is minimal. After 12 J/cm^2 of red light has been delivered there is a small loss of signal, which becomes noticeably less after 36 J/cm^2 has been given. After 84, 180, and 240 J/cm^2 the luminescence continues its dose-dependent decrease until after the highest dose of light (240 J/cm^2) there is hardly any detectable luminescence left and the loss of signal is >99% equivalent to more than two logs of bacterial killing.

This study was not designed to follow the survival of the mice, but we have published in the past (21) that PDT is capable of preventing the mice from dying of a systemic infection that develops from a localized wound infection on the back. When the PDT was able to kill 95% of the bacteria, the mice were saved from dying (*see* **Note 12**).

4. Notes

1. Sources and choice of microbiological strains. Defined strains of various species of microorganisms can be obtained from culture depositories or cell banks. ATCC (Manassas, VA) is the recognized vendor in the USA and many other worldwide collections are listed at http://www.bacterio.cict.fr/links.html. Stable bioluminescent bacteria are available from Caliper Life Sciences: http://www.caliperls.com/products/reagents/bioluminescent/light-producing-cells-and-microorganisms/microorganisms/
2. Antimicrobial PS. The area of PS structure is probably where the largest variation is possible. There are a relatively large number of compounds (tens) that have been reported to be antimicrobial PS in the scientific literature. Many if not most of these PS molecules are positively charged. In other words they are cationic molecules that have one or more quaternized nitrogen atoms. These molecules may be tetrapyrroles that are based on porphyrin (22, 23), phthalocyanine (20, 24), or chlorin (25) backbones. A second large group of compounds is composed of cationic synthetic dyes such as phenothiazinium dyes or triarylmethane dyes. In this chapter we have chosen to describe the easily available

MB in order to make it possible for most people to replicate the techniques described (26).

3. PS quality control. It is known that solutions of most PS are not stable indefinitely even when stored at 4°C in the dark. The dyes that are used can aggregate in aqueous solution and this is frequently not visible to the naked eye (i.e., there is no visible precipitate). However, aggregation does mean that the dyes can substantially lose effectiveness in producing photokilling of microbial cells. Visible absorption spectra can help to monitor the activity of these dyes.
4. Microbiological culture. The possibility of contamination is an ever-present danger in microbiology. Since rich growth media are used, stray microbial cells from the environment or from the laboratory can fairly easily grow in liquid media and, if care is not taken, can completely displace the desired species over time (in some cases without the experimenter realizing). Good aseptic technique will go a long way to avoid this occurrence. In addition it is useful to be able to recognize colony morphology of specific species on agar plates. A gram stain can be used to distinguish between Gram-positive and Gram-negative bacteria.

   It is sometimes necessary to distinguish between log-phase and stationary-phase cultures.
5. In vitro PDT. It is important to realize that there is a stoichiometric relationship between the number of microbial cells and the concentration of PS in the incubation mixture. In other words if the concentration of PS is increased then the fraction of bacteria killed will go up; similarly if the number of bacteria is decreased then the fraction killed will also go up. It is important to stir bacterial suspensions as the individual cells will settle to the bottom of the tube or well during illumination and when aliquots are withdrawn, the numbers of cells will steadily increase as the cell density rises as the total volume decreases. There is an upper limit to the concentration of PS that can be used if the compound is left in solution during the illumination. This is because of the self-shielding effect. This occurs when the dye in solution absorbs a significant proportion of the light falling on the bacterial suspension and prevents sufficient light reaching the PS-loaded cells. For many PSs this self-shielding happens when the concentration reaches about 300 μM.

   If several unknown PSs are to be tested for effectiveness in antimicrobial PDT, it may be preferable to use a set of different PS concentrations (for instance 0.1, 0.3, 1, 3, 10, 30, and 100 μM) and a single light fluence (for instance

10 J/cm^2 of the appropriate wavelength) instead of a single concentration and a set of fluences.

6. Serial dilutions. Bacteria have a pronounced tendency to stick together in buffers. This means that unless care is taken the actual numbers of CFU counted in the successive serial dilutions may not reflect the calculated numbers. To avoid this effect the microcentrifuge tubes should each be individually vortexed for several seconds before the next dilution is made. In the worst case small concentrations of detergents may need to be added to the PBS to encourage bacterial dissociation form clumps.
7. Animal models of infection. In order to create animal models of infection only certain microbial species (and even only certain strains within a single species) can be used. Bacteria are described as having varying degrees of virulence and pathogenicity. Moreover microbes that are highly pathogenic and virulent in humans may be markedly less so in mice (and vice versa). There have even been reports of differences in pathogenicity when a certain species and strain of microbe is tested for its ability to form an infection in two different strains of mice (27, 28).
8. Creation of mouse burn infection. The susceptibilities of different areas in the BALB/c mouse body to bacterial infection are variable. For example, the lower back is usually more susceptible to infection than the upper back. To ensure that the extent of infection is relatively consistent in different mice, it is recommended that the burns be made consistently on the lower half of the mouse back. When applying the bacteria solution to the mouse burns, it is also important to smear the solution evenly on the whole burned area to ensure an even extent of infection within each burn. Mouse burns can also be made by exposing the dorsal surface of mice with a template (1×2 cm^2 opening) to hot water bath (92–95°C) (29) or to the flame of an alcohol lamp (30). Bacteria can also be applied to the burn by subcutaneous injection of bacterial inoculum (31).
9. Alternative mouse infection models. It is possible to use excisional wounds as a basis for bacterial infections (21, 32). In some cases subcutaneous abscesses can be used as mouse models. In this case the bacterial suspension is injected under the skin and into the muscle (e.g., thigh muscle). Depending on the species of bacteria employed, temporary immune suppression of the mice using cyclophosphamide injection may be necessary to allow the bacteria to become established (33).

10. PDT of burn infections. The evaporation of the solvent (PBS) during PDT can cause non-PDT killing of bacteria. To prevent this artifact, it is recommended that aliquots of 10–15 μL PBS be added to the PDT-treated burns after each aliquot of light.

    Photobleaching of MB can impair the effectiveness of PDT and is a commonly encountered problem in PDT. The effect of photobleaching can be eliminated or reduced by applying MB in aliquots to the burns.

    Too much light (usually >350 J/cm^2) can impair the selectivity of killing of bacteria and cause non-specific host tissue damage by PDT.

11. Problem of regrowth. Bacterial regrowth after PDT is also a common problem. This is partially due to the fact that PDT is usually carried in the growing phase of the infection, which is usually from day 0 to day 3 after infection. For *P. aeruginosa* infection in mouse burns, bacterial regrowth can cause mortality of mice and subsequently failure of PDT. Repeated PDT (usually two to three times) or the combination of PDT with conventional antibiotics has shown to be a possible strategy to counteract the bacterial regrowth.

12. Progress course of burn infection. The main determinants of the severity of the burn infection and whether the rodents develop sepsis and die are as follows: the virulence of the particular strain, the number of bacteria applied to the burn, the size of the burn expressed as % of TBSA, whether the bacteria are applied to the surface or injected into or beneath the burn, and the length of time the heated object or liquid is in contact with the mouse skin. Without PDT, *P. aeruginosa* usually can invade through the burn into mouse bloodstream and subsequently induce fatal infection. In addition, a third-degree burn and superimposed infection can cause a deficiency of the gut barrier (34, 35), which can subsequently promote bacterial translocation from the gut (36).

References

1. Jesionek, A. and von Tappenier, H. (1903) Zur behandlung der hautcarcinomit mit fluorescierenden stoffen. *Muench Med Wochneshr*, **47**, 2042.
2. Raab, C. (1900) Über die Wirkung fluoreszierender Stoffe auf Infusoria. *Z Biol*, **39**, 524–546.
3. Bellin, J. S., Lutwick, L., and Jonas, B. (1969) Effects of photodynamic action on *E. coli*. *Arch Biochem Biophys*, **132**, 157–164.
4. Janikova, A. (1966) The photodynamic action of acridine orange and proflavine on the survival of *Escherichia coli* B and its capacity for phage T3. *Folia Biol*, **12**, 132–136.
5. Malik, Z., Ladan, H., and Nitzan, Y. (1992) Photodynamic inactivation of Gram-negative bacteria: problems and possible solutions. *J Photochem Photobiol B*, **14**, 262–266.
6. Malik, Z., Hanania, J., and Nitzan, Y. (1990) Bactericidal effects of photoactivated porphyrins – an alternative approach to

antimicrobial drugs. *J Photochem Photobiol B*, **5**, 281–293.
7. Bertoloni, G., Rossi, F., Valduga, G., Jori, G., and van Lier, J. (1990) Photosensitizing activity of water- and lipid-soluble phthalocyanines on *Escherichia coli*. *FEMS Microbiol Lett*, **59**, 149–155.
8. Hamblin, M. R. and Hasan, T. (2004) Photodynamic therapy: a new antimicrobial approach to infectious disease? *Photochem Photobiol Sci*, **3**, 436–450.
9. Merchat, M., Bertolini, G., Giacomini, P., Villanueva, A., and Jori, G. (1996) Meso-substituted cationic porphyrins as efficient photosensitizers of gram-positive and gram-negative bacteria. *J Photochem Photobiol B*, **32**, 153–157.
10. Merchat, M., Spikes, J. D., Bertoloni, G., and Jori, G. (1996) Studies on the mechanism of bacteria photosensitization by meso-substituted cationic porphyrins. *J Photochem Photobiol B*, **35**, 149–157.
11. Minnock, A., Vernon, D. I., Schofield, J., Griffiths, J., Parish, J. H., and Brown, S. T. (1996) Photoinactivation of bacteria. Use of a cationic water-soluble zinc phthalocyanine to photoinactivate both gram-negative and gram-positive bacteria. *J Photochem Photobiol B*, **32**, 159–164.
12. Minnock, A., Vernon, D. I., Schofield, J., Griffiths, J., Parish, J. H., and Brown, S. B. (2000) Mechanism of uptake of a cationic water-soluble pyridinium zinc phthalocyanine across the outer membrane of *Escherichia coli*. *Antimicrob Agents Chemother*, **44**, 522–527.
13. Hamblin, M. R., O'Donnell, D. A., Murthy, N., Rajagopalan, K., Michaud, N., Sherwood, M. E., and Hasan, T. (2002) Polycationic photosensitizer conjugates: effects of chain length and Gram classification on the photodynamic inactivation of bacteria. *J Antimicrob Chemother*, **49**, 941–951.
14. Moan, J. and Peng, Q. (2003) An outline of the hundred-year history of PDT. *Anticancer Res*, **23**, 3591–3600.
15. Demidova, T. N., Gad, F., Zahra, T., Francis, K. P., and Hamblin, M. R. (2005) Monitoring photodynamic therapy of localized infections by bioluminescence imaging of genetically engineered bacteria. *J Photochem Photobiol B*, **81**, 15–25.
16. Belmatoug, N. and Fantin, B. (1997) Contribution of animal models of infection for the evaluation of the activity of antimicrobial agents. *Int J Antimicrob Agents*, **9**, 73–82.
17. Jett, B. D., Hatter, K. L., Huycke, M. M., and Gilmore, M. S. (1997) Simplified agar plate method for quantifying viable bacteria. *Biotechniques*, **23**, 648–650.
18. Demidova, T. N. and Hamblin, M. R. (2005) Effect of cell-photosensitizer binding and cell density on microbial photoinactivation. *Antimicrob Agents Chemother*, **49**, 2329–2335.
19. Stevens, E. J., Ryan, C. M., Friedberg, J. S., Barnhill, R. L., Yarmush, M. L., and Tompkins, R. G. (1994) A quantitative model of invasive Pseudomonas infection in burn injury. *J Burn Care Rehabil*, **15**, 232–235.
20. Mantareva, V., Kussovski, V., Angelov, I., Borisova, E., Avramov, L., Schnurpfeil, G., and Wohrle, D. (2007) Photodynamic activity of water-soluble phthalocyanine zinc(II) complexes against pathogenic microorganisms. *Bioorg Med Chem*, **15**, 4829–4835.
21. Hamblin, M. R., Zahra, T., Contag, C. H., McManus, A. T., and Hasan, T. (2003) Optical monitoring and treatment of potentially lethal wound infections in vivo. *J Infect Dis*, **187**, 1717–1725.
22. Oliveira, A., Almeida, A., Carvalho, C. M., Tome, J. P., Faustino, M. A., Neves, M. G., Tome, A. C., Cavaleiro, J. A., and Cunha, A. (2009) Porphyrin derivatives as photosensitizers for the inactivation of Bacillus cereus endospores. *J Appl Microbiol*, **105**, 1986–1995.
23. Caminos, D. A., Spesia, M. B., Pons, P., and Durantini, E. N. (2008) Mechanisms of *Escherichia coli* photodynamic inactivation by an amphiphilic tricationic porphyrin and 5,10,15,20-tetra(4-N,N,N-trimethylammoniumphenyl) porphyrin. *Photochem Photobiol Sci*, **7**, 1071–1078.
24. Scalise, I. and Durantini, E. N. (2005) Synthesis, properties, and photodynamic inactivation of *Escherichia coli* using a cationic and a noncharged Zn(II) pyridyloxyphthalocyanine derivatives. *Bioorg Med Chem*, **13**, 3037–3045.
25. Schastak, S., Gitter, B., Handzel, R., Hermann, R., and Wiedemann, P. (2008) Improved photoinactivation of gram-negative and gram-positive methicillin-resistant bacterial strains using a new near-infrared absorbing meso-tetrahydroporphyrin: a comparative study with a chlorine e6 photosensitizer photolon. *Methods Find Exp Clin Pharmacol*, **30**, 129–133.
26. Wainwright, M., Phoenix, D. A., Laycock, S. L., Wareing, D. R., and Wright, P. A. (1998) Photobactericidal activity of phenothiazinium dyes against methicillin-resistant strains of *Staphylococcus aureus*. *FEMS Microbiol Lett*, **160**, 177–181.

27. Darville, T., Andrews, C. W., Jr., Laffoon, K. K., Shymasani, W., Kishen, L. R., and Rank, R. G. (1997) Mouse strain-dependent variation in the course and outcome of chlamydial genital tract infection is associated with differences in host response. *Infect Immun*, **65**, 3065–3073.
28. Wilson, K. R., Napper, J. M., Denvir, J., Sollars, V. E., and Yu, H. D. (2007) Defect in early lung defence against *Pseudomonas aeruginosa* in DBA/2 mice is associated with acute inflammatory lung injury and reduced bactericidal activity in naive macrophages. *Microbiology*, **153**, 968–979.
29. McVay, C. S., Velasquez, M., and Fralick, J. A. (2007) Phage therapy of *Pseudomonas aeruginosa* infection in a mouse burn wound model. *Antimicrob Agents Chemother*, **51**, 1934–1938.
30. Toliver-Kinsky, T. E., Varma, T. K., Lin, C. Y., Herndon, D. N., and Sherwood, E. R. (2002) Interferon-gamma production is suppressed in thermally injured mice: decreased production of regulatory cytokines and corresponding receptors. *Shock*, **18**, 322–330.
31. Barnea, Y., Carmeli, Y., Kuzmenko, B., Gur, E., Hammer-Munz, O., and Navon-Venezia, S. (2006) The establishment of a *Pseudomonas aeruginosa*-infected burn-wound sepsis model and the effect of imipenem treatment. *Ann Plast Surg*, **56**, 674–679.
32. Hamblin, M. R., O'Donnell, D. A., Murthy, N., Contag, C. H., and Hasan, T. (2002) Rapid control of wound infections by targeted photodynamic therapy monitored by in vivo bioluminescence imaging. *Photochem Photobiol*, **75**, 51–57.
33. Gad, F., Zahra, T., Francis, K. P., Hasan, T., and Hamblin, M. R. (2004) Targeted photodynamic therapy of established soft-tissue infections in mice. *Photochem Photobiol Sci*, **3**, 451–458.
34. Eaves-Pyles, T. and Alexander, J. W. (2001) Comparison of translocation of different types of microorganisms from the intestinal tract of burned mice. *Shock*, **16**, 148–152.
35. Gianotti, L., Alexander, J. W., Pyles, T., James, L., and Babcock, G. F. (1993) Relationship between extent of burn injury and magnitude of microbial translocation from the intestine. *J Burn Care Rehabil*, **14**, 336–342.
36. Manson, W. L., Coenen, J. M., Klasen, H. J., and Horwitz, E. H. (1992) Intestinal bacterial translocation in experimentally burned mice with wounds colonized by *Pseudomonas aeruginosa*. *J Trauma*, **33**, 654–658.

Chapter 13

Photodynamic Therapy of Bacterial and Fungal Biofilm Infections

Merrill A. Biel

Abstract

Biofilms have been found to be involved in a wide variety of microbial infections in the body, by one estimate 80% of all infections. Infectious processes in which biofilms have been implicated include common problems such as *urinary tract infections*, *catheter* infections, *middle-ear infections*, sinusitis, formation of *dental plaque*, *gingivitis*, coating *contact lenses*, *endocarditis*, infections in *cystic fibrosis*, and infections of permanent indwelling devices such as joint *prostheses* and *heart valves*. Bacteria living in a biofilm usually have significantly different properties from free-floating bacteria of the same species, as the dense and protected environment of the film allows them to cooperate and interact in various ways. One benefit of this environment is increased resistance to *detergents* and *antibiotics*, as the dense extracellular matrix and the outer layer of cells protect the interior of the community. In some cases antibiotic resistance can be increased 1000-fold. Also, the biofilm bacteria excrete toxins that reversibly block important processes such as translation and protecting the cell from bactericidal antibiotics that are ineffective against inactive targets. In the head and neck area, biofilms are a major etiologic factor in periodontitis, wound infections, oral candidiasis, and sinus and ear infections. For the past several decades, photodynamic treatment has been reported in the literature to be effective in eradicating various microorganisms using different photosensitizers, different wavelengths of light, and different light sources. PDT has been further studied to demonstrate its effectiveness for the eradication of both Gram-negative and Gram-positive antibiotic-resistant bacteria. This chapter will focus on the use of PDT in the treatment of antibiotic-resistant biofilms, antibiotic-resistant wound infections, and azole-resistant oral candidiasis using methylene blue-based photodynamic therapy.

Key words: Photodynamic therapy, wound infections, oral candidiasis, bacterial biofilms, candidal biofilms.

1. Introduction

A biofilm is a complex aggregation of microorganisms marked by the excretion of a protective and adhesive matrix. Biofilms are often characterized by surface attachment, structural

C.J. Gomer (ed.), *Photodynamic Therapy*, Methods in Molecular Biology 635,
DOI 10.1007/978-1-60761-697-9_13, © Springer Science+Business Media, LLC 2010

heterogeneity, genetic diversity, complex community interactions, and an extracellular matrix of polymeric substances.

Single-celled organisms generally exhibit two distinct modes of behavior. The first is the free floating, or planktonic, form in which single cells float or swim independently in some liquid medium. The second is an attached state in which cells are closely packed and firmly attached to each other and usually a solid surface. The change in behavior is triggered by many factors, including quorum sensing, as well as other mechanisms that vary between species. When a cell switches modes, it undergoes a phenotypic shift in behavior in which large suites of genes are up- and down-regulated.

Formation of a biofilm begins with the attachment of free-floating microorganisms to a surface. These first colonists adhere to the surface initially through weak, reversible van der Waals forces. If the colonists are not immediately separated from the surface, they can anchor themselves more permanently using cell adhesion molecules such as pili (1).

The first colonists facilitate the arrival of other cells by providing diverse adhesion sites and they begin to build the matrix that holds the biofilm together. Some species are not able to attach to a surface on their own but are often able to anchor themselves to the matrix or directly to earlier colonists. Once colonization has begun, the biofilm grows through a combination of cell division and recruitment.

Biofilms are usually found on solid substrates submerged in or exposed to some aqueous solution, although they can form as floating mats on liquid surfaces. Given sufficient resources for growth, a biofilm will quickly grow to be macroscopic. Biofilms can contain many different types of microorganism, e.g., bacteria, archaea, protozoa, and algae; each group performing specialized metabolic functions. However, some organisms will form monospecies films under certain conditions.

The biofilm is held together and protected by a matrix of excreted polymeric compounds called extracellular polymeric substance or exopolysaccharide (EPS). This matrix protects the cells within it and facilitates communication among them through biochemical signals. Some biofilms have been found to contain water channels that help distribute nutrients and signaling molecules.

Bacteria living in a biofilm usually have significantly different properties from free-floating bacteria of the same species, as the dense and protected environment of the film allows them to cooperate and interact in various ways. One benefit of this environment is increased resistance to detergents and antibiotics, as the dense extracellular matrix and the outer layer of cells protect the interior of the community. In some cases antibiotic resistance can be increased to 1000-fold (2). Kim Lewis of Northeastern University has discovered that a small fraction of cells within *Escherichia coli* biofilms are dormant within the biofilm and almost immune to the effects of antibiotics because of their very low level of metabolic activity. Once antibiotic levels drop, these dormant or "persister cells" become active and repopulate the biofilm. Persisters are not mutants, but phenotypic variants of the wild type (3). The biofilm bacteria excrete toxins that reversibly block important processes such as translation, protecting the cell from bactericidal antibiotics that are ineffective against inactive targets. These toxins promote the creation of the persister cells (1).

Biofilms have been found to be involved in a wide variety of microbial infections in the body, by one estimate 80% of all infections (3). Infectious processes in which biofilms have been implicated include common problems such as urinary tract infections, catheter infections, middle ear infections, sinusitis, formation of dental plaque, gingivitis, coating contact lenses, endocarditis, infections in cystic fibrosis, and infections of permanent indwelling devices such as joint prostheses and heart valves (4).

In the head and neck area biofilms are a major etiologic factor in periodontitis, wound infections, oral candidiasis, and sinus and ear infections. Biofilms have been demonstrated to be present on the removed tissue of patients undergoing surgery for chronic sinusitis (5–8). Patients with sinus biofilms were shown to have sinus mucosa that was denuded of cilia and goblet cells while normal controls without biofilms had normal cila and goblet cell morphology (5). Importantly, the species of bacteria from intraoperative cultures did not correspond to the bacteria species in the biofilm on the respective patient's tissue (6). Thus the biofilm, though a major cause of chronic sinusitis, was not present on routine culture and therefore was not treated. Due to the prevalence of biofilms as a cause of disease in the head and neck region and the significant bacterial resistance to conventional antibiotic therapies, new modalities of treatment are necessary to address this severe medical problem.

For the past several decades, photodynamic treatment has been reported in the literature to be effective in eradicating various microorganisms using different photosensitizers, different wavelengths of light, and different light sources (9–20). PDT has been further studied to demonstrate its effectiveness for the eradication of both Gram-negative and Gram-positive antibiotic-resistant bacteria (20). This chapter will focus on the use of PDT in the treatment of antibiotic-resistant wound infections and azole-resistant oral candidiasis.

2. Chronic Wounds

Chronic wounds afflict 18 million people in the United States annually and are a tremendous financial drain to our health-care system, accounting for tens of billions of dollars annually (21). The term chronic wound is a broad category that defines many conditions including cutaneous burns and several types of skin ulcers such as venous, decubitus, and diabetic. Wounds become chronic as a result of delayed or impaired healing usually caused by an underlying medical condition and/or by an infection. It is well established that significant bacterial bioburden and secondary infections delay healing, cause failure of healing, and even cause wound deterioration (22, 23). Most significantly, wound infections can result in sepsis and death (2). Antimicrobials have historically been the standard of care to combat infections. As reported by Parish, over 2200 topical and systemic antimicrobial preparations have been recommended for the treatment of ulcers to control infection (24). The fact that no standard for treatment is currently accepted by the health-care community indicates that none of these methods has enjoyed enduring success.

A chronic wound infection cannot be effectively managed without controlling the growth of biofilms. Certain bacteria commonly found in infected chronic wounds produce a polysaccharide and protein matrix known as a biofilm that protects the bacteria from antimicrobial treatment. Therefore, antimicrobial treatment of biofilm has proven to be clinically problematic (25–28). Biofilms are remarkably resistant to treatment with conventional topical and/or intravenous antimicrobial agents and use several resistance mechanisms to do so (25–33). Multiple resistance mechanisms of biofilm make it difficult for any individual antimicrobial agent with a single mechanism of action to be effective. Susceptibility tests with in vitro biofilm models have shown that clinically significant survival of bacterial biofilm occurs even after treatment with antibiotics at concentrations hundreds or one thousand times the normal clinical dose (27). In vivo testing has demonstrated that antibiotics might suppress symptoms of infection by killing free-floating bacteria shed from the attached population, but fail to eradicate those bacteria still embedded in the biofilm (26–28). When antimicrobial chemotherapy stops, the biofilm can act as a nidus for recurrence of infection. As a result biofilms have continued to be a cause of persistent infections even when clinical symptoms are controlled by antimicrobial treatment. Evaluation of new and improved methods to treat and eradicate wound biofilms has therefore been ongoing.

PDT, for the treatment of the microorganisms commonly found in cutaneous wound infections, has been proven to be effective by photochemists and clinicians for many years (9–13, 16, 18, 20). Investigators have also demonstrated PDT's effectiveness to successfully destroy viruses and fungi (14, 15, 17, 19). With the recent onset of antibiotic-resistant bacteria, studies have been reported using PDT to effectively eradicate antibiotic-resistant strains of bacteria (18, 20). In addition, PDT has been reported to be effective for the treatment of biofilms (34–37). Unlike the use of certain antiseptics and antibiotics, PDT has been proven to not adversely effect growth factors such as keratinocytes that are known to be responsible for promoting wound healing (38).

Lee et al. described the use of δ-aminolevulinic acid-based PDT to eradicate *Pseudomonas aeruginosa* planktonic forms and biofilms in vitro. They demonstrated that planktonic *Pseudomonas* was eradicated with 10 mM ALA at a light dose of 240 J/cm^2 and *Pseudomonas* biofilm was eradicated with ALA 20 mM and 240 J/cm^2, but this required two separate treatments to achieve complete eradication of the biofilm (39).

Hamblin and Hasan et al. performed a series of in vivo wound infection PDT studies with polylysine-chlorin e6 conjugate and methylene blue. These studies demonstrated a reduction of the pathogenic organisms *Staphylococcus aureus* and *P. aeruginosa* with PDT treatment at 40 J/cm^2 (40, 41).

Lin, Chen, and Huang performed an in vitro study of merocyanine 540- based PDT to treat *S. aureus* planktonic and biofilm cells. They demonstrated complete eradication of the biofilm with 15 μg of merocyanine 540 and 600 J/cm^2 of light (42).

2.1. Methods

Biel, Teichert, and Usacheva performed a series of in vitro and in vivo biofilm wound experiments to demonstrate the efficacy of methylene blue-mediated PDT to eradicate wound biofilms (43). The in vitro biofilm studies were performed to demonstrate the drug and light dose response of the combination of methylene blue, benzalkonium chloride, and polymyxin B sulfate for the treatment of antibiotic-resistant *S. aureus* and mixed *Staphylococcus* and *Pseudomonas* biofilms using 664 nm light. These studies demonstrated that dense tenacious mixed organism antibiotic-resistant biofilms grown for 24 h were greatly reduced (75%) after a one-time PDT treatment with a double light dose treatment (**Table 13.1**). Any remaining culture positive biofilm contained only *Pseudomonas. S. aureus* biofilms were more easily treated than the mixed *Staphylococcus* and *Pseudomonas* biofilms. Importantly, treatment of the biofilms with MB alone, polymyxin B sulfate, or gentamicin did not result in any reduction of the microbial biofilms when compared to the non-treated controls. Based on these studies, the optimal light dose to treat mixed biofilms was determined to be at a dose rate of 400 mW/cm and a total light dose of 100 J/cm.

Table 13.1
Photodestruction of artificially generated biofilms with methylene blue, polymyxin B sulfate, and benzalkonium chloride

Biofilm	Dose rate (mW/cm)	Light dose	Kill (%) Total	Near complete	Partial	No effect
S. aureus	300	Single	6	31	6	57
S. aureus	300	Double	57	31	6	6
S. aureus	400	Single	13	38	0	49
S. aureus	400	Double	49	38	0	13
P. aeruginosa + *S. aureus*	300	Single	0	0	0	100
P. aeruginosa + *S. aureus*	300	Double	25	0	0	75
P. aeruginosa + *S. aureus*	400	Single	0	0	0	100
P. aeruginosa + *S. aureus*	400	Double	25	25	25	25

An in vivo study by Biel et al. was performed to demonstrate the efficacy of PDT to eradicate methicillin-resistant *S. aureus* infections in an albino guinea pig model using methylene blue as the photosensitizing agent (44). In this study statistical comparisons were made of bacterial growth (log CFU), photosensitizer concentration (μg/ml), total light dose (J/cm^2), and dose rate (mW/cm^2) groups. Bacterial counts were averaged for each animal, i.e., right- and left-sided wounds.

2.2. Results

Statistically significant observations for PDT methylene blue treatment of *S. aureus* tissue infection were as follows:

- Groups 9 and 10 (photosensitizer concentration and/or light dose = 0) had significantly more bacteria than all groups with a concentration of methylene blue greater than 150 μg/ml.
- Groups 6, 7, and 8 with the highest concentration of methylene blue (>200 μg/ml) had fewer bacteria than groups with concentrations under 150 μg/ml or a light dose of 0.
- Group 6 had the lowest bacterial growth, with a concentration of methylene blue of 250 μg/ml. This group was significantly different than all groups with the concentration of methylene blue less than 250 μg/ml. Concentrations greater than 250 μg/ml did not appear to offer any benefit in terms of bacterial reduction.

- Comparing groups 3 and 5 (concentration 150 μg/ml and total light dose 60 J/cm^2) demonstrated that the light dose rate of 150 versus 100 mW/cm^2 was not significant.
- It was difficult to evaluate the effect of increasing the total light dose from 30 to 60 J/cm^2 since these two doses were not used while holding the photosensitizer concentration and dose rate constant.

In summary, the optimal methylene blue concentration, total light dose, and dose rate required to maximally and significantly reduce ($p < 0.05$) the bacterial growth (3.49 log CFU reduction) in a methicillin-resistant *Staphylococcus* wound infection was methylene blue 250 μg/ml at a total light dose of 60 J/cm^2 at a dose rate of 150 mW/cm^2 (**Table 13.2**). Furthermore, the percent elimination of Staphylococcal bacteria from the wounds at this methylene blue concentration and light dose compared to the control group was 99.98%.

Table 13.2
Statistical comparison of different groups[a]

Group	MB (μg/ml)	Light dose (J/cm^2)	Dose rate (mW/cm^2)	Mean log CFU (SD)	Significant difference[b]
1	50	30	100	5.62 (0.709)	6,7,8
2	100	30	100	5.55 (0.566)	6,7,8
3	150	60	100	4.35 (0.531)	6,9,10
4	200	60	100	4.29 (0.192)	6,9,10
5	150	60	150	4.78 (0.805)	6,8
6	250	60	150	2.57 (0.552)	1,2,3,4,5,9,10
7	340	60	150	3.51 (0.154)	1,2,9,10
8	400	60	150	2.99 (0.368)	1,2,5,9,10
9	250	0	0	5.93 (0.242)	3,4,6,7,8
10	0	0	0	6.06 (0.102)	3,4,6,7,8

[a]The one-way ANOVA for the difference between the mean bacterial growth for the 10 groups was significant with a *p value* = 0.001.
[b]The group numbers indicated are those that are significantly different for this group ($p < 0.05$) using Tukey's method of adjusting for multiple comparisons in order to maintain an overall α of 0.05.

The gross morphologic observations demonstrated no evidence of clinical infection in wounds that cultured less than 3 log CFU bacteria. This is consistent with the findings in the literature that wound cultures with less than 5 log CFU bacteria do not demonstrate clinical infection or pus (45–49). There was no gross evidence of skin or muscle tissue necrosis. The histologic evaluation, using hematoxylin and eosin staining, of all the photodynamically treated and non-photodynamically treated wounds demonstrated no difference. There was no evidence of microscopic wound tissue necrosis to the skin, muscle, or fascia related to the action of methylene blue and light activation.

These in vitro and in vivo studies of the use of PDT to treat wound infections and sterilize wound biofilms demonstrate the significant potential for PDT to provide a substantial advance in the treatment of difficult-to-treat wound infections and promote healing of non-healing wounds.

3. Oral Candidiasis

Oropharyngeal candidiasis is an opportunistic mucosal infection caused by *Candida albicans* in over 85% of cases. The four main types of oropharyngeal candidiasis are (1) pseudomembranous (thrush), comprising white discrete plaques on an erythematous background, located on the buccal mucosa, throat, tongue, or gingivae; (2) erythematous, comprising smooth red patches on the hard or soft palate, dorsum of tongue or buccal mucosa; (3) hyperplastic, comprising white firmly adherent patches or plaques, usually bilateral on the buccal mucosa; (4) denture-induced stomatitis, presenting as either a smooth or granular erythema confined to the denture bearing area of the hard palate. Symptoms vary, ranging from none to a sore, painful mouth with a burning tongue and altered taste, which can impair speech, nutritional intake, and quality of life.

Candida species are commensals in the gastrointestinal tract. Transmission occurs directly between infected people or on fomites. *Candida* is found in the mouth of 31–60% of healthy people (50). Oropharyngeal candidiasis affects 15–60% of people with hematological or oncological malignancies during period of immunosuppression (51). Oropharyngeal candidiasis occurs in 7–48% of people with HIV infection and in over 90% of those with advanced disease. In severely immunosuppressed people, relapse rates are high (30–50%) and usually occur within 14 days of treatment cessation (52).

Risk factors associated with symptomatic oropharyngeal candidiasis include local or systemic immunosuppression, hematological disorders, broad-spectrum antibiotic use, inhaled or systemic steroids, xerostomia, diabetes and wearing dentures, obturators or orthodontic appliances. The same strain may persist for months or years without overt evidence of clinical infection (53).

Mucocutaneous oropharyngeal candidiasis is one of the most common manifestations of HIV infection. In one prospective study, 84% of HIV-infected patients had oropharyngeal colonization by *Candida* species on at least one occasion and 55% developed clinical thrush (54). The recent use of protease inhibitors to treat HIV patients has resulted in a decrease in the frequency of oral candidiasis but the incidence of oral candidiasis remains high in the HIV patient population (55). While other yeasts may occasionally cause clinical disease, *C. albicans* is the organism isolated from most patients (54, 56). *Candida* species normally colonize the gastrointestinal tract of healthy adults, and most infections in HIV-infected patients are endogenously acquired. In some cases, candidal strains can be transmitted from person to person (54).

During the course of HIV infection, patients appear to be colonized with one or a few dominant strains, which tend not to change over time. Powderly and colleagues isolated the same strain of *C. albicans* in 11 of 17 patients with recurrent yeast infection by DNA probe analysis (56). In another study, using contour-clamped homogeneous electric field electrophoresis, Sangeorzan et al. found that 60% of patients were colonized with one dominant strain of C. *albicans.* In 74% of these patients, recolonization with the same strain occurred after antifungal therapy (54). Using biotyping and restriction fragment length polymorphism analysis of 25 S ribosomal DNA, Whelan and colleagues found that strains of *C. albicans* isolated from 24 patients with AIDS were not significantly different from strains from 23 patients without HIV infection (57). Thus, the candidal strains causing disease in patients with HIV infection appear to be the same as those colonizing patients without HIV infection and, in most patients, do not change over time.

In immunosuppressed and HIV-infected patients, candidiasis is virtually always mucocutaneous, involving the oropharynx, the esophagus, and the vagina. HIV infection by itself is not associated with the syndrome of disseminated candidiasis, which is characterized by candidemia, endophthalmitis, and multiple organ involvement. The precise immunologic processes that control candidal infection in HIV-infected patients are not known. However, mucocutaneous candidiasis is clearly related to the development of clinical cellular immunodeficiency. In fact, oropharyngeal candidiasis is an independent predictor of immunodeficiency in patients with AIDS (58). Moreover, a CD4 lymphocyte count <200/μl is a major risk factor for the development of clinical thrush in HIV-infected persons (54).

Although oropharyngeal candidiasis is frequent in men, recurrent vaginal candidiasis is a common early manifestation of HIV infection in women. The location and severity of candidiasis in women with HIV infection appear to be closely associated with the degree of cellular immunodeficiency, based on the peripheral blood CD4 lymphocyte count. In a study of 66 women, mucocutaneous candidiasis developed in more than half of the women over a median of 14 months of follow-up, vaginal candidiasis, with a mean CD4 lymphocyte count of 506/μl, developed only in 10, while oropharyngeal candidiasis, with a mean count of 230/μl, developed in 16, and esophagitis, with a mean count of 30/μl, developed in 9(59).

Mucocutaneous candidiasis can be treated either topically or with systemic antifungal agents (54, 60), but such therapy does not eradicate colonization (54). A variety of agents are effective for the treatment of oropharyngeal candidiasis with factors such as the extent and severity of disease, patient adherence, and the pharmacokinetic properties of the drug influencing the clinical response. Reported response rates range from 34 to 100% (61–65), and in general, there are few significant differences in response rates between topical and systemic therapies or between the different systemic therapies. Classes of antifungal agents include the azoles including the imidazoles (clotrimazole) and triazoles (ketoconazole, itraconazole, and fluconazole), the polyenes (nystatin and amphotericin B), and pyrimidine synthesis inhibitors, including 5-fluorocytosine. The first-line therapy for the treatment of oropharyngeal candidiasis is with topical administration of nystatin, clotrimazole, or amphotericin B four to five times per day for a period of 14 days. Clinical cure rates are 34–72%. Chronic use of these agents has resulted in development of candidal resistance. Side effects related to nystatin and clotrimazole include diarrhea, nausea, vomiting, and rash in 5.2% and abnormal liver function tests in 15% of patients. Fluconazole is the most commonly prescribed treatment after failure of topical nystatin and clotrimazole. In general, toxicities associated with ketoconazole, itraconazole, and fluconazole are similar, the most common being headache, dyspepsia, diarrhea, nausea, vomiting, hepatitis, and skin rash (66). Prolonged administration may require surveillance of liver enzymes and patients receiving polypharmacy should be monitored for drug interactions.

Refractory oropharyngeal candidiasis has been increasingly reported since 1990 (67–74). Disease refractory to fluconazole has received particular attention because of significant morbidity, the typical requirement for the use of parenteral agents, and widespread use of fluconazole. Refractory disease tends to occur in persons with advanced HIV disease, i.e., CD4+ cell counts <50 cells/mm^3, who have been exposed to antifungal therapy on a chronic basis (75). Recently, several reports have noted the failure of azole drugs, particularly fluconazole, to treat recurrent cases of oropharyngeal candidiasis (54, 76). In a recent study comparing the effects of different fluconazole prophylaxis treatment regimens on the development of acquired *Candida* azole resistance during an 11 month treatment period, 56% developed antifungal resistance on the continuous fluconazole therapy and 46% developed antifungal resistance on the intermittent fluconazole prophylaxis therapy (77). Another study has demonstrated the emergence of *C. albicans* resistance to Clotrimazole in HIV-infected children that results in cross resistance to other azoles resulting in mucosal candidasis refractory to medical therapy (78). Furthermore, transmission of azole-resistant strains of *C. albicans* has been demonstrated among HIV-infected family members with oropharyngeal candidiasis (79). While factors such as diminishing cellular immunity, drug interactions, or decreased drug absorption may account for some of these treatment failures, increasing evidence suggests that *Candida* organisms are developing drug resistance and that the drug resistance can be transmitted among susceptible immunosuppressed individuals.

In the past, a lack of consensus on the methods for performing antifungal susceptibility tests made it difficult to establish whether clinical failure of antifungal therapy was due to resistance of the organism. However, the National Committee for Clinical Laboratory Standards (NCCLS) has now developed reference methods allowing for uniform testing of yeast isolates (80). Using an NCCLS method, Sangeorzan et al. found that the MIC of fluconazole for *Candida* isolates increased over time among patients who had received fluconazole compared with those who received clotrimazole. Clinical resistance to fluconazole was associated with an increased MIC required by the isolate as well as the patient's low CD4 lymphocyte count (54). These data strongly suggest that continued use of antifungal agents, particularly fluconazole, leads to both clinical treatment failure and antifungal resistance, especially in highly immunodeficient patients. A study by Johnson confirmed these results with up to 81% of AIDS patients on chronic azole drug therapy having azole-resistant *C. albicans* (81).

PDT has been found to eradicate azole-resistant *Candida* in vitro and in vivo. This treatment modality has the advantages of ease of treatment at home or in an outpatient office setting, repeatability, and low morbidity related to the therapy. As this treatment has a different mechanism of action than topical and systemic antifungal antibiotics, it would also reduce the significant problem of developing fungal drug resistance in an at-risk patient population.

The photodynamic mechanism of fungal cell destruction is by perforation of the cell wall and membrane with PDT-induced singlet oxygen and oxygen radicals thereby allowing the dye to be further translocated into the cell. Subsequently, the photodynamic dye in its new sites photodamages inner organelles such as the nucleus and induces cell death (82, 83). The significance of this mechanism of fungal cell death is that it is completely different from that of the oral and systemic antifungal agents. Therefore, it would be effective against antifungal agent-resistant *Candida*, as well as help to prevent the development of resistant *Candida* by providing for another means of *Candida* eradication.

3.1. Methods

Teichert and Biel performed an in vivo experiment to demonstrate the efficacy of methylene blue-mediated photodynamic therapy (PDT) treatment of azole-resistant oropharyngeal candidiasis in an immunodeficient mouse model that simulates the immunosuppression of AIDS patients (19).

In this experiment a patient isolate azole-resistant *C. albicans* was used. Experimental severe combined immunodeficiency disease (SCID) beige nude mice were challenged three times a week by swabbing the oral cavity with a *C. albicans* inoculated Calgis type 4 swab for a period of 4 weeks. In addition drinking water was inoculated at a McFarland Standard of 3, which corresponds to 9×10^8/ml.

The SCID beige nude mice were divided into 15 groups. Controls consisted of mice inoculated with *C. albicans* and no treatment received (M–L–) and mice receiving MB but without light activation (M+L–). Mice were anesthetized using 0.1 ml of ketamine:xylazine (20:2.5 mg/ml) by intraperitoneal injection. Control and experimental mice were cultured for baseline growth using Calgis type 4 swabs into 1 ml of saline for determining CFU. Next MB (87% MB, Sigma-Aldrich, St. Louis, MO) was added topically at the following concentrations: 250, 275, 300, 350, 400, 450, and 500 μg/ml to experimental mice. After waiting for 10 min the mice underwent PDT using 664 nm of diode laser light (Miravant Systems, Inc., Santa Barbara, CA) with a 1 cm cylindrical diffuser (PDT Systems, Santa Barbara, CA) at 275 J/cm fiber length at 400 mW. Upon completion of PDT, mice were cultured again for CFU. Mice were killed in a CO_2 chamber. After killing, the tongues were surgically removed and placed into vials containing 10% formalin for histopathologic studies. CFU specimens were diluted, plated on standard plate count agar (Remel Microbiology Products, Lenexa, Kansas), and grown at 37°C for 24 h, and counted.

Histopathologic evaluation was performed using standard hematoxylin and eosin staining methods. Histologic silver staining was performed to determine the presence of candidal elements on the surface of the tissue as well as any candidal tissue invasion.

3.2. Results

This study demonstrated that all groups, regardless of the MB concentration (250–500 μg/ml), exhibited a decrease in the *C.albicans* population after having received light activation (M+L+) (**Table 13.3**). This decrease in the CFU between the M–L– and M+L+ stages correlated well with an increase in the concentration of MB. This pattern was adhered to with only a few exceptions but even then the overall progression was an increase in *C. albicans* eradication with an increase in MB concentration. The most effective and highly statistically significant total eradication of *C. albicans* occurred with MB concentrations of 450

Table 13.3
Log_{10} reductions in CFU between different treatment stages and MB concentrations

MB conc. μg/ml	Treatment stage M–L–[a]	M+L–[b]	M+L+[c]
250	2.50853	2.372912	1.625312
275	2.305351	2.232149	1.761003
300	2.122762	2.40002	1.457377
350	1.963788	2.170262	0.970037
400	2.158362	1.80618	1.146128
450	2.546543	2.614897	0
500	2.748188	2.365488	0

[a]No MB, no light.
[b]MB, no light.
[c]MB and light.

and 500 μg/ml. Both 450 and 500 μg/ml were able to *totally* eradicate *C. albicans* from the oral cavity with light activation. A reduction from 2.54 log_{10} to 0 was obtained using 450 μg/ml. A volume of 500 μg/ml reduced fungal CFU from 2.74 log_{10} to 0. All of the concentrations of MB with light activation resulted in a dose- or concentration-dependent curve (**Fig. 13.1**).

Teichert and Biel performed further studies combining other agents with MB to enhance the phototoxic effect of PDT and

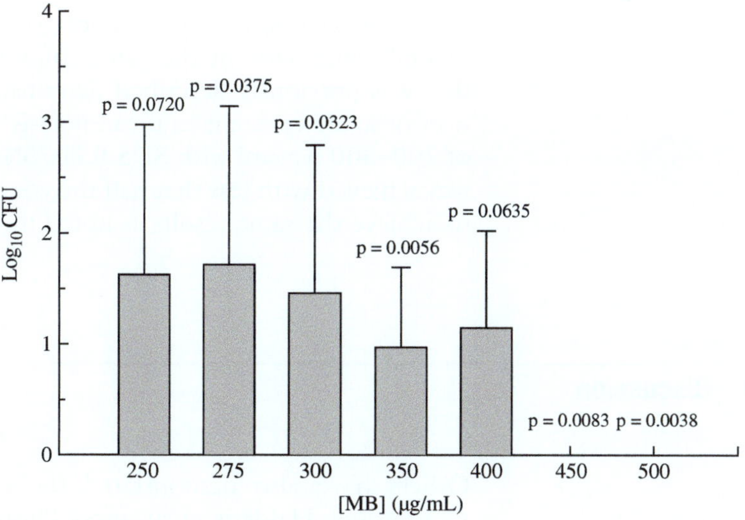

Fig. 13.1. *Candida* CFU after PDT light treatment.

demonstrated that the combination of MB and SDS enhances the phototoxic effect of PDT on azole-resistant *C. albicans* in vitro and in preliminary in vivo experiments (84). In vitro PDT treatment of a solution of azole-resistant *C. albicans* (9×10^8/ml) using different concentrations of methylene blue with or without different concentrations of SDS demonstrated that the addition of SDS resulted in a much improved eradication of *Candida* in solution at lower concentrations of MB. The optimal dose of MB/SDS in vitro was MB 100 μg/ml with 0.0075% SDS (**Table 13.4**).

Table 13.4
In vitro MB/SDS Candidiasis PDT

Tube	1	2	3	4	5
Description	Ca+MB	Ca+MB+SDS	Ca+MB+SDS	Ca+MB+SDS	Ca+MB+SDS
MB (conc.) (μg/ml)	100	100	100	100	100
SDS (%)	0	0.003	0.005	0.0075	0.01
Light dose (J/cm^2)	60	60	60	60	60
Dose rate (mW)	150	150	150	150	150
Time (s)	400	400	400	400	400
Results					
L−	4	4	4	4	4
L+	4	3	3	0	1
2L+	2	0	1	0	0

4 = 301+ colonies L− is no light administered, 3 = 101–300 colonies L+ is 664 nm light administered, 2 = 6–100 colonies 2L+ is 664 nm light administered × 2, 1 = 1–5 colonies
0 = 0 colonies

An in vivo study of the effect of MB/SDS PDT treatment of oral candidiasis in the same immunodeficient mouse model that was previously described demonstrated a complete eradication of azole-resistant oral candidiasis using MB concentrations of 200–300 μg/ml with SDS 0.0075% (**Table 13.5**). This result was achieved with less that half the concentration of MB required to achieve the same results as noted in the previous study results.

4. Discussion

Others have also demonstated the efficacy of PDT to treat *C. albicans*. Haidaris et al. used Photofrin-based PDT to treat

Table 13.5
In vivo *Candida* CFU with MB/SDS PDT treatment

Mouse	MB (μg/ml)	SDS (%)	CFU		
			M–L–a	M+L–b	M+L+c
1	450	0	1.2×10^3	1.2×10^3	4×10^3
2	450	0	4×10^2	2×10^1	4×10^1
3	100	0.0075	2×10^1	n/a	0
4	100	0.0075	0	1×10^2	4×10^1
5	100	0.0075	2×10^2	8×10^1	4×10^1
6	200	0.0075	0	2×10^1	0
7	200	0.0075	2.4×10^2	8×10^2	4×10^1
8	200	0.0075	0	2×10^2	0
9	200	0.0075	2×10^1	6×10^1	4×10^2
10	200	0.0075	2×10^2	4×10^2	6×10^1
11	200	0.0075	2×10^2	6×10^1	0
12	300	0.0075	4×10^1	2×10^2	0
13	300	0.0075	8.6×10^2	1.6×10^2	8×10^1
14	300	0.0075	8×10^2	1.6×10^2	0
15	300	0.0075	4×10^1	1×10^2	0
16	300	0.0075	2×10^2	6×10^1	0
17	300	0.0075	4×10^1	0	0
18	400	0.0075	3.8×10^2	3.4×10^3	1.2×10^2
19	400	0.0075	2×10^1	8×10^1	6×10^1
20	400	0.0075	2×10^1	2×10^1	0

[a]No methylene blue or light activation.
[b]Methylene blue only.
[c]Methylene blue and light activation.
n/a = not available.

and eradicate *C. albicans* (85). They demonstrated that the mechanisms microorganisms use to subvert either antimicrobial oxidative defenses or antimicrobial therapy are not operative during PDT treatment of *C. albicans.*

In conclusion, PDT treatment of oral candidiasis is a potential viable treatment alternative to traditional antifungal drug therapy. Since PDT utilizes a different fungal cell death mechanism than traditional antifungals, it can be effectively used against antifungal agent-resistant *Candida* and may be used as a first line of therapy for mucocutaneous oropharyngeal candidiasis to prevent further development of resistance. Additionally this method of topical treatment of mucocutaneous oropharyngeal candidiasis would be a non-toxic, simple, inexpensive, and repeatable therapy without the risk of fungal resistance that exists with present conventional pharmaceutical therapies. Further studies and clinical trials are required to further demonstrate the efficacy of this therapy.

5. Conclusion

Although the use of PDT to treat infections and biofilms is in its infancy, it has great potential as a means to treat many different sites in the body where biofilms are the cause of significant morbidity with resistance to standard antibiotic therapies. Multiantibiotic-resistant bacteria is a rapidly growing and alarming problem and alternative methods of treatment of localized infections are urgently needed. In addition, in many localized infections, oral or systemically administered antibiotics are not particularly effective either because the bacteria are infecting tissue that is not well perfused or because the bacteria are present in a biofilm and are resistant to standard doses of antibiotics. In addition, the increase in the number of immunosuppressed organ transplant, cancer, and AIDS patients has led to increasing rates of intractable infections.

PDT in the future could be used to treat otherwise hard to treat localized infections. The photosensitizer is capable of local, topical, or intracavitary administration into the infected area and after a period of time, the appropriate light dose could be administered to the infected area using direct illumination or via specialized fiberoptic probes. This repeatable method of treatment has the ability to eradicate biofilms and antibiotic-resistant microorganisms and may someday replace antibiotics as the first-line treatment of localized infections.

Acknowledgments

These research studies were funded by National Institutes of Health Grants R44DE014511, R44NR009189, R43AI047461 and R44AI041866.

References

1. Allison, D. G., Gilbert, P., Lappin-Scott, H. M., and Wilson, M. (eds.) (2001) Community Structure and Cooperation in Biofilms. Cambridge: Cambridge University Press. ISBN 0-521-79302-5.
2. Stewart, P. S. and Costerton, J. W. (2001) Antibiotic resistance of bacteria in biofilms. *The Lancet*, **358**, 135–138.
3. Lewis, K. (2001) Riddle of biofilm resistance. *Antimicrob Agents Chenother*, **45**, 999–1007.
4. Parsek, M. R. and Singh, P. K. (2003) Bacterial biofilms: an emerging link to disease pathogenesis. *Annu Rev Microbiol*, **57**, 677–701.
5. Sanclement, J. P., Webster, P., Thomas, J., and Ramadan, H. H. (2005) Bacterial biofilms in surgical specimens of patients with chronic rhinosinusitis. *Laryngoscope*, **115**, 578–582.
6. Ramadan, H. H., Sanclement, J. A., and Thomas, J. G. (2005) Chronic rhinosinusitis and biofilms. *Otolaryngol Head Neck Surg*, **132**, 414–417.
7. Bendouah, Z., Barbeau, J., Hamad, W. A., and Desrosiers, M. (2006) Biofilm formation by *Staphylococcus aureus* and *Pseudomonas aerugenosa* is associated with unfavorable evolution after surgery for chronic sinusitis and nasal polyposis. *Otolaryngol Head Neck Surg*, **134**, 991–996.
8. Sanderson, A. R., Leid, J. G., and Hunsaker, D. (2006) Bacterial biofilms on the sinus mucosa of human subjects with chronic rhinosinusitis. *Laryngoscope*, **116**, 1121–1126.
9. Malik, Z., Hanania, J., and Nitzan, Y. (1990) Bactericidal effects of photoactivated porphyrins – an alternative approach to antimicrobial drugs. *J Photochem Photobiol B*, **5**, 281– 293.
10. Hamblin, M. R., Zahra, T., Contag, C. H., McManus, A. T., and Hasan, T. (2003) Optical monitoring and treatment of potentially lethal wound infections in vivo. *J Infect Dis*, **187**, 1717–1725.
11. Soukos, N. S., Ximenez-Fyvie, L. A., Hamblin, M. R., Socransky, S. S., and Hasan, T. (1998) Targeted antimicrobial photochemotherapy. *Antimicrob Agents Chemother*, **42**, 2595–2601.
12. Embleton, M. L., Nair, S. P., Cookson, B. D., and Wilson, M. (2002) Selective lethal photosensitization of methicillin-resistant *Staphylococcus aureus* using an IgG-tin (IV) chlorin e6 conjugate. *J Antimicrob Chemother*, **50**, 857–864.
13. Wainwright, M., Phoenix, D. A., Laycock, S. L., Wareing, D. R., and Wright, P. A. (1998) Photobacteriocidal activity of phenothiazinium dyes against methicillin-resistant strains of *Staphylococcus aureus*. *FEMS Microbiol Lett*, **160**, 177–181.
14. Smijs, T. G. and Schuitmaker, H. J. (2003) Photodynamic inactivation of the dermatophyte *Trichophyton rubrum*. *Photochem Photobiol*, 77, 556–560.
15. Friedberg, J. S., Skema, C., Baum, E. D., Burdick, J., Vinogradov, S. A., Wilson, D. F., Horan, A. D., and Nachamkin, I. (2001) In vitro effects of photodynamic therapy on *Aspergillus fumigatus*. *J Antimicrob Chemother*, **48**, 105–107.
16. Zeina, B., Greenman, J., Purcell, W. M., and Das, B. (2001) Killing of cutaneous microbial species by photodynamic therapy. *Br J Dermatol*, **144**, 274–278.
17. Wainwright, M. (2003) Local treatment of viral disease using photodynamic therapy. *Int J Antimicrob Agents*, **21**, 510–520.
18. Sharma, M., Bansal, H., and Gupta, P. K. (2002) Photodynamic inactivation of antibiotic resistant strain of *Pseudomonas aeruginosa* by porphyrins induced by delta-aminolaevulinic acid. *Indian J Med Res*, **116**, 99–105.
19. Teichert, M. C., Jones, J. W., Usacheva, M. N., and Biel, M. A. (2002) Treatment of oral candidiasis with methylene blue-mediated photodynamic therapy in an immunodeficient murine model. *Oral Surg Oral Med Oral Pathol Oral Radiol Endod*, **93**, 155–160.
20. Usacheva, M. N., Teichert, M. C., and Biel, M. A. (2001) Comparison of the methylene blue and toluidine blue photobactericidal efficacy against gram-positive and gram-negative microorganisms. *Lasers Surg Med*, **29**, 165–173.
21. Swanson, L. (1999) Solving stubborn wound problems could save millions. *JAMC*, **160**, 536.
22. Singer, A. J., and Clark, R. A. F. (1999) Cutaneous wound healing. *New Eng J Med*, **341**, 738–745.
23. Dow, G., Browne. A., and Sibbald, R. G. (1999) Infection in chronic wounds: controversies in diagnosis and treatment. *Ost/Wound Manang*, **45**, 23–40.
24. Parish, L. C., Witkowski, J. A., and Crissey, J. T. (1993) The Decubitus Ulcer. Chicago: Year Book Medical Publishers.
25. Gilbert, P., Allison, D. G., McBain, A. J. (2002) Biofilms in vitro and in vivo: do

singular mechanisms imply cross-resistance? *J Appl Microbiol*, **92**, 98S–110S.

26. Drenkard, E., Ausubel, F. M. (2002) Pseudomonas biofilm formation and antibiotic resistance are linked to phenotypic variation. *Nature*, **416**, 740–743.
27. Gotz, F. (2002) Staphylococcus and biofilms. *Mol Microbiol*, **43**, 1367–1378.
28. Stewart, P. S. and Costerton, J. W. (2001) Antibiotic resistance of bacteria in biofilms. *Lancet*, **358**, 135–138.
29. McBain, A. J., Allison, D., and Gilbert, P. (2000) Emerging strategies for the chemical treatment of microbial biofilms. *Biotechnol Genet Eng Rev*, **17**, 267–279.
30. Drosou, A., Falabella, A., and Kirsner, C. (2003) Antiseptics on wounds: an area of controversy. *Wounds*, **15**, 149–166.
31. US Food and Drug Administration. Antibiotic Resistance-Fact Sheet. (2003) www.fda.gov/oc/opacom/hottopics/anti_resist.html
32. National Institute of Allergy and Infectious Disease. Antimicrobial Resistance. (2003) www.niaid.nih.gov/factsheets/antimicro.htm.
33. Bowler, P. G. and Davies, B. J. (1999) The microbiology of acute and chronic wounds. *Wounds*, **11**, 72–78.
34. Biel, M. A. and Teichert, M. (2008) Phototherapy of antibiotic resistant wound infections. Unpublished results, NIH Grant R43AI47461.
35. Biel, M. A., Teichert, M., Usacheva, M., and Sievert, C. (2008) PDT treatment of periodontal biofilms. Unpublished results. Supported NIH Grant R44AI041866.
36. Metclaf, D., Robinson, C., Devine, D., and Wood, S. (2006) Enhancement of erythrosine-mediated phtodynamic therapy of Streptococcus mutant biofilms by light fractionation. *J Antimicrob Chemother*, **58**, 190–192.
37. Zanin, I. C., Lobo, M. M., and Rodrigues, L. K. (2006) Photosensitization of in vitro biofilms by toluidine blue O combined with light emitting diode. *Europ J Oral Sci*, **114**, 64–69.
38. Zeina, B., Greenman, J., Corry, D., and Purcell, C. (2003) Antimicrobial photodynamic therapy: assessment of genotoxic effects on keratinocytes in vitro. *Br J Dermatol*, **148**, 229–232.
39. Lee, C. F., Lee, C. J., Chen, C. T., and Huang, C. T. (2004) Delta-aminolaevulinic acid mediated photodynamic chemotherapy on *Pseudomonas aerugenosa* planktonic and biofilm cultures. *J Photochem Photobiol B-Biol*, **75**, 21–25.
40. Hamblin, M. R., O'Donnell, D. A., Murthy, N., Contag, C. H., and Hasan, T. (2002) Rapid control of wound infections by targeted photodynamic therapy monitored by in vivo bioluminescence imaging. *Photochem Photobiol*, **75**, 51–57.
41. Gad, F., Zahra, T., Hasan, T., and Hamblin, M. R. (2004) Effects of growth phase and extracellular slime on photodynamic inactivation of gram-positive pathogenic bacteria. *Antimicrob Agent Chemother*, **48**, 2173–2178.
42. Lin, H. Y., Chen, C. T., and Huang, C. T. (2004) Use of merocyamine 540 for photodynamic inactivation of *Staphylococcus aureus* planktonic and biofilm cells. *Appl Enviroment Microbio*, **70**, 6453–6458.
43. Biel, M. A., Teichert, M., and Usacheva, M. (2008) Photodynamic therapy of Staphylococcus infections. Unpublished results, NIH Grant R43AI04866.
44. Biel, M. A., Teichert, M., and Usacheva, M. (2008) PDT of wound infections. Unpublished results, NIH Grant R44NR009189.
45. Robson, M. and Heggers, J (1969) Bacterial quantification of open wounds. *Mulit Med*, **134**, 19–24.
46. Robson, M. C. (1997) Wound infection: a failure of wound healing caused by an imbalance of bacteria. *Surg Clin N Am*, **77**, 637–650.
47. Robson, M. C., Krizek, T. K., and Heggers, J. P. (1993) Biology of surgical infection. In: Ravich M. M. (ed.) Current Problems in Surgery. Chicago, IL: Yearbook Medical Publishers, 1–62.
48. Bendy, R., Nuccio, P., and Wolfe, E. (1964) Relationship of quantitative wound bacterial counts to healing of decubitii: effect of topical gentamicin. *Antimicrob Agents Chemother*, **4**, 147–155.
49. Krizek, T., Robson, M., and Kho, E. (1967) Bacterial growth and skin graft survival. *Surg Forum*, **18**, 518–519.
50. Webb, B. C., Thomas, C. J., and Willcox, M. D. (1998) Candida-associated denture stomatitis. Aetiology and management: a review. Part 3. Treatment of candidosis. *Aust Dent J*, **43**, 244–249.
51. Ninane, J. A. (1994) Multicentre study of fluconazole versus oral polyenes in the prevention of fungal infection in children with hematological or oncological malignancies. Multicentre study group. *Eur J Clin Microbiol Infect Dis*, **13**, 330–337.
52. Philips, P., Zemcov, J., and Mahmood, W. (1996) Itraconazole cyclodextrin solution for fluconazole-refractory oropharyngeal candidiasis in AIDS: correlation of

clinical response with in vitro susceptibility. *AIDS*, **10**, 1369–1376.

53. Pankhurst, C. (2000) Oropharyngeal candidiasis. *Clin Evid*, **4**, 761–773.
54. Sangeorzan, J. A., Bradley, S. F., Re, X., and Zarins, L. T. (1994) Epidemiology of oral candidiasis in HIV-infected patients. *Am J Med*, **97**, 339–346.
55. Diz Dios, P., Ocampo, A., Miralles, C., Otero, I., Iglesias, I., and Rayo, N. (1999) Frequency of oropharyngeal candidiasis in HIV-infected patients on protease inhibitor therapy. *Oral Surg Oral Med Oral Pathol*, **87**, 437–441.
56. Powderly, W. G., Robinson, K., and Keath, E. J. (1993) Molecular epidemiology of recurrent oral candidiasis in human immunodeficiency virus-positive patients: evidence for two patterns of recurrence. *J Infect Dis*, **168**, 463–466.
57. Whelan, W. L., Kirsch, D. R., Kwon-Chung, K. J., and Wahl, S. M. (1990) *Candida albicans* in patients with acquired immunodeficiency syndrome: absence of a novel or hypervirulent strain. *J Infect Dis*, **162**, 513–518.
58. Klein, R. S., Harris, C. A., Butkus-Small, C., and Moll, B. (1984) Oral candidiasis in high-risk patients as the initial manifestation of the acquired immunodeficiency syndrome. *N Engl J Med*, **311**, 354–358.
59. Imam, N., Carpentar, C. C., Mayer, K. H., and Fisher, A. (1990) Hierarchical pattern of mucosal *Candida* infections in HIV-seropositive women. *Am J Med*, **89**, 142–146.
60. Stevens, D. A., Greene, S. I., and Lang, O. S. (1991) Thrush can be prevented in patients with acquired immunodeficiency syndrome and the acquired immunodeficiency syndrome-related complex: randomized, double blind, placebo-controlled study of 100-mg oral fluconazole daily. *Arch Intern Med*, **151**, 2458–2464.
61. Pons, V. G., Greespan, D., Koletar, S., and the Multicenter Study Group. (1993) Comparative study of fluconazole and clotrimazole troches for the treatment of oral thrush in AIDS. *J AIDS*, **6**, 1311–1316.
62. Lim, S. G., Lee, C. A., and Hales, M. (1991) Fluconazole for oropharyngeal candidiasis in anti-HIV positive hemophiliacs. *Aliment Pharmacol Ther*, **5**, 199–205.
63. De Wit, S., Goosens, H., and Weerts, D. (1989) Comparison of fluconazole and ketoconazole for oropharyngeal candidiasis in AIDS. *Lancet*, **101**, 746–747.
64. Koletar, S., Russell, J. A., and Fass, R. J. (1990) Comparison of oral fluconazole and clotrimazole troches as treatment for oral candidiasis in patients infected with human immunodeficiency virus. *Antimicrob Agents Chemother*, **34**, 2267–2268.
65. De Repentigny, L. and Ratelle, J. (1996) Comparison of itraconazole and ketoconazole in HIV-positive patients with oropharyngeal or esophageal candidiasis. *Chemotherapy*, **42**, 374–383.
66. Munoz, P., Moreno, S., and Berenguer, J. (1991) Fluconazole-related hepatotoxicity in patients with acquired immunodeficiency syndrome. *Arch Intern Med*, **151**, 1020–1021.
67. Heinic, G. S., Stevens, D. A., and Greenspan, D. (1993) Fluconazole-resistant *Candida* in AIDS patients. *Oral Surg Oral Med Oral Pathol*, **76**, 711–715.
68. Quereda, C., Polanco, A. M., and Giner, C. (1996) Correlation between in vitro resistance to fluconazole and clinical outcome of oropharyngeal candidiasis in HIV-infected patients. *Eur J Clin Microbiol Infect Dis*, **15**, 30–37.
69. Maenza, J. R., Merz, W. G., and Romagnoli, M. J. (1993) Infection due to fluconazole-resistant *Candida* in AIDS patients: prevalence and microbiology. *Clin Infect Dis*, **24**, 28–34.
70. Hitchcock, C. A. (1993) Resistance of *Candida albicans* to antifungal agents. *Biochem Soc Trans*, **132**, 1039–1047.
71. Baily, G. G., Perry, F. M., and Denning, D. W. (1994) Fluconazole-resistant candidosis in an HIV cohort. *AIDS*, **8**, 787–792.
72. Newman, S. L., Flanigan, T. P., and Fisher, A. (1994) Clinically significant mucosal candidiasis resistant to fluconazole treatment in patients with AIDS. *Clin Infect Dis*, **19**, 684–686.
73. White, A. and Goetz, M. B. (1994) Azole-resistant *Candida albicans*: reports of two cases of resistance to fluconazole and review. *Clin Infect Dis*, **19**, 687–692.
74. Sanguineti, A., Carmichael, J. K., and Campbell, K. (1993) Fluconazole-resistant *Candida albicans* after long-term suppressive therapy. *Arch Intern Med*, **153**, 1122–1124.
75. Maenza, J. R. (1996) Risk factors for fluconazole-resistant candidiasis in human immunodeficiency virus-infected patients. *J Infect Dis*, **173**, 219–225.
76. Redding, S., Smith, J., Farinacci, G., and Rinaldi, M. (1994) Resistance of *Candida albicans* to fluconazole during treatment of oropharyngeal candidiasis in a patient with AIDS: documentation by in vitro susceptibility testing and DNA subtype analysis. *Clin Infect Dis*, **18**, 240–242.

77. Revankar, S. G., Kirkpatrick, W. R., and McAtee, R. K. (1998) A randomized trial of continuous or intermittent therapy with fluconazole for oropharyngeal candidiasis in HIV-infected patients: clinical outcomes and development of fluconazole resistance. *Am J Med*, **105**, 7–11.
78. Pelletier, R., Peter, J., and Antin, C. (2000) Emergence of resistance of *Candida albicans* to Clotrimazole in human immunodeficiency virus-infected children: in vitro and clinical correlations. *J Clin Microbiol*, **38**, 1563–1568.
79. Müller, F. M. C., Kasal, M., and Francesconi, A. (1999) Transmission of an azole-resistant isogenic strain of *Candida albicans* among human immunodeficiency virus-infected family members with oropharyngeal candidiasis. *J Clin Microbiol*, **37**, 3405–3408.
80. Rex, J. H., Pfaller, M. A., Rinaldi, M. G., and Polack, A. (1993) Antifungal susceptibility testing. *Clin Microbiol Rev*, **6**, 357–381.
81. Johnson, E. M., Warnock, D. W., Luker, J., Porter, S. R., and Scully, C. (1995) Emergence of azole drug resistance in *Candida* species from HIV-infected patients receiving prolonged fluconazole therapy for oral candidiasis. *J Antimicrob Chemother*, **35**, 103–114.
82. Ladan, H., Nitzan, Y., and Malik, Z. (1993) The antibacterial activity of haemin compared with cobalt, zinc and magnesium protoporphyrin and its effect on potassium and ultrastructure of *Staphylococcus aureus. FEMS Micrbiol Lett*, **12**, 173–177.
83. Stenstrom, K., Moan, J., Brunborg, G., and Eklund, T. (1980) Photodynamic inactivation of yeast cells sensitized by hematoporphyrin. *Photochem Photobiol*, **32**, 349–352.
84. Teichert, M. and Biel, M. A. (2008) Treatment of AIDS-related oral candidiasis. Unpublished results, NIH Grant R44DE14511.
85. Chabrier-Rosello, Y., Foster, T. H., Perez-Nazario, N., Mitra, S., and Haidaris, C. G. (2005) Sensitivity of *Candida albicans* germ tubes and biofilms to photofrin-mediated phototoxicity. Antimicrob Agent Chemotherap **49**, 4288–4295.

Chapter 14

Calculation of Cellular Oxygen Concentration for Photodynamic Therapy In Vitro

Michael S. Patterson and Emma Mazurek

Abstract

In vitro photodynamic therapy experiments are usually performed by irradiating cells in confluent or nearly confluent monolayer cultures. Oxygen is consumed in the monolayer by photodynamic reactions and cellular respiration and is supplied by diffusion from the overlying medium. Calculations of oxygen concentration by numerical solution of the time-dependent diffusion equation show that hypoxia can be induced in the monolayer under typical PDT conditions and that this will limit the total treatment effect. There is an optimum fluence rate at which the greatest singlet oxygen dose can be delivered before hypoxia becomes limiting. It is recommended that researchers use these calculations to avoid hypoxia or confirm that fortuitous oxygen transport by other mechanisms (e.g., convection) is adequate to prevent it.

Key words: Photodynamic therapy, oxygen, diffusion, hypoxia, monolayer.

1. Introduction

Much of our basic understanding of photodynamic therapy (PDT) and its development for clinical application have resulted from studies performed in vitro. Although multicell spheroids and cells in suspension have been used, the most common technique is to culture cells in a monolayer, incubate that monolayer with medium containing the photosensitizer, replace with fresh medium, and then irradiate the cells with light of the appropriate wavelength. One disadvantage of this method, as we will show in this chapter is the potential for hypoxia to be induced in the monolayer by the combination of metabolic and photodynamic oxygen consumption. Failure to account for this possibility

C.J. Gomer (ed.), *Photodynamic Therapy*, Methods in Molecular Biology 635,
DOI 10.1007/978-1-60761-697-9_14, © Springer Science+Business Media, LLC 2010

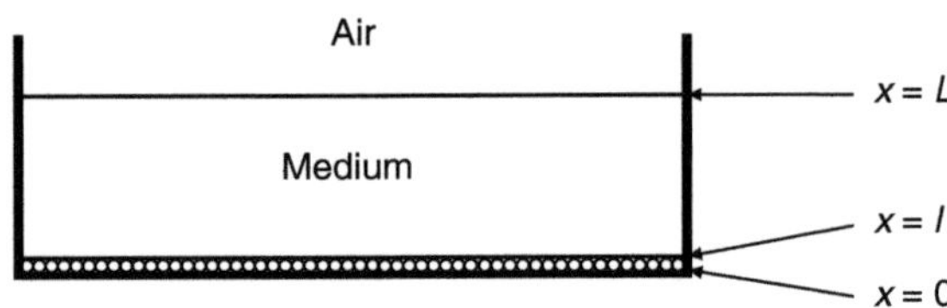

Fig. 14.1. Schematic diagram of cell monolayer geometry for the calculation of $C(x, t)$.

could lead to the misinterpretation of assays performed on the cells after PDT.

The geometry of the problem is illustrated in **Fig. 14.1**. The cells are plated on the bottom of the flask or well at $x = 0$. The cell monolayer thickness is l and we assume the cells form a confluent homogeneous layer. The top surface of the medium covering the cells at $x = L$ is exposed to air. We assume that the concentration of oxygen in the cells and medium is a function of time t and x and that diffusion is the only process that transports oxygen (*see* **Note 4**). Within the monolayer, the following partial differential equation describes $C(x, t)$, the concentration of oxygen,

$$\frac{\partial C(x,t)}{\partial t} = D_c \frac{\partial^2 C(x,t)}{\partial x^2} - \Gamma(x,t), \tag{1}$$

where D_c is the diffusion coefficient for oxygen within the cell and $\Gamma(x, t)$ is the local rate at which oxygen is consumed. Both normal cell metabolism and photodynamic therapy consume oxygen, so

$$\Gamma(x,t) = \Gamma_{\mathrm{met}}(x,t) + \Gamma_{\mathrm{PDT}}(x,t). \tag{2}$$

As described by Georgakoudi et al. (1), the dependence of these consumption rates on the local oxygen concentration can be expressed as

$$\Gamma(x,t) = \frac{\Gamma^0_{\mathrm{met}} C(x,t)}{k_{\mathrm{met}} + C(x,t)} + \frac{\Gamma^0_{\mathrm{PDT}} C(x,t)}{k_{\mathrm{PDT}} + C(x,t)}, \tag{3}$$

where Γ^0_{met} is the rate of metabolic consumption under well oxygenated conditions and Γ^0_{PDT} is the corresponding photodynamic consumption rate. Assuming that the PDT oxygen consumption rate is equal to the singlet oxygen production rate, we can write

$$\Gamma^0_{\mathrm{PDT}} = \frac{E_0 \lambda [S_0] \sigma \phi_\Delta}{hc}, \tag{4}$$

where E_0 is the treatment fluence rate, λ is the wavelength, $[S_0]$ is the intracellular photosensitizer concentration, σ is the molecular ground state absorption cross-section at wavelength λ, ϕ_Δ is the singlet oxygen quantum yield, h is Planck's constant, and c is the speed of light. At oxygen concentration k_{met} the metabolic consumption rate falls to half of Γ^0_{met}, and k_{PDT} is the corresponding oxygen concentration for PDT. Note that when Γ_{PDT} decreases, the production of singlet oxygen falls as well. Thus Equation [3] also represents the dependence of PDT efficacy (per unit light fluence) on oxygen concentration. In the medium outside the cell monolayer, an equation similar to Equation [1] applies, except that the consumption term is zero and the diffusion coefficient for water, D_w, is used.

In order to solve for $C(x, t)$ the boundary conditions for the problem must also be specified. We assume that fresh medium is added at time zero so that $C(x, t = 0) = 240\ \mu M$, the concentration of oxygen in air saturated water at room temperature. The concentration at the surface is maintained at this value so $C(x = L, t) = 240\ \mu M$. We also require the oxygen concentration and flux to be continuous at $x = l$, the interface between the cells and the medium, so that

$$C(x = l^-,t) = C(x = l^+,t) \tag{5}$$

and

$$D_c \frac{\partial C(x = l^-,t)}{\partial x} = D_w \frac{\partial C(x = l^+,t)}{\partial x}. \tag{6}$$

Finally, as there is no flux of oxygen into the plate, we can specify that

$$D_c \frac{\partial C(x = 0,t)}{\partial x} = 0. \tag{7}$$

2. Methods

A simple analytical solution can be found to Equation [1] when the oxygen consumption rate in the cell monolayer is constant and when equilibrium has been established (i.e., the transport of oxygen across the air-medium boundary compensates for consumption in the monolayer). In general, this equilibrium is not established over the PDT treatment time and the consumption rate is not constant (*see* Equation [3]). Hence we must

Table 14.1
Values for parameters in the diffusion calculations. More detail regarding these choices is provided in Notes 1, 3, and 5

Parameter	Numerical value	Source (*see* Notes 1, 3, and 5)
Γ^0_{met}	15.1 μM s^{-1}	Weston and Patterson (5)
k_{met}	0.5 μM	Georgakoudi et al. (1)
Γ^0_{PDT}	0–100 μM s^{-1}	Typical conditions
k_{PDT}	8.7 μM	Mitra and Foster (12)
D_w	1.9×10^{-5} cm^2 s^{-1}	O'Loughlin et al. (6)
D_c	3.8×10^{-6} cm^2 s^{-1}	O'Loughlin et al. (6)
l	15 μm	MLL cell diameter
L	3 mm	L > 3 mm gives same results
$C(x = L, t)$	240 μM	Nichols and Foster (14)

rely on numerical solutions of the diffusion equation. We used a standard finite difference method (2) in which the time and space variables are discretized. This leads to a system of coupled equations that can be solved at each time step using the distribution found for the previous step. The parameter values used in the solution are summarized in **Table 14.1** and discussed in **Notes 1, 3,** and **5**. In **Table 14.2** we show typical values of the parameters in Equation [4] for the sensitizers Photofrin and meso-tetra(hydoxyphenyl)chlorin (mTHPC), a so-called "second generation" drug with a higher absorption cross-section. Based on the values in **Table 14.2** and the range of parameters in the literature, the initial PDT oxygen consumption rate was varied from 0 to 100 μM/s.

Table 14.2
Typical initial PDT oxygen consumption rates for cells incubated with Photofrin or mTHPC. The results can be scaled for different incubation concentrations and fluence rates. The absorption cross-sections were obtained from Mitra (15) and the intracellular concentrations from Dysart and Patterson (4) and Dysart et al. (3)

Sensitizer	λ (nm)	σ (cm^2)	Incubation (μg ml^{-1})	$[S_0]$ (μM)	ϕ_Δ	Γ^0_{PDT} (μM s^{-1}) for $E_0 = 10$ mW cm^{-2}
Photofrin	630	7.4×10^{-18}	1.0 for 18 h	39	0.5	4.6
mTHPC	652	2.0×10^{-16}	0.15 for 18 h	16	0.5	53

3. Results

The typical characteristics of the oxygen distribution can be appreciated from the results in **Fig. 14.2** calculated for $\Gamma^0_{PDT} =$

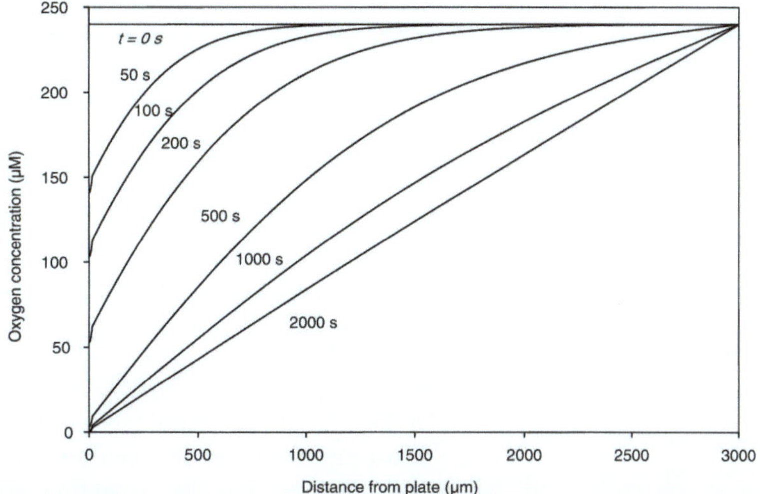

Fig. 14.2. Oxygen concentration versus distance from the plate surface at various times during a PDT treatment. $\Gamma^0_{met} = 15.1$ μM s^{-1}, $\Gamma^0_{PDT} = 20$ μM s^{-1}, $l = 15$ μm, $L = 3$ mm.

20 μM s^{-1}. At time zero the concentration is 240 μM at all depths, but the oxygen consumption rate exceeds the supply of oxygen from the medium so that by 500 s the cells are hypoxic and PDT efficacy (per unit fluence) is significantly reduced. At 2,000 s the distribution is almost in equilibrium as the flux of oxygen (proportional to the gradient) is the same at all depths outside the monolayer. The depth of the medium plays a key role in determining cellular hypoxia and the time required to reach equilibrium. In **Fig. 14.3** we have recalculated the results in **Fig. 14.2** for $L = 0.1, 0.5, 1, 2$ mm and have plotted C at $x = 0$ as functions of time. When only 85 μm of medium covers the cells, equilibrium is established within 20 s and the cellular oxygenation stabilizes at about 210 μM. The curve for $L = 2$ mm is essentially the same as for $L = 3$ mm, so there is a critical thickness at which the time course of oxygenation at $x = 0$ is insensitive to further increases. This thickness depends on the oxygen consumption rate in the cell monolayer. For $\Gamma^0_{met} = 15.1$ μM s^{-1} and $\Gamma^0_{PDT} = 0$ (the lowest total consumption rate) the results are insensitive to increases in L beyond 3 mm, so that value has been used in all calculations except **Fig. 14.3**.

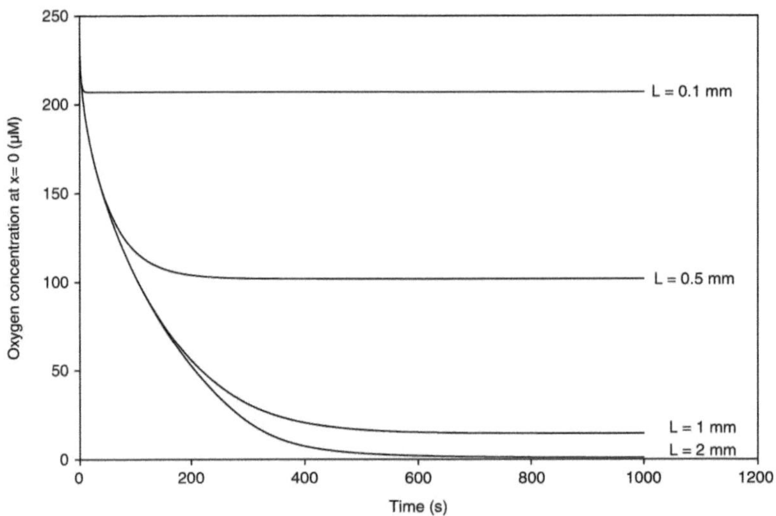

Fig. 14.3. Oxygen concentration at plate surface versus time for various amounts of overlying medium. $\Gamma^0_{met} = 15.1$ $\mu M\ s^{-1}$, $\Gamma^0_{PDT} = 20\ \mu M\ s^{-1}$, $l = 15\ \mu m$.

In **Fig. 14.4** we examine the effect of different PDT oxygen consumption rates on the time course of C at $x = 0$. From **Fig. 14.2** we see that the oxygen concentration is not a strong function of x within the cell, so the value at $x = 0$ gives a reasonable indication of cellular oxygenation. As might be expected, the higher the PDT oxygen consumption rate, the faster the cell layer becomes hypoxic. Even if the only oxygen consumption is metabolic, $C\ (0)$ falls below 10 μM after 1600 s. At first glance

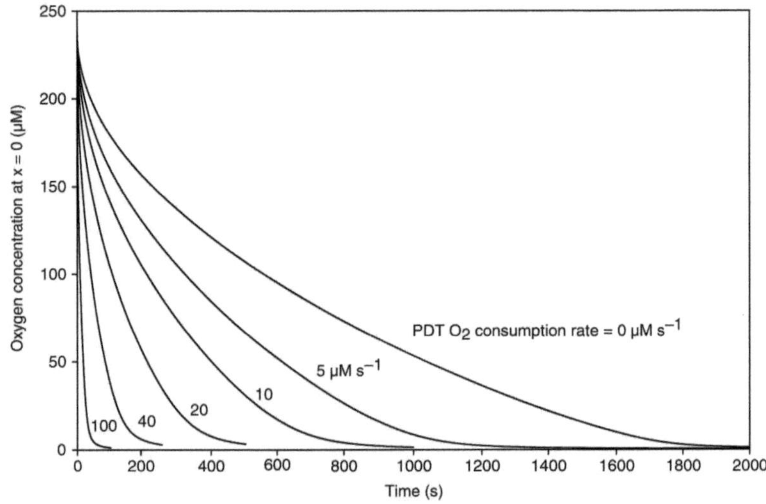

Fig. 14.4. Oxygen concentration at plate surface versus time for various initial photodynamic therapy oxygen consumption rates. $\Gamma^0_{met} = 15.1\ \mu M\ s^{-1}$, $l = 15\ \mu m$, $L =$ 3 mm.

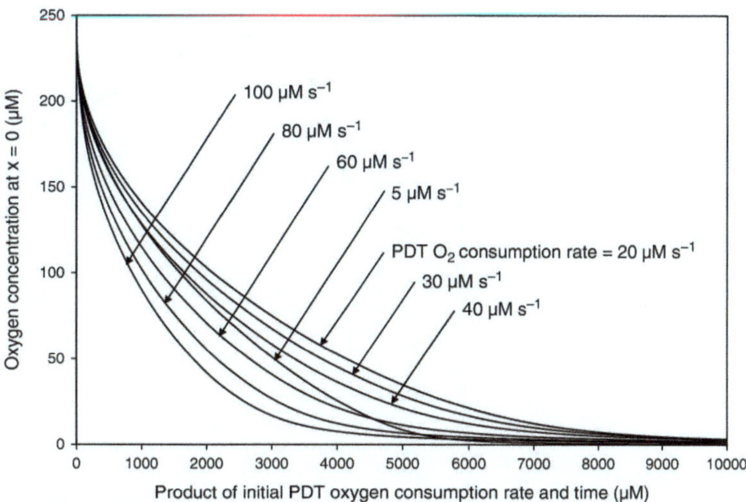

Fig. 14.5. Oxygen concentration at plate surface plotted against the product of initial PDT oxygen consumption rate and treatment time. $\Gamma^0_{\mathrm{PDT}} = 20\ \mu\mathrm{M\ s}^{-1}$ allows the largest production of singlet oxygen before hypoxia is induced. $\Gamma^0_{\mathrm{met}} = 15.1\ \mu\mathrm{M\ s}^{-1}$, $l = 15\ \mu\mathrm{m}$, $L = 3$ mm.

Fig. 14.4 might suggest that PDT be performed at a very low fluence rate to avoid hypoxia, but at a low fluence rate it takes longer to deliver a given PDT "dose." A more useful way to look at the data is shown in **Fig. 14.5** where we have plotted $C(0)$ versus the product of Γ^0_{PDT} and time. This product is proportional to fluence and is indicative of the PDT effect – at least until hypoxia comes into play. From **Fig. 14.5** it is evident that there is an optimum PDT oxygen consumption rate (or fluence rate) where the maximum PDT effect can be achieved before hypoxia becomes limiting. For the parameters used in these calculations the optimum is about 20 μM s^{-1}. At higher consumption rates hypoxia develops at lower fluence and at lower consumption rates metabolic consumption is the major cause of hypoxia. To emphasize this point, we select $C = k_{\mathrm{PDT}}$ as a marker of hypoxia. For each value of Γ^0_{PDT} we then calculate (from **Fig. 14.5**) the value of $\Gamma^0_{\mathrm{PDT}}\,t$ at which $C(0) = k_{\mathrm{PDT}}$. This is a measure of the PDT "dose" that can be delivered before hypoxia severely limits treatment efficacy. Note that the units of this product are μM; this is a measure of the total amount of singlet oxygen produced per unit volume in the cell (*see* **Note 6**). This is plotted against Γ^0_{PDT} in **Fig. 14.6** to illustrate that the maximum dose can be delivered at $\Gamma^0_{\mathrm{PDT}} = 20\ \mu\mathrm{M\ s}^{-1}$. This would correspond to fluence rates of 43 and 3.8 mW cm^{-2} for cells incubated in Photofrin and mTHPC, respectively, using the concentrations in **Table 14.2**. Interestingly, the maximum "dose" in **Fig. 14.6** is about 7.7 mM of singlet oxygen. This is comparable to the dose required to

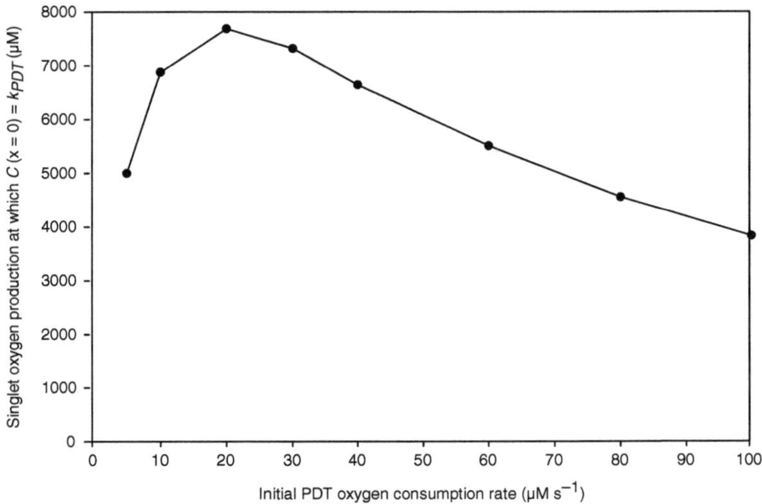

Fig. 14.6. Total intracellular singlet oxygen production achieved before hypoxia (defined as $C = k_{PDT}$) is induced plotted versus initial PDT oxygen consumption rate. There is an optimum rate (and corresponding excitation light fluence rate) at which the largest PDT dose can be delivered. $\Gamma^0_{met} = 15.1\ \mu M\ s^{-1}$, $l = 15\ \mu m$, $L = 3$ mm.

perform clonogenic cell survival assays with these sensitizers (3, 4).

It is useful to compare these results for PDT of cell monolayers to those obtained for stirred cell suspensions. The formalism is the same as described above except that the diffusion equation is written in spherical co-ordinates with the origin at the center of a spherical cell of radius 7.5 μm. Because the suspension is stirred, we impose the boundary condition that $C\ (r,\ t) = 240$ μM at $r = 100$ μm – a distance comparable to the average intercellular distance in suspensions. **Figure 14.7** shows the oxygen concentration as a function of radial distance 10 s after the initiation of PDT at an oxygen consumption rate of 1,000 μM s^{-1}. Even though this rate is an order of magnitude higher than that used for the monolayer geometry calculations, an equilibrium is established in which the cell remains well oxygenated. Very high fluence rates and/or photosensitizer concentrations are required to produce intracellular hypoxia in stirred cell suspensions at typical (around 10^6 cells per ml) concentrations. As shown in **Fig. 14.7**, the intracellular diffusion coefficient has a significant effect on the oxygen distribution in this case.

In summary, unless there is transport of oxygen by physical mixing of the medium (*see* **Note 4**), hypoxia in cell monolayers undergoing PDT is possible under typical conditions. This may limit the efficacy of the treatment itself or may have other effects on the cells if maintained for sufficient time.

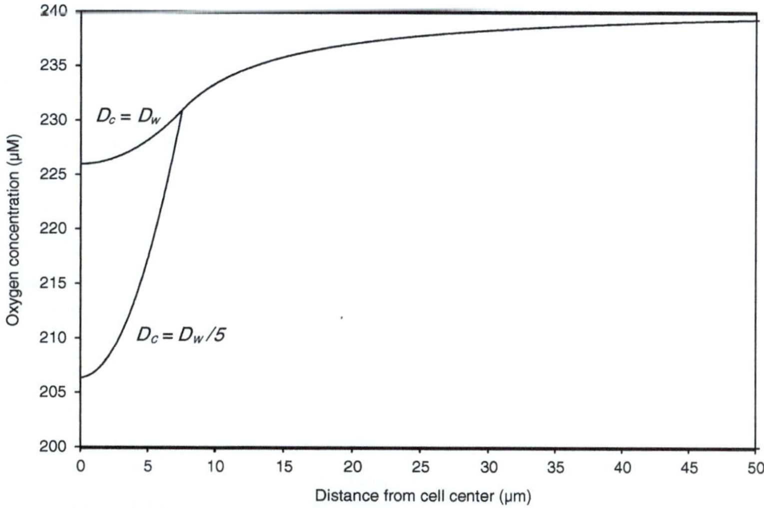

Fig. 14.7. Calculated oxygen concentration versus distance from the center of a spherical cell of radius 7.5 μm 10 s after initiation of PDT. It is assumed that stirring maintains the oxygen concentration at 240 μM at 100 μm from the cell center. Results are shown for two different values of the intracellular oxygen diffusion coefficient, D_c. Γ^0_{met} = 15.1 μM/s, Γ^0_{PDT} = 1,000 μM s^{-1}.

4. Notes

1. We used Γ^0_{met} = 15.1 μM s^{-1}, the value we measured in our lab for Mat-LyLu (MLL) cells (5). The metabolic consumption rates reported in the literature range from about 5 to 30 μM s^{-1} depending on the cell line and estimated cell volume.
2. We assumed that metabolic oxygen consumption was "turned on" at the same time as PDT. Obviously, if cells are left in fresh medium for some time before PDT is performed, there is the potential for significant deoxygenation that would reduce the excitation light fluence required for cellular hypoxia.
3. We used $D_W = 1.9 \times 10^{-5}$ cm^2 s^{-1} for oxygen in water at room temperature (6). Literature data range from about 1.8 to 2.1 × 10^{-5} cm^2 s^{-1}, although the temperature is not clearly stated in some papers. Data for D_c are sparse and somewhat inconsistent, but the majority of reports suggest that D_c is three to five times lower than D_W (6–8). In practice, the results for the monolayer geometry are not very sensitive to the exact value used for the intracellular diffusion coefficient.

4. It is important to note that we have assumed that diffusion is the only mechanism of oxygen transport in the medium. There is experimental evidence to show that this can be the case. Direct measurement with a microelectrode in monolayer culture showed that intracellular oxygen concentration dropped below 10 μM about half an hour after medium replacement due to normal cellular respiration (9). Microelectrode measurements in the medium have also shown the linear concentration versus depth behavior predicted in **Fig. 14.2** (10). However, vertical mixing of the liquid due to thermal gradients for example could fortuitously reoxygenate the cells. Mitra et al. (11) measured oxygen concentrations just above monolayers during PDT and reported no significant hypoxia – presumably due to vertical mixing. It is recommended that researchers either use the calculations in this chapter to avoid hypoxia or confirm by independent measurement that it is not a concern.
5. For simplicity we used a single value for k_{PDT} measured for mTHPC by Mitra and Foster (12). The values reported in the literature for Photofrin are slightly higher (1, 13) but this would not have a significant impact on the results.
6. We stated above that the total amount of singlet oxygen generated per unit volume in the cell is equal to Γ^0_{PDT} t as long as $C > k_{PDT}$ at time t. This is not exactly true, as the yield of singlet oxygen is a monotonically decreasing function of C. One should actually perform a numerical integration over the production rate, but the added complexity would obscure the argument and not affect the conclusions.

Acknowledgments

The authors wish to thank Tom Farrell for his assistance with the finite difference calculations. This work was supported by the Canadian Institute for Photonic Innovations (CIPI).

References

1. Georgakoudi, I., Nichols, M. G., and Foster, T. H. (1997) The mechanism of Photofrin photobleaching and its consequences for photodynamic dosimetry. *Photochem Photobiol*, **65**, 135–144.
2. Mathews, J. H. and Fink, K. D. (1999) Numerical Methods Using MATLAB. Upper Saddle River, NJ: Prentice-Hall.
3. Dysart, J. S., Singh, G., and Patterson, M. S. (2005) Calculation of singlet oxygen dose from photosensitizer fluorescence and photobleaching during mTHPC photodynamic therapy of MLL cells. *Photochem Photobiol*, **81**, 196–205.
4. Dysart, J. S. and Patterson, M. S. (2005) Characterization of Photofrin

photobleaching for singlet oxygen dose estimation during photodynamic therapy of MLL cells in vitro. *Phys Med Biol*, **50**, 2597–2616.

5. Weston, M. A. and Patterson, M. S. (2009) Simple photodynamic therapy dose models fail to predict the survival of MLL cells after HPPH-PDT in vitro. *Photochem Photobiol*, **85**, 750–759.
6. O'Loughlin, M. A., Whillans, D. W., and Hunt, J. W. (1980) A fluorescence approach to testing the diffusion of oxygen into mammalian cells. *Rad Res*, **84**, 477–495.
7. Hatz, S., Poulsen, L., and Ogilby, P. R. (2008) Time-resolved singlet oxygen phosphorescence measurements from photosensitized experiments in single cells: effect of oxygen diffusion and oxygen concentration. *Photochem Photobiol*, **84**, 1284–1290.
8. Kuimova, M. K., Yahioglu, G., Levitt, J. A., and Suhling, K. (2008) Molecular rotor measures viscosity of live cells via fluorescence lifetime imaging. *J Am Chem Soc*, **130**, 6672–6673.
9. Wolff, M., Fandrey, J., and Jelkmann, W. (1993) Microelectrode measurements of pericellular pO_2 in erythropoietin-producing human hepatoma cell cultures. *Am J Physiol Cell Physiol*, **265**, C1266–C1270.
10. Mamchaoui, K. and Saumon, G. (2000) A method for measuring the oxygen consumption in intact cell monolayers. *Am J Physiol Lung Cell Mol Physiol*, **278**, L858–L863.
11. Mitra, S., Cassar, S. E., Niles, D. J., Puskas, J. A., Frelinger, J. G., and Foster, T. H. (2006) Photodynamic therapy mediates the oxygen-independent activation of hypoxia-inducible factor 1α. *Mol Cancer Ther*, **5**, 3268–3274.
12. Mitra, S. and Foster, T. H. (2005) Photophysical parameters, photosensitizer retention and tissue optical properties completely account for the higher photodynamic efficacy of meso-tetra-hydroxyphenyl-chlorin vs Photofrin. *Photochem Photobiol*, **81**, 849–859.
13. Moan, J. and Sommer, S. (1985) Oxygen dependence of the photosensitizing effect of hematoporphyrin derivative in NHIK 3025 cells. *Cancer Res*, **45**, 1608–1610.
14. Nichols, M. G. and Foster, T. H. (1994) Oxygen diffusion and reaction kinetics in the photodynamic therapy of multicell tumour spheroids. *Phys Med Biol*, **39**, 2161–2181.
15. Mitra, S. (2004) *Photodynamic therapy: biophysical mechanisms and molecular responses*, Ph.D. thesis, University of Rochester.

Chapter 15

Fluorescent Molecular Imaging and Dosimetry Tools in Photodynamic Therapy

Brian W. Pogue, Kimberley S. Samkoe, Summer L. Gibbs-Strauss, and Scott C. Davis

Abstract

Measurement of fluorescence and phosphorescence in vivo is readily used to quantify the concentration of specific species that are relevant to photodynamic therapy. However, the tools to make the data quantitatively accurate vary considerably between different applications. Sampling of the signal can be done with point samples, such as specialized fiber probes or from bulk regions with either imaging or sampling, and then in broad region image-guided manner. Each of these methods is described below, the application to imaging photosensitizer uptake is discussed, and developing methods to image molecular responses to therapy are outlined.

Key words: Fluorescence, measurement, quantification, molecular, fluorescent, photosensitizer, imaging, instrumentation, system, fiber, spectroscopy.

1. Introduction

Fluorescence measurements from tissue have been a part of research in photodynamic therapy for several decades, but now with the advent of increased molecular reporters, they take on some expanded roles. This chapter focuses on the methods for measurement of fluorescence and the applications of what these measurements can be used for.

The first fluorescence-based measurements of photosensitizer uptake in tissue during photodynamic therapy with Photofrin occurred more than 30 years ago (1); and at that time fluorescence measurements of tissue constituents like NADH were

C.J. Gomer (ed.), *Photodynamic Therapy*, Methods in Molecular Biology 635,
DOI 10.1007/978-1-60761-697-9_15, © Springer Science+Business Media, LLC 2010

being sampled by UV/blue fluorescence (2). The latter studies were focused on diagnostically assessing tissue oxygenation and health with this type of sampling, and later examining response to therapy (3). Since that time, thousands of papers have examined both these areas, and in more recent times, there are very mature systems being examined for detection of dysplasia (4–6) and advanced photodynamic therapy dosimetry (7–9). While only a few clinically viable systems have been generated from all this work, there has been a widespread maturation of the technology, leading to better designs, such that optical systems can be better tailored to the constraints of particular niche areas. This maturation is very important, because the wide array of optical source, delivery systems, and detection methods can lead to considerable confusion about which optical system is optimal for which application. It is common to see competing optical technologies for niche applications where there is good commercial potential.

In the past decade there has been an explosion of work in small animal imaging, focusing on molecular imaging and reporting of tissue health, response to therapy, or presence of certain genetic or proteomic expression (10, 11). Since this time, there have been widespread commercial successes in preclinical systems for imaging, microscopy, and fluorescence sampling of tissues, allowing large growth in the areas of molecular diagnostics and molecular medicine and therapy. In addition, commercial success in clinical applications such as surgery (12) have led the way for future use of molecular probes in tissue.

While all these developments have led to considerable excitement, it is important to recognize that the range of technologies available leads to confusion about what the term “fluorescence measurement” means. In this chapter, we take a top-level overview of what fluorescence measurement systems are available both in the commercial and in the research stages, and then examine the range of applications and commercially available probes which can be used for cancer therapy, with a particular focus on photodynamic therapy response.

2. Materials

The conceptual framework of the tools that can be used is shown in **Fig. 15.1.** The workhorse of invasive sampling, shown in **Fig. 15.1a**, is tissue extraction via biopsy to then liquefy and sample the fluorescence in dilute solvent. While this process has historically been the main way to proceed, there are inherent problems with this which make it less attractive for PS that tend to aggregate or those that have low fluorescent yields.

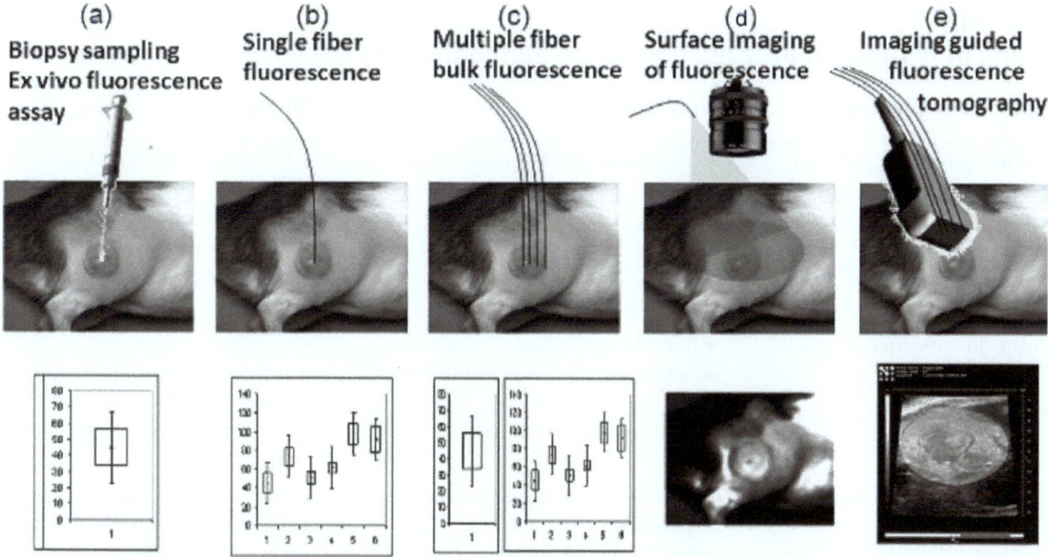

Fig. 15.1. Illustration of the four methods of sampling fluorescence discussed here, including (**a**) the routine biopsy/tissue extraction approach; (**b**) the use of a single fiber probe; (**c**) the use of multiple fibers to sample bulk tissue; (**d**) surface imaging using a broad beam source and sensitive CCD imager; and (**e**) the concept of image-guided fluorescence quantification as applied to surface or sub-surface imaging.

Also, when the biopsy sampling will affect outcome, this method becomes problematic. The three non-invasive methods illustrated in **Fig. 15.1b–e** will be discussed in further detail below, as well as the strengths and limitations of each being summarized in **Table 15.1**.

2.1. Small Fiber Probe or Point Measurements

Several systems for fiber-based sampling have been developed over the years, dating back to nearly the first fluorescence measurements in vivo (**Fig. 15.1b**). Improvements in diode lasers, robust detectors for compact spectrometers and avalanche photodiodes, and filter technology have all contributed to better fluorescence detection at dramatically less expense than earlier versions. Still most advanced systems do some form of filtering or spectral fitting to the data and capture as much of the emitted spectrum as possible.

The choice of fiber diameter has a significant effect upon the signal, as previously studied (13). As the fiber size decreases below the average scattering length in tissue, the detected signal becomes one which is not significantly scattered when detected. Thus the signal is more dependent upon the scatter coefficient than anything else, but also linearly related to the fluororphore concentration. Since typical scatter length distances in tissue are near 100 μm, then fibers larger than a few hundred microns are detecting light that is not just fluorescent but also has an inherent scatter component within it. This is not a problem, and indeed leads to higher signals, but must be interpreted carefully, because

Table 15.1
Listing of photosensitizer quantification methodologies based upon fluorescence

Methods to quantify PS	Limitations	Strengths
Tissue extraction and assay fluorescence in solution	• Volumetric errors in handling • Single time point sampling	• Direct measurement of tissue • Most established • Single time point only • Limited ability for multiple points
Point fluorescence in vivo	• Sample individual points only • Insertion of fibers sometimes needed • Multipoint sampling takes time	• In vivo • Potentially real time, multi-point sampling possible • Track photobleaching in situ
Bulk fluorescence assay in vivo	• Non-linearity from tissue-fiber geometry • Model-based interpretation of data	• Obtain whole organ data • Thick tissue sampling • Direct measure during therapy • Integrate with online dosimetry
Surface imaging of fluorescence	• Non-linearity of signal from geometry and tissue properties • Limited penetration of signal • Surface weighted • Higher cost	• Several commercial systems • Ease of use • Intuitive image display • Fast • Multiple point data (surface)
Image-guided fluorescence sampling	• Non-linearity from geometry • Model-based interpretation • Imaging system required • Higher cost	• Obtain whole animal/ organ data • Thick tissue sampling • Visualize anatomy with signal • Integration into clinical workflow

simple things like pressure on the tissue can decrease the signal due to inducing higher blood volume around the fiber tip. Changes in measurement site can also affect the signal because of local changes in tissue absorption or scattering coefficient.

There have been many interstitial studies, where the fluorescence is captured to sample the photosensitizer concentration prior to therapy. Prostate studies using this technique have been ongoing in a few sites (14).

2.2. Multifiber or Multipoint Model-Based Bulk Sampling

Measurement of fluorescence from larger volumes has been a goal for many researchers for over a decade (**Fig. 15.1c**). The most common approach to try and quantify concentrations in bulk tissue has been to model the light propagation, and use a model-based interpretation of the fluorescence to quantify the signal intensity. This approach would have the benefits of sampling the active photosensitizer concentration in vivo and directly sampling a large fraction of the tumor volume. Modeling is possible with either diffusion theory or Monte Carlo, where the diffusion approach is viable over larger distances with relative data (15–20). The Monte Carlo approach is more accurate but also requires more accurate structure and optical property information to achieve this increased level of accuracy (21, 22) and because of large computational time requirements has been used mostly in smaller geometries. The most common use of this approach now is in the Caliper small animal tomography system where the IVIS 200 system (discussed in the next section) originally designed for surface imaging has added in capabilities for transmission fluorescence tomography. Similarly, the ART Inc system completes a surface scan over the animal with rasterization, and the source and detector are not collocated, so it effectively deeply samples the tissue by a millimeter or so.

Outside of small animal imaging, examples of this approach tend to be situation specific, because a clear knowledge of the tissue surface geometry are important parts of the system design. The most complete scientific design of such a system was developed for fluorescence tomography in situ to allow dosimetry of photosensitizer distribution in bulk tissues (14).

The drawbacks of this approach are obvious in that the ability to quantify heterogeneity and local changes in variation are not possible. However, the key to success in this approach is to measure the transmitted excitation signal as well as the remitted fluorescence signal, and when the normalized value of fluorescence to transmittance is used, this can match most homogeneous models with reasonable accuracy. Application of analytic or numerical diffusion theory to bulk tissue signal recovery is feasible, and could be an area of future development (20).

In vivo fluorescence molecular tomography was developed as an offshoot of these studies, as pioneered by Ntziachristos et al. (23, 24), and since that time dramatic improvements in diffuse tomography have been used to make niche systems for small animal tomography.

2.3. Surface Imaging

Imaging and image-guided measurement of luminescence signals are readily achieved, although mostly with customized instrumentation at this point in time (**Fig. 15.1d**). There has been an explosion of preclinical systems here, based upon simple broad-beam light excitation and filtered, cooled CCD detectors. Imaging systems for fluorescence of surfaces have of course been studied for many years, and endoscopically coupled systems for fluorescence bronchoscopy and laryngeal screening of malignancy have been studied extensively by Xillix Inc. (6, 25), and competing systems (26). Experimental systems for colonoscopy

(27, 5), esophageal studies (28, 29), and intrasurgical use have all be developed. The intrasurgical systems have been stimulated by the approval of fluorescence guided resection techniques for Glioma tumors (12, 30, 31).

2.4. Image-Guided Fluorescence Sampling

It has only been within the last few years that systems have been created to test the concept of image-guided fluorescence sampling (**Fig. 15.1e**). This approach uses optical fibers or an imaging system embedded with or onto a standard imaging system. The goal is to provide both anatomical and fluorescent molecular information that is localized from deeper within the tissue. Imaging systems that have been combined with fluorescence are ultrasound, magnetic resonance, microCT, and optical coherence tomography. At the current time, these are largely experimental, although human studies are likely not far away. When combined with ultrasound, the fibers must be beside the transducer array, allowing either simultaneous or sequential measurement of the same volume. In the MRI, a prototype custom design for a rodent body coil was produced and tested in a 3T Philips Achieva system (32, 33). In combination with MicroCT, this has been done in a sequential manner several years ago, and a hybrid system was recently produced to allow sequential in vivo scanning where the animal is not moved off the subject bed, but is translated directly from the MicroCT into the fluorescence tomography scanner. This process allows overlay and has been used to show the first deep tissue tomography of glioma tumor in a mouse cranium (34, 35).

3. Methods

3.1. Small Fiber Probe or Point Measurements

Photosensitizer dosimetry is an important part of photodynamic therapy, especially considering that the interplay between the photosensitizing agent, oxygen and light is highly variable and not fully understood. Here, point measurements on the surface of a tumor are used to determine the uptake of photosensitizing drug prior to performing photodynamic therapy (**Figs. 15.2** and **15.3**). This is especially important in tumors with a high variability in vascular distribution, such as pancreatic cancer.

A laparotomy is performed, exposing the pancreas tumor (Panc-1 in this case) and the liver (**Fig. 15.3a**). The Aurora Dosimeter (**Fig. 15.3b**) was used to take alternating point measurements between the pancreas and liver. Pre-injection measurements, illustrated as negative time (**Fig. 15.3c**), are taken prior to photosensitizer injection. Verteporfin for injection (1 mg/kg) was administered via the tail vein after which measurements were

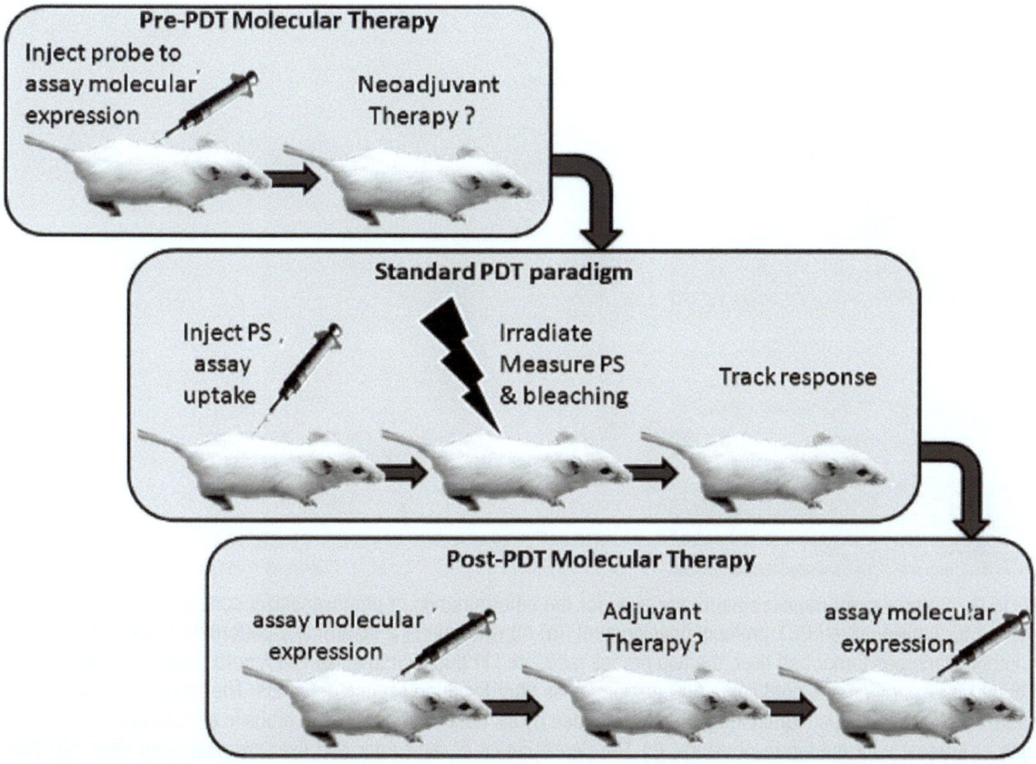

Fig. 15.2. The regimes in which fluorescence signals might need to be measured can be thought of as pre-PDT where neoadjuvant therapy may be beneficial based upon a measurement of the tumor molecular signals. Then during PDT, there is a clear need for PS dosimetry and possibly photobleaching dosimetry if significant. Then after PDT, adjuvant therapies are typically required, and again may be chosen based upon molecular expression, which could be measured via fluorescent probes.

immediately started and were continued for 30 min. The tumor had an immediate increase in fluorescence and then decayed slightly followed by a plateau for the duration of the 30 min. On the other hand, the liver had a more prominent increase in fluorescence but also plateaued within 5 min. A much higher signal in the liver was expected because it is part of the metabolic degradation pathway of verteporfin.

Using point measurements is a quick method of determining photosensitizer concentration within a tumor prior to PDT and allows alteration in the PDT protocol (i.e., light dose) to accommodate differences between patients for individualized therapy. The draw back to this type of measurement is that the photosensitizer concentration is highly heterogeneous within the tumor, especially in the central region that is typically necrotic. Taking surface point measurements only samples a few microns into the tissue, thus assuming that photosensitizer concentration is homogeneous throughout the entire sample.

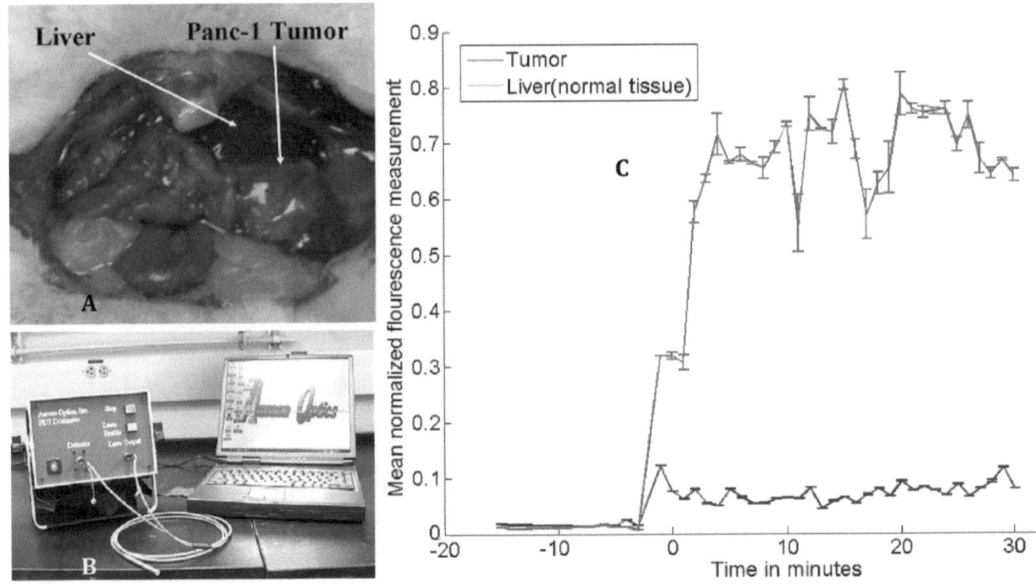

Fig. 15.3. Surface point measurements are used for the determination of photosensitizer concentration within a tumor allowing for individualized PDT protocol development. (**a**) An example of a laparotomy performed to expose the Panc-1 orthotopic pancreas tumor and liver, the two organs measured in this example. (**b**) The Aurora dosimeter uses blue light (405 nm) for excitation and contains a 600 nm long pass filter for fluorescence detection. The probe is made from fiber bundle containing a single illuminating fiber, surrounded by six collection fibers. The probe is directly placed against the organ of interest with moderate pressure. (**c**) The fluorescence of the tumor and liver are measured after injection of verteporfin (1 mg/kg). This graph is an average of four mice.

3.2. Bulk Sampling

Measuring fluorescence in vivo in a large sample of tissue can provide important information regarding the presence, general location, and changes in status of a tumor. The example presented here detects the presence of a brain tumor in a mouse using diffuse fluorescence tomography. Bulk sampling can be used as a method of non-invasive imaging to determine the presence of a tumor or stratify animals into treatment groups.

A mouse implanted with an orthotopic brain tumor (U251) was injected with LI-COR IRDye 800 CW EGF optical probe 48 h prior to imaging of the head (i.e., bulk tissue). The mouse was anesthetized and placed into a mouse holder, specifically made to image the brain, which accepts optical fibers used for tomography (**Fig. 15.4a**). The fibers were placed directly on the skin of the mouse in the plane of the tumor. Successive fluorescence and transmission measurements were made from the eight fibers surrounding the mouse head. A fluorescence map of the mouse head was then created using the NIRFAST reconstruction protocols (**Fig. 15.4b**).

In bulk measurements such as these, the presence and location of the tumor (high fluorescence to the left of the head) can be identified; however, specific information such as delineation of

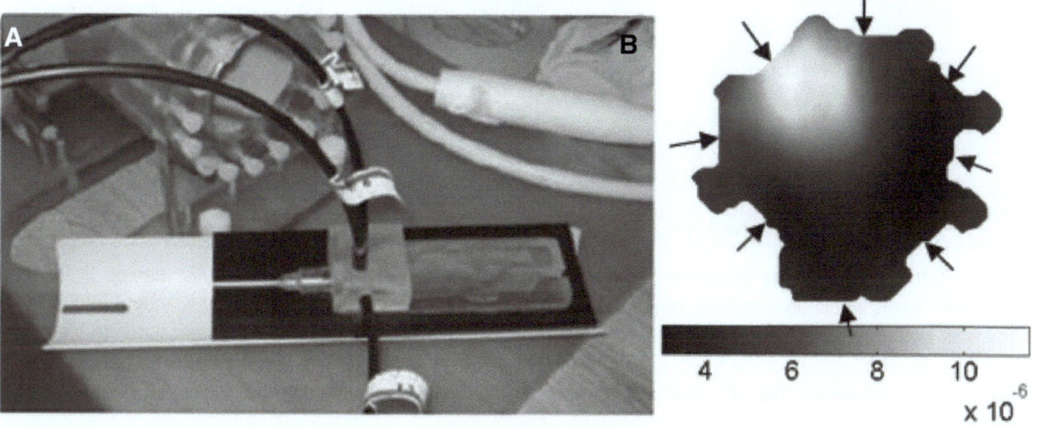

Fig. 15.4. Bulk fluorescence measurements to determine the presence and location of a tumor can be performed with diffuse fluorescence tomography. In this photograph at *left*, the fibers are inserted into a mouse holding apparatus, and fluorescence transmission data is accumulated between fibers, allowing estimation with diffusion theory of the fluorescence signal origin, as shown in the diffuse tomography reconstruction at *right*. This is the fluorescence from a tracer agent localized within the glioma tumor of a mouse model (shown further in Fig. **15.6**).

the tumor border or distribution of the molecular marker within the tumor is limited due to the diffuse nature of bulk imaging.

3.3. Surface Imaging

Surface imaging can be used with a general photosensitizing agent, such as the aminolevulinic acid–protoporphyrin IX system in surgical brain resections, or a specific molecular probe, such as epidermal growth factor (EGF). Surface imaging can give you information regarding where a tumor is, its metabolic function, and even the success of treatment (i.e., PDT).

In this case, ex vivo tissue samples of a mouse brain are imaged to determine the location and growth factor status. Rat brain tumors transfected with green fluorescent protein (9L-GFP) were implanted into nude mice and allowed to develop for approximately 3 weeks. The mice were injected with EGF fluorescently labeled with the LI-COR IRDye 800CW via the tail vein 48 h prior to the experimental endpoint. The brains were removed, sliced, and imaged on the LI-COR Odyssey® Near-Infrared Imaging System (**Fig. 15.5a**). The brain slice was then imaged for the GFP fluorescence using the GE Healthcare Typhoon scanner (**Fig. 15.5b**). Both of these fluorescent images can be compared to the H&E histology section (**Fig. 15.5c**) taken from the surface of the brain slice. The GFP fluorescence arising directly from the tumor corresponds very closely with the H&E section; however, the EGF-IRDye is not evenly distributed across the entirety of the tumor. Instead, it appears that only the most actively growing regions on the edge of the tumor display increased epidermal growth factor levels.

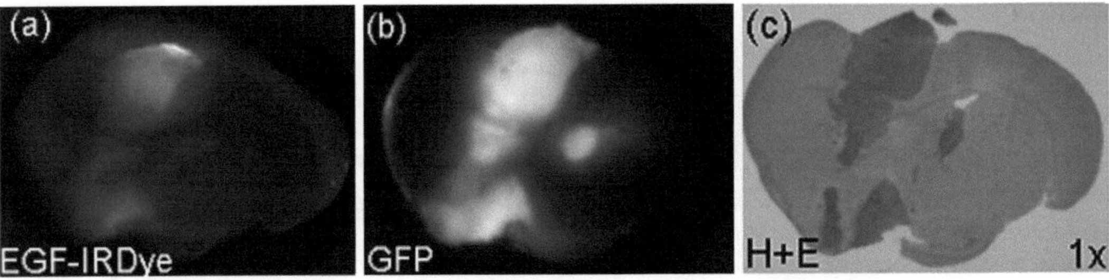

Fig. 15.5. Tumor status can be determined using surface imaging of a fluorescence molecular marker. In this case, growth factor levels within an orthotopic brain tumor in a mouse can be determined ex vivo by scanning for EGF-IRDye (**a**) that was injected 48 h prior to killing. The tissue sample can then be scanned for GFP fluorescence to identify the entire tumor (**b**). The location of the tumor is confirmed with H&E staining of a fixed tissue slice taken directly from the surface of the slice imaged. The GFP and H&E images correlate very well, while the EGF molecular marker indicates areas of growth.

One can imagine using surface measurements such as these to determine success of PDT, cancer, antibody, or combination therapies. The drawback of surface imaging is that the fluorescence profile of a tumor changes three dimensionally making multiple measurements or predictive assumptions necessary. Additionally, surface imaging is used best as an ex vivo technique or as an invasive surgical technique, limiting its use in fluorescence monitoring.

3.4. Image - Guided Fluorescence Sampling

Image-guided fluorescence sampling can provide very detailed in vivo information regarding tissue structure, metabolic activity, or tumor status for diagnosis or therapeutic monitoring. In this example magnetic resonance (MR)-guided near-infrared diffuse fluorescence tomography is used to assess the local distribution of growth factors within a brain tumor, thus providing more detailed information than the bulk sampling technique explored in **Section 3.2** and allowing for in vivo visualization complimentary to the ex vivo imaging described in **Section 3.3**.

A mouse implanted with an orthotopic U251 brain tumor was intravenously injected with EGF-IRDye 48 h prior to imaging. The mouse was anesthetized and placed into a small animal RF coil that accommodates optical fibers (**Fig. 15.6a**). MR images were collected on a 3.0T Achieva MR machine (Philips) while fluorescence and transmission data were collected simultaneous with a multi-spectral tomography system (**Fig. 15.6b**) [Davis, 2008 #4865]. The MR images of the mouse were subsequently segmented for the entire head, brain, gadolinium highlighting and non-highlighting regions. The fluorescence tomography images in **Fig. 15.6c,d** were created by using the segmented regions as spatial hard priors and spatial soft priors, respectively. These images illustrate that the distribution of fluorescently labeled growth factor is not homogeneous throughout

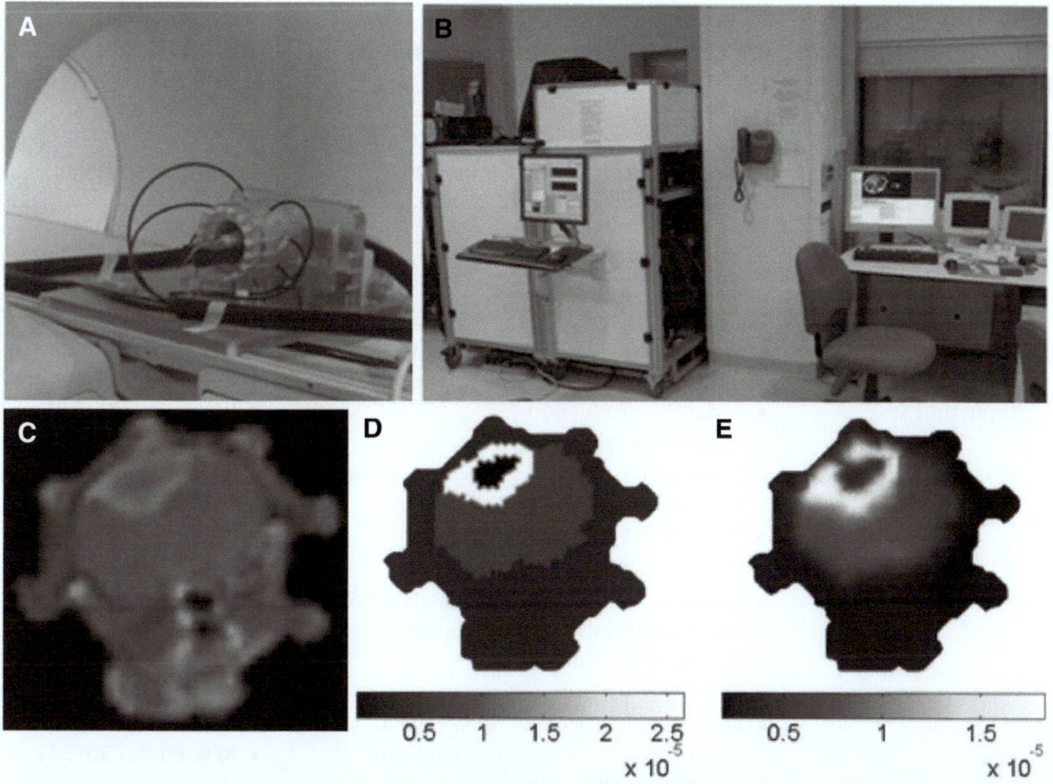

Fig. 15.6. Magnetic resonance (MR)-guided near-infrared diffuse optical tomography is used to illustrate how functional information can be obtained in vivo. A specially designed small animal RF coil accommodates optical fibers (**a**) so that fluorescence tomography can be performed simultaneously with MR imaging (**b**) (33). A T1-weighted gadolinium enhanced MR image (**c**) of a mouse with a U251 brain tumor is depicted. The corresponding fluorescence tomography images are illustrated in **d** and **e** using the image segmentation as spatial hard and soft priors, respectively.

the tumor and that the contrast enhanced regions of the MR image correlates with the actively growing region of the tumor.

The tomography image in **Fig. 15.4b** represents the same mouse without any spatial priors from the MR images (i.e., bulk sampling); thus, adding image guidance to the tomographic process allows information regarding the tumor to be elucidated in addition to the spatial parameters.

4. Notes

The focus of this chapter has been on identifying the methods available to the researcher or clinician who has an interest in PDT. The tools are present and readily available for creation in any lab or for purchase from a number of technology vendors.

Table 15.2
Photosensitizers used in clinical PDT and their needs in terms of fluorescence dosimetry

Generic name and photosensitizer name	Fluorescence signal	Photobleaching important?	Excitation/emission
Photofrin, hematoporphyrin derivative	• Should be measured • Permeability limited delivery	• Likely important	• Soret 350–420 nm • Q-band 625–640 nm • Emission 600–700 nm • Reference (44)
Levualn, aminolevulinic acid, inducing protoporphyrin IX	• Needs to be measured • Variable production between tumors.	• Critically important	• Soret 400–440 nm • Q-band 630–640 nm • Emission 620–720 nm • Reference (45)
Verteporfin, benzoporphyrin derivative	• Needs to be measured • Permeability limited delivery	• Not clear how important	• Soret 400–440 nm • Q-band 680–695 nm • Emission 690–705 nm • References (46, 47)
Foscan, mTHPC	• Complex fluorescence in vivo • Permeability limited delivery	• Not clear how important	• Soret 380–440 nm • Q-band 645–660 nm • References (48, 49)
WST11	• May not need to be measured • Vascular therapy only	• Not likely important	• Q-band 755–770 nm • References (50, 51)

The primary application in PDT has been to quantify the PS concentration or activity in situ immediately prior to therapy. The drugs available for clinical use are several, and are summarized in **Tables 15.2 and 15.3**, with a focus on whether the fluorescence signal would have value in measurement or dosimetry in PDT. Some photosenstizers that have been in use for many years, such as Photofrin, are routinely assayed ex vivo through tissue biopsy sampling. In vivo measurement of fluorescence is complicated in this compound by having a multicomponent mixture of hematoporphyrins which have different photosensitivies, localization, and fluorescence levels (36). In addition, photobleaching of Photofrin has been shown to be complex due to the bleaching rate having more than one component, which was attributed to oxygen and non-oxygen mechanisms (37), making fluorescence signal complex to interpret for therapy efficacy quantification. Photosensitizing compounds that are more dominated by a single component, such as benzoporphyrin derivative, are easier to quantify and track with fluorescence because the signal seems to be linear with active photosensitizer and predictive of dose deposition (38). The endogenously generated drug protoporphyrin IX is known to

Table 15.3
General classes of fluorescent reporters and their uses available

Molecular probes	Example names	Companies
Blood flow/vascular	• Fluorescein • Indocyanine Green	• Akorn Inc. • Sigma-Aldrich
Vascular permeability	• Methylene blue • Varying sized dextran bound with fluorophore	• Sigma • Invitrogen
Receptor/ligand binding	• Monocolonal antibodies • Antibody fragments • Peptides • Deoxyglucose	• Invitrogen • LI-COR
Transfection-based reporters	• Bioluminescence reporters • Fluorescent proteins	• Caliper Biosciences • Anticancer Inc. • Promega
Activatable probes	• Activated by cathepsin, matrix metalloprotease,	• VisEn Inc.

photobleach rapidly and so sampling its fluorescence is thought to be quite important for tracking the response to therapy, and for interpreting dose rate effects, which can confound the therapy (39–43).

Acknowledgments

The authors would like to acknowledge important discussions with Tayyaba Hasan, Ph.D. (Harvard Medical School), Keith D. Paulsen Ph.D. (Dartmouth), Julie A. O'Hara, Ph.D. (Dartmouth), and P. Jack Hoopes, D.V.M. Ph.D. (Dartmouth), and experimental work by Timothy Monahan, M.S. (Dartmouth). This work has been funded through NIH grants P01CA84203 and R01CA109558.

References

1. Kelly, J. F. and Snell, M. E. (1976) Hematoporphyrin derivative: a possible aid in the diagnosis and therapy of carcinoma of the bladder. *J Urol*, **115**(2), 150–151.
2. Ji, S., Chance, B., Stuart, B. H., and Nathan, R. (1977) Two-dimensional analysis of the redox state of the rat cerebral cortex in vivo by NADH fluorescence

photography. *Brain Res*, **119**(2), 357–373.

3. Schantz, S. P. and Alfano, R. R. (1993) Tissue autofluorescence as an intermediate endpoint in cancer chemoprevention trials. [Review]. *J Cell Biochem – Suppl*, **17F**, 199–204.
4. Gillenwater, A., Jacob, R., and Richards-Kortum, R. (1998) Fluorescence spectroscopy: a technique with potential to improve the early detection of aerodigestive tract neoplasia. *Head Neck*, **20**(6), 556–562.
5. DaCosta, R. S., Wilson, B. C., and Marcon, N. E. (2000) Light-induced fluorescence endoscopy of the gastrointestinal tract. *Gastrointest Endosc Clin N Am*, **10**(1), 37–69.
6. Weigel, T. L., Yousem, S., Dacic, S., Kosco, P. J., Siegfried, J., and Luketich, J. D. (2000) Fluorescence bronchoscopic surveillance after curative surgical resection for non-small-cell lung cancer. *Ann Surg Oncol*, 7(3), 176–180.
7. Andersson-Engels, S., Klinteberg, C., Svanberg, K., and Svanberg, S. (1997) In vivo fluorescence imaging for tissue diagnostics. *Phys Med Biol*, **42**(5), 815–824.
8. Svanberg, K., af Klinteberg, C., Nilsson, A., Wang, I., Andersson-Engels, S., and Svanberg, S. (1998) Laser-based spectroscopic methods in tissue characterization. *Ann N Y Acad Sci*, **838**, 123–129.
9. Svanberg, K., Wang, I., Colleen, S., Idvall, I., Ingvar, C., Rydell, R., Jocham, D., Diddens, H., Bown, S., Gregory, G., Montan, S., Andersson-Engels, S., and Svanberg, S. (1998) Clinical multi-colour fluorescence imaging of malignant tumours – initial experience. *Acta Radiol*, **39**(1), 2–9.
10. Ntziachristos, V., Ripoll, J., Wang, L. V., and Weissleder, R. (2005) Looking and listening to light: the evolution of whole-body photonic imaging. *Nat Biotech*, **23**(3), 313–320.
11. Campo, M. A. and Lange, N. (2006) Fluorescence diagnosis using enzyme-related metabolic abnormalities of neoplasia. *J Environ Pathol, Toxic Oncol*, **25**(1–2), 341–372.
12. Stummer, W., Pichlmeier, U., Meinel, T., Wiestler, O. D., Zanella, F., and Reulen, H.-J., and A.L.-G.S. Group, (2006) Fluorescence-guided surgery with 5-aminolevulinic acid for resection of malignant glioma: a randomised controlled multicentre phase III trial.[see comment]. *Lancet Oncol*, 7(5), 392–401.
13. Pogue, B. W., Chen, B., Zhou, X., and Hoopes, P. J. (2005) Analysis of sampling volume and tissue heterogeneity upon the in vivo detection of fluorescence. *J Biomed Opt*, **10**(4), 041206.
14. Finlay, J. C., Zhu, T. C., Dimofte, A., Stripp, D., Malkowicz, S. B., Busch, T. M., and Hahn, S. M. (2006) Interstitial fluorescence spectroscopy in the human prostate during motexafin lutetium-mediated photodynamic therapy. *Photochem Photobiol*, **82**(5), 1270–1278.
15. Durkin, A. J., Jaikumar, S., Ramanujam, N., and Richards-Kortum, R. (1994) Relation between fluorescence spectra of dilute and turbid samples. *Appl Opt*, **33**(3), 414–423.
16. Wu, J., Feld, M. S., and Rava, R. P. (1993) An analytical model for extracting intrinsic fluorescence in turbid media. *Appl Opt*, **32**, 3585–3595.
17. Patterson, M. S. and Pogue, B. W. (1994) Mathimatical model for time-resolved and frequency-domain fluorescence spectroscopy in biological tissues. *Appl Opt*, **33**(10), 1963–1974.
18. Durkin, A. J. and Richards-Kortum, R. (1996) Comparison of methods to determine chromophore concentrations from fluorescence spectra of turbid samples. *Lasers Surg Med*, **19**(1), 75–89.
19. Welch, A. J., Gardner, C., Richards-Kortum, R., Chan, E., Criswell, G., Pfefer, J., and Warren, S. (1997) Propagation of fluorescent light. *Lasers Surg Med*, **21**(2), 166–178.
20. Hyde, D. E., Farrell, T. J., Patterson, M. S., and Wilson, B. C. (2001) A diffusion theory model of spatially resolved fluorescence from depth-dependent fluorophore concentrations. *Phys Med Biol*, **46**(2), 369–383.
21. Wang, L. and Jacques, S. (1992) *Monte Carlo Modeling of Light Transport in Multi-Layered Tissues in Standard C.*
22. Vishwanath, K., Pogue, B., and Mycek, M. A. (2002) Quantitative fluorescence lifetime spectroscopy in turbid media: comparison of theoretical, experimental and computational methods. *Phys Med Biol*, **47**(18), 3387–3405.
23. Ntziachristos, V., Bremer, C., Graves, E. E., Ripoll, J., and Weissleder, R. (2002) In vivo tomographic imaging of near-infrared fluorescent probes. *Mol Imaging*, **1**(2), 82–88.
24. Ntziachristos, V., Bremer, C., and Weissleder, R. (2003) Fluorescence imaging with near-infrared light: new technological advances that enable in vivo molecular imaging. *Eur Radiol*, **13**(1), 195–208.
25. Zargi, M., Fajdiga, I., and Smid, L. (2000) Autofluorescence imaging in the diagnosis of laryngeal cancer. *Eur Arch Oto-Rhino-Laryngol*, **257**(1), 17–23.

26. Zellweger, M., Grosjean, P., Goujon, D., Monnier, P., van den Bergh, H., and Wagnieres, G. (2001) In vivo autofluorescence spectroscopy of human bronchial tissue to optimize the detection and imaging of early cancers. *J Biomed Opt*, **6**(1), 41–51.
27. Haringsma, J., Tytgat, G. N., Yano, H., Iishi, H., Tatsuta, M., Ogihara, T., Watanabe, H., Sato, N., Marcon, N., Wilson, B. C., and Cline, R. W. (2001) Autofluorescence endoscopy: feasibility of detection of GI neoplasms unapparent to white light endoscopy with an evolving technology. *Gastrointest Endosc*, **53**(6), 642–650.
28. Endlicher, E., Knuechel, R., Hauser, T., Szeimies, R.-M., Schölmerich, J., and Messmann, H. (2001) Endoscopic fluorescence detection of low and high grade dysplasia in Barrett's oesophagus using systemic or local 5-aminolaevulinic acid sensitisation. *Gut*, **48**(3), 314–319.
29. Stepinac, T., Felley, C., Jornod, P., Lange, N., Gabrecht, T., Fontolliet, C., Grosjean, P., vanMelle, G., van den Bergh, H., Monnier, P., Wagnieres, G., and Dorta, G. (2003) Endoscopic fluorescence detection of intraepithelial neoplasia in Barrett's esophagus after oral administration of aminolevulinic acid. *Endoscopy*, **35**(8), 663–668.
30. Stummer, W., Reulen, H. J., Novotny, A., Stepp, H., and Tonn, J. C. (2003) Fluorescence-guided resections of malignant gliomas – an overview. *Acta Neurochir – Suppl*, **88**, 9–12.
31. Stepp, H., Beck, T., Pongratz, T., Meinel, T., Kreth, F.-W., Tonn, J. C., and Stummer, W. (2007) ALA and malignant glioma: fluorescence-guided resection and photodynamic treatment. *J Environ Pathol Toxic Oncol*, **26**(2), 157–164.
32. Davis, S. C., Pogue, B. W., Dehghani, H., and Paulsen, K. D. (2005) Contrast-detail analysis characterizes diffuse optical fluorescence tomography image reconstruction. *J Biomed Opt*, **10**(5), 050501-1-3.
33. Davis, S. C., Springett, R., Leussler, C., Mazurkewitz, P., Tuttle, S., Gibbs-Strauss, S. L., Dehghani, H., Pogue, B. W., and Paulsen, K. D. (2008) Magnetic resonance-coupled fluorescence tomography scanner for molecular imaging of small animals and human breasts. *Rev Sci Instr* (submitted).
34. Kepshire, D., Gibbs-Strauss, S. L., O'Hara, J. A., Hutchins, M., Mincu, N., Leblond, F., Khayat, M., Dehghani, H., Srinivasan, S., and Pogue, B. W. (2008) Imaging of glioma tumor with endogneous fluoresence tomography coupled to MicroCT. *J Biomed Opt*, **14**(3), 030501–030503.
35. Kepshire, D., Mincu, N., Hutchins, M., Gruber, J., Dehghani, H., Hypnarowski, J., Leblond, F., Khayat, M., and Pogue, B. W. (2009) A MicroCT guided fluorescence tomography system for small animal molecular imaging. *Rev Sci Instr*, **80**, 043701.
36. Braichotte, D. R., Wagnieres, G. A., Bays, R., Monnier, P., and van den Bergh, H. E. (1995) Clinical pharmacokinetic studies of photofrin by fluorescence spectroscopy in the oral cavity, the esophagus, and the bronchi. *Cancer*, **75**(11), 2768–2778.
37. Finlay, J. C., Mitra, S., Patterson, M. S., and Foster, T. H. (2004) Photobleaching kinetics of Photofrin in vivo and in multicell tumour spheroids indicate two simultaneous bleaching mechanisms. *Phys Med Biol*, **49**(21), 4837–4860.
38. Zhou, X., Pogue, B. W., Chen, B., Demidenko, E., Joshi, R., Hoopes, P. J., and Hasan, T. (2006) Pre-treatment photosensitizer dosimetry reduces variation in treatment response. *Int J Rad Oncol Biol Phys*, **64**(4), 1211–1220.
39. Robinson, D. J., de Bruijn, H. S., van der Veen, N., Stringer, M. R., Brown, S. B., and Star, W. M. (1998) Fluorescence photobleaching of ALA-induced protoporphyrin IX during photodynamic therapy of normal hairless mouse skin: the effect of light dose and irradiance and the resulting biological effect. *Photochem Photobiol*, **67**(1), 140–149.
40. Finlay, J. C., Conover, D. L., Hull, E. L., and Foster, T. H. (2001) Porphyrin bleaching and PDT-induced spectral changes are irradiance dependent in ALA-sensitized normal rat skin in vivo. *Photochem Photobiol*, **73**(1), 54–63.
41. Star, W. M., Aalders, M. C. G., Sac, A., and Sterenborg, H. J. C. M. (2002) Quantitative model calculation of the time-dependent protoporphyrin IX concentration in normal human epidermis after delivery of ALA by passive topical application or lontophoresis. *Photochem Photobiol*, **75**(4), 424–432.
42. Boere, I. A., Robinson, D. J., de Bruijn, H. S., Kluin, J., Tilanus, H. W., Sterenborg, H. J. C. M., and de Bruin, R. W. F. (2006) Protoporphyrin IX fluorescence photobleaching and the response of rat Barrett's esophagus following 5-aminolevulinic acid photodynamic therapy. *Photochem Photobiol*, **82**(6), 1638–1644.
43. Sheng, C., Hoopes, P. J., Hasan, T., and Pogue, B. W. (2007) Photobleaching-based dosimetry predicts deposited dose in ALA-PpIX PDT of Rodent Esophagus. *Photochem Photobiol*, **83**, 738–748.

44. Ramponi, R., Sacchi, C. A., and Cubeddu, R. (1991) Present status of research on hematoporphyrin derivatives and their photophysical properties. In: M. L. Wolbarsht (ed.) Laser Applications in Medicine. New York: Springer.
45. Brancaleon, L. and Moseley, H. (2002) Effects of photoproducts on the binding properties of protoporphyrin IX to proteins. *Biophys Chem*, **96**(1), 77–87.
46. Aveline, B., Hasan, T., and Redmond, R. W. (1994) Photophysical and photosensitizing properties of benzoporphyrin derivative monoacid ring A (BPD-MA). *Photochem Photobiol*, **59**(3), 328–335.
47. Aveline, B. M., Hasan, T., and Redmond, R. W. (1995) The effects of aggregation, protein binding and cellular incorporation on the photophysical properties of benzoporphyrin derivative monoacid ring A (BPDMA). *J Photochem Photobiol. B Biol*, **30**(2–3), 161–169.
48. Ma, L. W., Moan, J., and Berg, K. (1994) Evaluation of a new photosensitizer, meso-tetra-hydroxyphenyl-chlorin, for use in photodynamic therapy – a comparison of its photobiological properties with those of 2 other photosensitizers. *Int J Cancer*, **57**(6), 883–888.
49. Glanzmann, T., Hadjur, C., Zellweger, M., Grosiean, P., Forrer, M., Ballini, J. P., Monnier, P., van den Bergh, H., Lim, C. K., and Wagnieres, G. (1998) Pharmacokinetics of tetra(m-hydroxyphenyl)chlorin in human plasma and individualized light dosimetry in photodynamic therapy. *Photochem Photobiol*, **67**(5), 596–602.
50. Borle, F., Radu, A., Monnier, P., van den Bergh, H., and Wagnieres, G. (2003) Evaluation of the photosensitizer Tookad (R) for photodynamic therapy on the Syrian golden hamster cheek pouch model: Light dose, drug dose and drug-light interval effects. *Photochem Photobiol*, **78**(4), 377–383.
51. Koudinova, N. V., Pinthus, J. H., Brandis, A., Brenner, O., Bendel, P., Ramon, J., Eshhar, Z., Scherz, A., and Salomon, Y. (2003) Photodynamic therapy with Pd-Bacteriopheophorbide (TOOKAD): successful in vivo treatment of human prostatic small cell carcinoma xenografts. *Int J Cancer*, **104**(6), 782–789.

Chapter 16

Bifunctional Agents for Imaging and Therapy

Ravindra K. Pandey, Nadine S. James, Yihui Chen, Joseph Missert, and Munawar Sajjad

Abstract

Multiple, complementary techniques for tumor detection, including magnetic resonance, nuclear and optical imaging, are under active development; each approach has particular strengths and advantages. Efforts are also currently underway to develop bifunctional agents, so that a single molecule can be used for imaging, therapy, and monitoring the long-term tumor response. This chapter is mainly focused on illustrating the utility of certain tumor-avid photosensitizers in developing agents for tumor imaging [fluorescence, magnetic resonance imaging (MRI), positron emission tomography (PET)] and photodynamic therapy. Recent approaches for developing target-specific agents for photodynamic therapy (PDT) and in vivo tumor imaging are also briefly discussed.

Key words: Photodynamic therapy (PDT), positron emission tomography (PET), photosensitizers (PS), near-infrared (NIR), magnetic resonance imaging (MRI), food and drug administration (FDA), field of view (FOV).

1. Introduction

1.1. Basics of Photodynamic Therapy

Photodynamic therapy (PDT), also referred as phototherapy, involves the localization of certain therapeutic agents called photosensitizers (PS) in tumors upon systemic administration (1–5). It is known that PDT is a non-invasive treatment used for several types of cancers worldwide; however, its use is not limited to oncology. It is also used to treat cardiovascular, dermatological, and ophthalmic diseases (6). There are certain key steps involved in PDT (7, 8). The first step requires administration (intravenous or topical) and delivery of the PS to the target malignant tissue.

C.J. Gomer (ed.), *Photodynamic Therapy*, Methods in Molecular Biology 635,
DOI 10.1007/978-1-60761-697-9_16, © Springer Science+Business Media, LLC 2010

Upon selective uptake of PS, the tumor tissue is then irradiated with an appropriate wavelength of visible or near-infrared (NIR) light. Photoexcitation of the PS enables its activation and leads to transfer of its excess energy to the surrounding molecular oxygen, resulting in the generation of reactive oxygen species (ROS), namely, singlet oxygen ($^1O_2$), free radicals, superoxides, and peroxides. These species lead to the irreversible destruction of diseased tissue without significantly affecting surrounding healthy tissue (2, 5, 8).

It is noteworthy that there are three essential components required for photodynamic interactions to occur. These are the PS, light of the appropriate wavelength, and oxygen. Immediately following light absorption, the PS is initially excited from its ground state (PS) to a short-lived singlet state ($^1PS^*$) and is later converted to a long-lived excited triplet state ($^3PS^*$).

The triplet state of PS can generate ROS via two processes, type I and/or II shown in **Fig. 16.1** (9–11). Type I is the process whereby reactive free radicals, superoxides, and peroxides are generated via electron or hydrogen transfer reaction with water or biomolecules. Type II mediates the evolution of the highly reactive singlet oxygen species from the reaction of the triplet state PS and molecular oxygen in the tissue, (7, 8, 10). Generally, type II

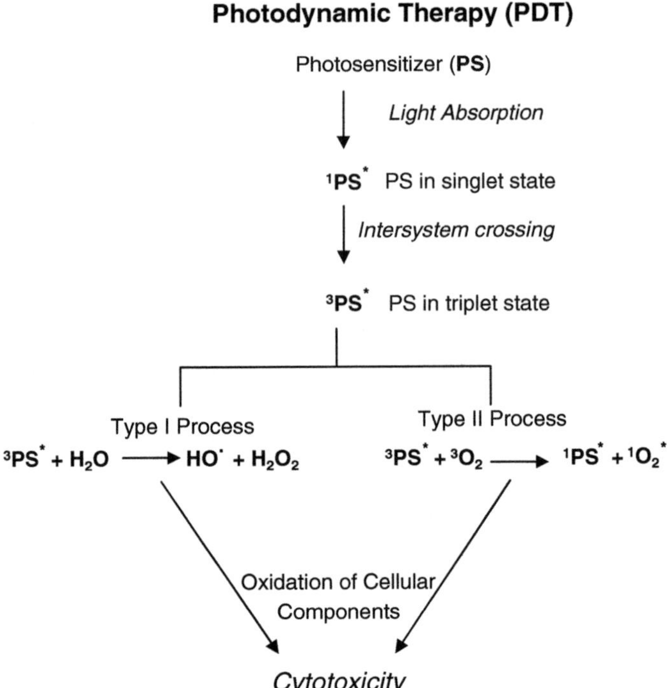

Fig. 16.1. Mechanism of PDT cytotoxicity.

reactions occur more frequently in photodynamic therapy via the generation of cytotoxic singlet oxygen. Studies have shown that singlet oxygen mainly obliterates tumors by causing damage to membranes through oxidation. Some components oxidized by singlet oxygen are amino acids (tryptophan, cysteine, histidine, methionine, phenylalanine, and guanine), unsaturated fatty acids, and cholesterol (9).

1.2. Structural Features of Tetrapyrrole-Based Photosensitizers

Tetrapyrrole-based photosensitizers (porphyrin, chlorin, and bacteriochlorin) consist of four pyrrole subunits linked together by four methine bridges as shown in **Fig. 16.2**. Insertion of nitrogen at the meso-positions of the tetrapyrrole unit produces phthalocyanines with long-wavelength absorptions near 700 nm. In general, the characteristics for an ideal photosensitizer are that it should be non-toxic, selectively retained in tumor tissue in high concentrations, water soluble, have long-wavelength absorptions in the far- and near-infrared regions and show minimal skin phototoxicity with a high singlet oxygen producing efficiency (7, 12–20).

It is noteworthy that chlorins and bacteriochlorins (the mono- or di-pyrroles reduced form of porphyrins, respectively), and phthalocyanines tend to absorb light at wavelengths higher than porphyrins. As a result long-wavelength photosensitizer may be able to exhibit the advantages of deeper light penetration in tumors. Although, certain porphyrin-based compounds show tumor avidity, the mechanism associated with their preferential accumulation in tumor is still evasive and currently under investigation. However, it is hypothesized that several characteristics associated with the tumor environment contribute to this phenomenon, namely, high number of LDL receptors, low interstitial pH, reduced lymphatic drainage, large interstitial space, and leaky vasculature (21). As a result, porphyrin derivatives are believed to selectively accumulate within tumors because of their affinity for proliferating endothelium, high tumor vascular permeability, and lack of lymphatic drainage (21). Photofrin (a hematoporphyrin derivative developed at Roswell Park Cancer Institute) is the first generation PS approved by the FDA for the treatment of several cancers, namely actinic keratoses, high-grade

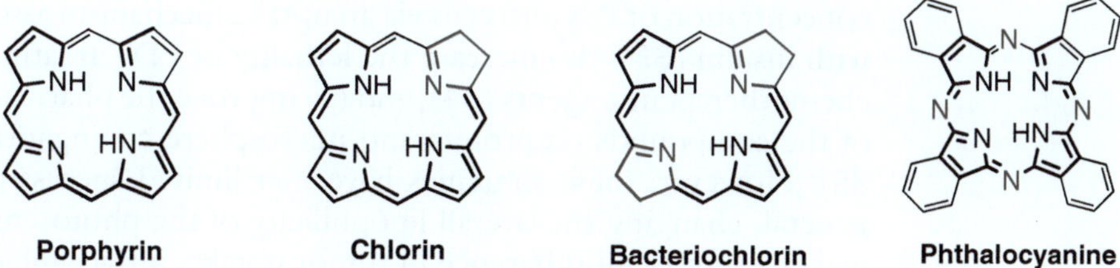

Fig. 16.2. Core structure of some porphyrin-based photosensitizers.

dyplasia in Barrett's esophagus, early-stage lung cancer, and non-small cell lung cancer. However, it is known that the clinical use of Photofrin has several disadvantages, such as its complex chemical nature, and poor selectivity in terms of tumor to normal tissue ratio. Additionally, its weak absorption at long-wavelength region (630 nm) requires the administration of large amounts of the drug. Furthermore, its long-wavelength absorption maxima falls at 630 nm, which results in poor tissue penetration (4, 5). Another disadvantage associated with Photofrin is that it tends to accumulate in the skin leading to prolonged photosensitivity which may last for 4–6 weeks after the light treatment (3, 5, 22). Therefore, to overcome these drawbacks and improve the treatment efficacy several strategies have been employed for the development of more tumor-selective agents with reduced skin phototoxicity.

In recent years several tetrapyrrole-based photosensitizers (e.g., HPPH (23), BPD-MA (24), m-THPC (25), ALA (26), NPe6 (Talaporfin) (27), TOOKAD (28), Purpurinimide (drug 277) (29), bacteriopurpurinimide (drug 605) (29), and phthalocyanine (PC-4) (30)) are at the various stages of preclinical or advanced clinical trials. The FDA-approved benzoporphyrin derivative monoacid (BPD-MA or verteporfin), meso-tetrahydroxphenyl-chlorin (m-THPC), and protoporphyrin IX derived in situ from a natural biosynthetic process that occurs when the topically administered prodrug δ-aminolevulinic acid (ALA) is taken up by cells. Other second generation PSs currently under investigation are talaporphin (NPe6), HPPH, purpurinimide (drug 277), TOOKAD, bacteriopurpurinimide (drug 605), and the phthalocyanine (PC-4) (**Fig. 16.3**). Among these analogs the HPPH, talaporphin, and purpurinimide (drug 277) were derived from chlorophyll-*a* and exhibit their long-wavelength absorption in the range of 660–700 nm, whereas the TOOKAD and bacteriopurpurinimide (drug 605) were obtained from bacteriochlorophyll-*a*, which in turn was isolated from naturally occurring *Rhodobacter sphaeroides.*

Several attempts have been made to deliver PSs to known cellular targets via conjugation to ligands specific for those targets. Some examples of the conjugates developed were designed to (i) improve localization to the cell via cholesterol (31), (ii) direct PSs to specific tumor antigens via antibodies (32), (iii) target high concentration of PSs into cells via an uptake mechanism associated with insulin (33), (iv) increase the lethality of PDT treatment via chemotherapeutic agents (34), and (v) improve the pharmacology of the compounds via protein and microsphere conjugation (31, 35). However, these strategies have met limited success (7). In general, changing the overall lipophilicity of the photosensitizers makes a significant difference in tumor uptake, intracellular localization, and PDT efficacy. This approach (SAR and QSAR) has

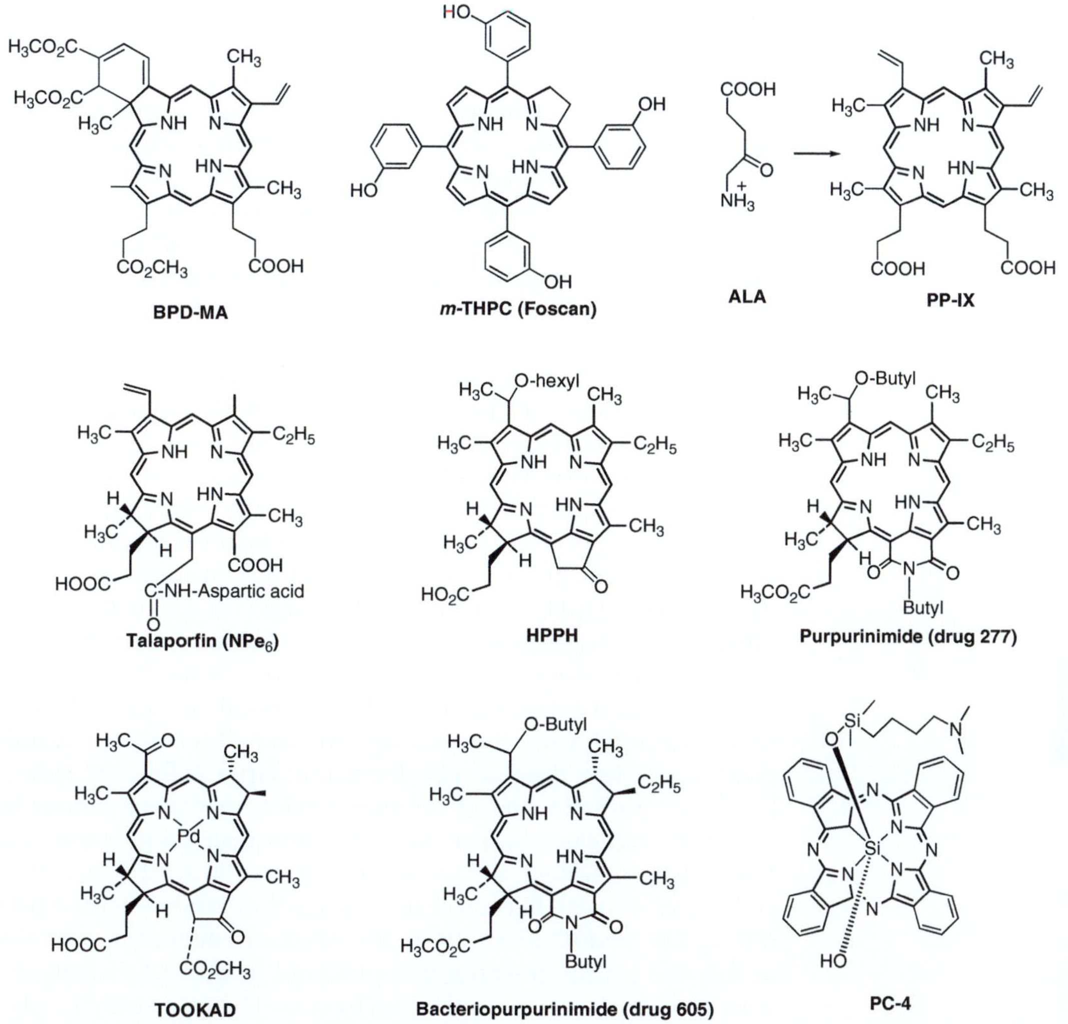

Fig. 16.3. Structures of the tetrapyrrole-based photosensitizers approved by various health organizations or are at the various stages of advanced clinical and preclinical trials.

been extremely useful in developing the improved PDT agents (36).

1.3. Porphyrin-Based Compounds in Fluorescence Imaging

The biomedical use of fluorescence-based techniques is increasing. Frequently used techniques are fluorescence microscopy, flow cytometry, and cell sorting. These techniques are frequently based on fluorescence marking, utilizing externally added fluorophores, which selectively bind to specific targets in tissues. Many drugs investigated for their photodynamic activity in the field of photodynamic therapy (PDT) have properties of interest for fluorescence tissue diagnostics. Fluorophore used must somehow alter the fluorescence characteristics of the bulk tissue examined. This difference might be found in the fluorescence excitation or emission spectrum or in the fluorescence lifetime. The difference may be due to a change in concentration of the fluorophore between the lesion and surrounding normal tissue, but it might also be due to an alteration in the fluorescence properties of that fluorophore due to variations in the microenvironment. The development of exogenous fluorophores as tumor markers for fluorescence diagnostics is closely associated with that of photodynamic therapy (PDT), a tumor treatment modality utilizing production of cytotoxic agents in photoinitiated chemical reactions. Experiments related to in vivo biodistribution with fluorescent substances were first performed at the very end of the nineteenth century by Raab and coworkers (37). The first quantitative study of fluorescence in vivo with exogenous fluorophores was performed by Winkelman and Rasmussen-Taxdal (38) using fluorometry and spectrophotometry of porphyrins chemically extracted from tissue. In the same year, Lipson and Baldes (39) reported on a derivative of hematoporphyrin (HpD) as a fluorescent tumor marker and photosensitizer of malignant tumors. HpD was first tested clinically in 15 patients with bronchial or esophageal tumors and in a further 51 patients, 31 of whom had malignant lesions of cervix or vagina. All bronchial and esophageal tumors and 29 of the cervical or vaginal lesions were examined with the unaided eye and observed to exhibit positive reddish fluorescence from the HpD following violet-light excitation. In one of the two cervical or vaginal lesions in which no red fluorescence was seen, the malignant lesion was found histopathologically to be covered with normal tissue. Several other clinical fluorescence visualization studies with HpD during the period 1964–1976 also showed encouraging results as follows: (a) fluorescence was observed in 80% of 35 patients with bronchial or esophageal carcinomas; (b) in a study involving 226 patients, of whom 173 had malignant lesions of various types, positive HpD fluorescence was obtained in 77% of 132 patients and 22% of 53 patients with benign lesions also showed positive fluorescence; (c) epithelial carcinomas of the mouth, hypopharynx, larynx, or trachea all showed HpD fluorescence in a study involving 40 patients; (d) 18 of 23 patients with invasive or in situ cervical cancer showed positive HpD fluorescence; (e) all 12 patients with carcinoma in situ or dysplasia of the cervical uterus and 3 of 4 patients with squamous metaplasia showed reddish fluorescence in the lesions; (f) in a study of bladder carcinoma, lesions of 11 patients showed HpD fluorescence, and no normal tissue showed any HpD fluorescence, although a slight fluorescence was observed in the edematous submucosa around the tumors in 3 patients. By the end of the 1970s the use of HpD as a tumor marker for fluorescence diagnostics was growing rapidly, largely due to the breakthrough in the use of HpD as a photosensitizer for photodynamic therapy by Dougherty and coworkers (40, 41). However, there also exist several drawbacks with this substance. Due to chemically complex nature of Photofrin, it is difficult to fully characterize. Furthermore, it has a low-fluorescence yield, a poor selectivity for malignant tissue during the first 24 h after the drug administration, and the patient may suffer from skin sensitivity up to several weeks afterward. For these reasons alternative drugs have been examined as tumor markers for fluorescence diagnostics have been considered. As previously mentioned most of the photosensitizers currently under investigation as PDT agents are tetrapyrrole-based structures due to their ability to make singlet oxygen and tumor avidity.

Phthalocyanines are interesting, as many of them have a much stronger fluorescence than HpD and at longer wavelengths with less overlap with the tissue autofluorescence. Some of the compounds in this series have also shown tumor specificity and one of the photosensitizers (PC-4) is at phase I clinical trials. Other PDT drugs examined for fluorescence tumor marking capabilities include chlorins mono-aspartyl chlorin e6 (MACE) (42), di-aspartyl chlorin e6 (DACE), meso-tetra hydroxyphenyl chlorin (m-THPC), and benzoporphyrin derivatives. They all show high singlet oxygen producing efficiency, but some of them show long-term skin phototoxicity. Several rhodamine-based photosensitizers have also been reported. The binding of these dyes to tissue is partly attributed to the positive charge on the molecule leading to attraction to transformed cells.

The introduction of δ-aminolevulinic acid (ALA), a precursor to heme in the heme cycle has also created quite-a-bit of attention. Following administration of ALA, an excess amount of protoporphyrin IX (PPIX), the intermediate product just before heme in the intracellular chain reaction called the heme cycle, will build up in the tissue. Several advantages were found with this fluorescence tumor-marking technique. First, both ALA and PPIX are substances normally present in the body, making the toxicity issue less critical. Furthermore, the drug can conveniently be administered orally or applied topically. The ALA molecule is itself a small non-photoactive substance, quickly metabolized to PPIX in tissue with a high selectivity to malignant tissue. The photophysical properties of PPIX are similar to those of HpD. Research is also being pursued in various laboratories to develop fluorescence agents without an ability to generate singlet oxygen. For example, certain tumor-avid porphyrins and chlorins are conjugated with carotenes in which the singlet oxygen produced by the excitation of the photosensitizers with an appropriate wavelength of light is quenched by the carotene moiety (43), thus the skin phototoxicity can be eliminated.

2. Materials

2.1. NIR Fluorescence Imaging

As stated before, most porphyrins fluoresce and their fluorescent property have been exploited and used for the detection of early-stage cancers in the lung, bladder, and other sites. However, photosensitizers are not optimal fluorophores for tumor detection because they have a small difference between their long-wavelength absorption band and the fluorescence wavelength (Stokes shift), which makes it technically difficult to separate the fluorescence from an excitation wavelength <800 nm, which is not optimal for deep tissue penetration by light.

The use of near-infrared (NIR) light to interrogate deep tissues has enormous potential for molecular-based imaging when coupled with NIR excitable dyes (44). More than a decade has now passed since the initial proposals for NIR optical tomography (45) for breast cancer screening using time-dependent measurements of light propagation in the breast. Much accomplishment in the development of optical mammography has been demonstrated, most recently in the application of time-domain, frequency-domain, and continuous-wave measurements that depend on endogenous contrast owing to angiogenesis and increased hemoglobin absorbance for contrast. Although exciting and promising, the necessity of angiogenesis-mediated absorption contrast for diagnostic optical mammography minimizes the potential for using NIR techniques to assess sentinel lymph node staging, metastatic spread, and multifocality of breast disease, among other applications. Many efforts to design fluorescent NIR contrast agents have recently appeared. Although photodynamic agents are typically designed to exhibit triplet states that will form cytotoxic products in the presence of oxygen, several exhibit radiative relaxation from the singlet state, or fluorescence. Indeed, we have modified our experimental photodynamic agent, hexylpyropheophorbide (HPPH), with a carotene moiety that suppresses the triplet state and renders the therapeutic agent ineffective while preserving its diagnostic fluorescence contrast agent abilities. Using the same instrumentation and animal model, Sevick-Muraca's group (43, 46) assessed the photodynamic agent HPPH-car **(Fig. 16.4)**. Injected into the canine model, the dye was excited at 660 nm and its fluorescence was collected at 710 nm. With an extinction coefficient of 45,000 M^{-1} cm^{-1}, a lifetime of 3.6 ns, and quantum efficiency of 0.11, the maximum absorption and emission wavelengths of HPPH-car fall within the melanin and hemoglobin absorbance maxima, making the dye less diagnostically effective. Nonetheless, the pharmacokinetics show HPPH-car to be selectively taken up by an adenocarcinoma of the canine, owing presumably to the

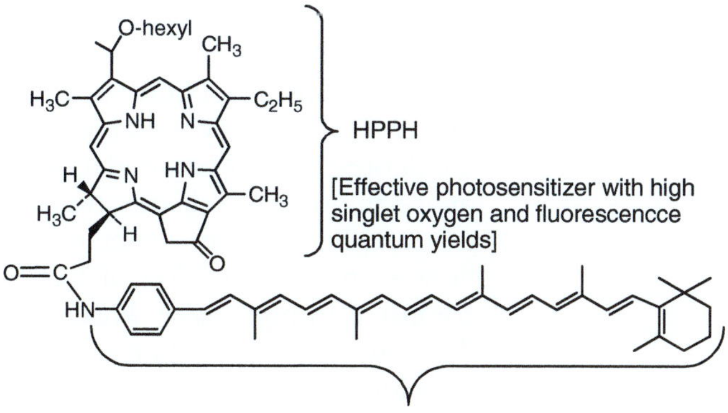

Fig. 16.4. Structure of HPPH–carotene conjugate, a fluorescence-imaging agent for tumor detection. The singlet oxygen produced by exciting the HPPH moiety is quenched by the carotene molecule, which eliminates the PDT efficacy and skin phototoxicity.

dye's association with low-density lipoproteins (LDL) within the plasma and the overexpression of LDL receptors on cancer cells. The use of PDT agents and their modified, non-therapeutic forms has long been used for identification of lesions using continuous-wave techniques. With the development of newer red-shifted agents, great opportunities exist for employing them as fluorescent diagnostic agents in deep tissues with the potential benefit of added therapeutic action. Several other efforts to design fluorescent NIR contrast agents that target the overexpression of proteases or membrane receptors in pathogenesis can also be found in the literature. For example, Tung and colleagues conjugated a cyanine dye (Cy 5.5) onto a peptide with specificity for cathepsin D that is an enzyme common to many neoplasms (47). Upon conjugation of several dye–peptide dimers to methoxy polyethylene glycol, the fluorescence of the Cy 5.5 dyes was quenched due to their close proximity in the complex. However, upon enzymatic cleavage, the dyes were released from the conjugated compound and radiatively re-emitted. The Cy 5.5 dyes also tend to be outside the optimal range for fluorescence near-infrared imaging exhibiting an absorbance maximum of 670 nm and emission maximum at 700 nm. Nonetheless, the group demonstrated the efficacy of their fluorescent agent in cultured cells and millimeter-sized lesions in tumor-bearing mice. The excitation/emission of the Cy 5.5 dyes may be suitable for small-tissue volume imaging, as in the case of a mouse, but may be restricted from imaging larger tissue volumes as in the case of mammographic imaging.

2.2. Development of Bifunctional Agents

As discussed previously photosensitizers generate cytotoxic singlet oxygen upon irradiation with light of a particular wavelength (48, 49). Additionally, they also tend to exhibit fluorescence. Recently Olivo et al. investigated the utility of naturally occurring chlorins, consisting of a complex of the trisodium salt chlorin e6 (Ce6) and the hydrophilic polymer polyvinylpyrrolidone (PVP) for its potential clinical application as an imaging and PDT agent for cancer diagnosis and therapy (50, 51). These studies evaluated the fluorescence of accumulation in human bladder tumor, determined fluorescence distribution of Ce6–PVP using tissue extraction and fluorescence imaging techniques, and subsequently the fluorescence distribution of Ce6, Ce6–PVP, and Photofrin was compared in nude mice. From these studies they concluded that the Ce6–PVP formulation seemed to be a promising photosensitizer for fluorescence imaging and PDT (51–53).

In another study, Jiang et al. (54) improved the cellular uptake of the cationic porphyrin, meso-tetrakis(*N*-methylpyridinium-4-yl)porphyrin (H_2TMPyP) by increasing it hydrophobicity through the synthesis of an amphiphilic bis-porphyrin, **Fig. 16.5** (21). In this complex Yb^{III} ion is coordinated with the porphyrin macrocycle, TMPyP, which upon irradiation at 514 nm transfers the triplet-excited state to the metal. The metal then dissipates this energy by emitting strongly in the NIR region at 1000 nm. Precaution was taken to ensure the integrity of the complex and prevented the activation and/or quenching of the NIR fluorescence capability of the Yb by encapsulating the Yb^{III} ion within an anionic tripodal ligand, L_{OMe}^- [(cyclopentadienyl) tris(dimethylphosphito)-cobaltate].

Jiang et al. demonstrated that Yb-bis-porphyrin exhibited substantial PDT activity toward the rat tumor cell model sarcoma 180 and fluoresced strongly in NIR region upon uptake by cells. The results achieved from their experiments alongside the DNA photocleavage and $^1O_2$-generating activity of the complex suggested that the complex may serve as a "see and treat" bifunctional agent (21). However, no in vivo data were reported. Although numerous researchers have demonstrated that porphyrin-based photosensitizers can be used in a dual capacity as fluorescence imaging and PDT agents (9, 21, 51, 53, 55–71), these agents generally exhibit weak fluorescence and a small wavelength difference between their absorption and emission bands (Stokes shift), which limits their application in optical imaging. Pandey et al. recently developed bifunctional agents possessing both tumor-avid photosensitizers and imaging probes that can be used as PDT and tumor-imaging agents (57, 61, 72); *see* **Fig. 16.6**.

2.3. Molecular Imaging and Its Importance

Molecular imaging can be defined as the visual representation, characterization, and quantification of biological processes at the cellular and subcellular levels within intact living organisms (73). The term "molecular imaging" represents the merger of a variety of subject disciplines such as basic cell/molecular biology, chemistry, medicine, pharmacology, medical physics,

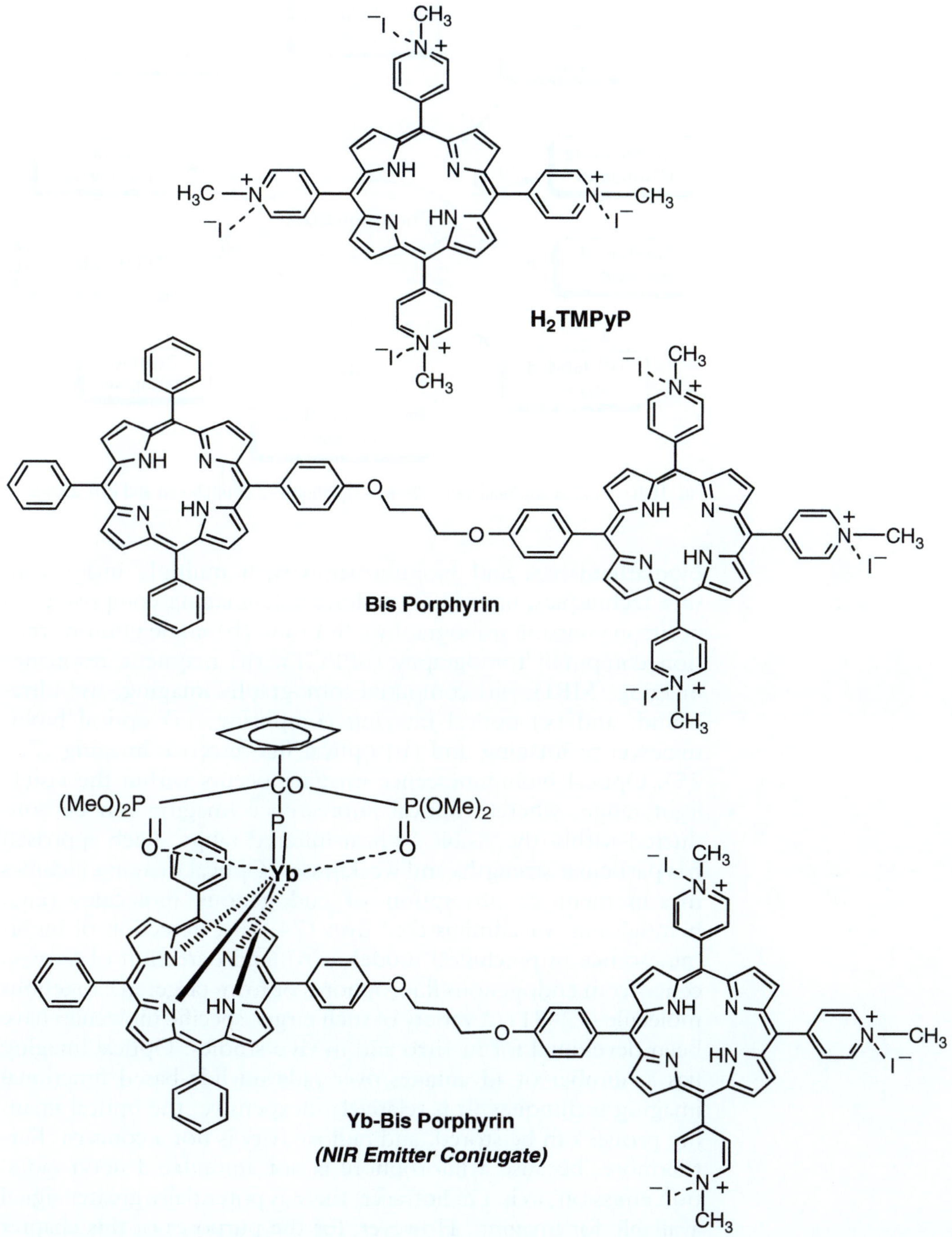

H_2TMPyP

Bis Porphyrin

Yb-Bis Porphyrin
(NIR Emitter Conjugate)

Fig. 16.5. Structures of H_2TMPyP, the amphiphilic bisporphyrin, and the Yb-bisporphyrin (NIR emitter) as bifunctional agent for fluorescence imaging and PDT.

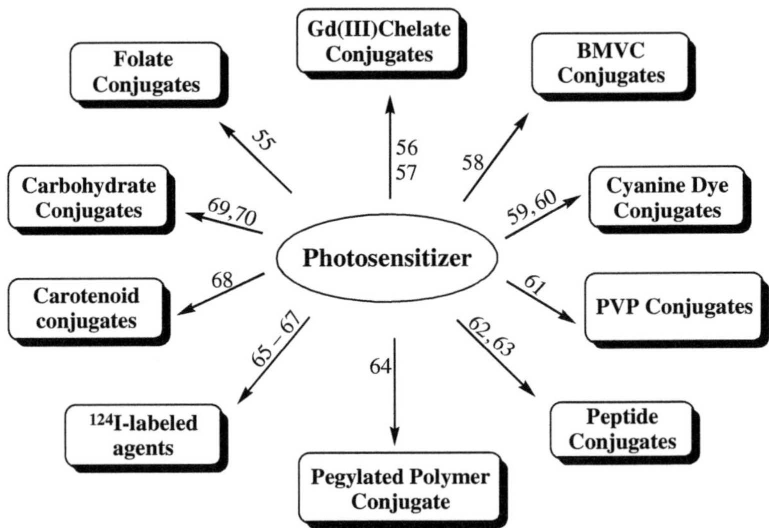

Fig. 16.6. Various approaches for developing improved bifunctional and PDT agents.

biomathematics, and bioinformatics with multiple image capture techniques, namely, (i) radionuclide imaging comprising (a) positron emission tomography (PET) and (b) single photon emission computed tomography (SPECT), (ii) magnetic resonance imaging (MRI), (iii) computed tomography imaging, (iv) ultrasound, and (v) optical imaging comprising: (a) optical bioluminescence imaging and (b) optical fluorescence imaging (73–75). Optical bioluminescence imaging occurs within the visible light range, whereas optical fluorescence imaging can be conducted within the visible or near-infrared range. Each approach has particular strengths and weaknesses. Optical imaging includes measurement of absorption of endogenous molecules (e.g., hemoglobin) or administered dyes (74, 75), detection of bioluminescence in preclinical models (76), and detection of fluorescence from endogenous fluorophores or from targeted exogenous molecule (77–81). A variety of such target-specific molecules have been developed for in vitro and in vivo studies. Optical imaging has a number of advantages over radionuclide-based functional imaging techniques. It is relatively inexpensive, the optical imaging probes can be stored, and radioactivity is not a concern. Furthermore, because a fluorophore is not annihilated upon radiation emission, as is a radiotracer, there is potentially greater signal available for imaging. However, for the purposes of this chapter we will be discussing the utility of near-infrared (NIR) fluorescence in conjunction with photodynamic therapy (PDT).

2.4. Characteristics of Near-Infrared (NIR) Fluorescence

NIR fluorescence imaging techniques have advanced considerably over the past few years, and as such are increasingly being investigated for more challenging biotechnology and biomedical applications (82) One such application is the in vivo imaging of biological targets and disease (83). The emergence of this application has enabled in vivo imaging of physiological, metabolic, and molecular function (83–86). NIR fluorescence techniques are advantageous because they are (i) highly sensitive – in that, a minute quantity of fluorochromes can be detected in live and dead cells and data-processing techniques are available for quantitative and real-time NIR imaging, (ii) cost effective, and (iii) use non-ionizing radiation (21, 73, 85). Fluorescence, which involves absorption of light and re-emission at a longer wavelength is highly sensitive, a typical cyanine dye with a lifetime of 0.6 ns can emit up to 10^{32} photons/s/mol (87). A sensitive optical detector can image $<10^3$ photons/s. Thus even with low-excitation power, low concentrations of fluorescent molecular beacons can be detected. Optical imaging instruments may be simpler and less expensive to operate than those required for other imaging technologies, thus facilitating their future incorporation in less specialized medical centers. Therapeutically (especially, in applications such as endoscopic examination), fluorescence imaging can allow precise assessment of the location and size of a tumor and provide information on its invasiveness. During debulking surgery, where malignant loci can be difficult to identify, the presence of a fluorescent signal might assist the surgeon in identifying the diseased site.

However, NIR fluorescent systems give planar images and are not quantitative, that is, anything closer to the surface will appear brighter compared with deeper structures (73). As a result, researchers have devised another approach to visualize the fluorescent probes within tissue volumes of deeper structures using a technique called optical tomography. In vivo NIR fluorescence imaging is usually conducted within the "NIR window," also known as the "diagnostic window" of 700–900 nm. This is because light scattering is minimized and tissues and body fluids, such as oxy- and deoxyhemoglobin, lipids, and water, the major endogenous absorbers of visible and infrared light, respectively, exhibit their lowest absorption coefficients in the NIR region (73, 88, 89), *see* **Fig. 16.7**. Imaging within this range minimizes tissue autofluorescence, allowing photons to propagate further into tissue thus enabling the detection of fluorochromes deep within tissue resulting in substantial enhancement of target/background ratios (21, 73, 89).

As previously mentioned, fluorescence techniques are attractive because they are highly sensitive and they enable the detection of picomoles of light-emitting fluorophores in heterogenous mediums. As a result, aberrant molecular events that indicate early manifestation of diseases can be assessed by tissue-specific fluorescent biomolecules. A variety of exogenous probes belonging to a family of polymethine cyanine-based fluorophores are in

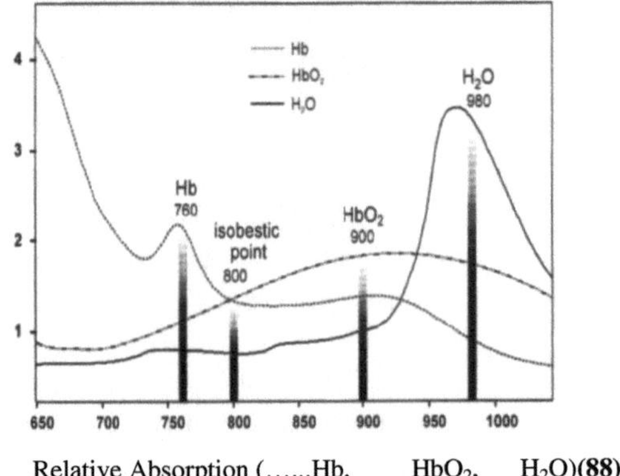

Relative Absorption (……Hb, _ _ _HbO$_2$,___H$_2$O)(**88**)

Fig. 16.7. Indicates the near-infrared (650–1100 nm) spectra of deoxyhemoglobin (Hb), oxyhemoglobin (HbO$_2$), and water (H$_2$O) (88).

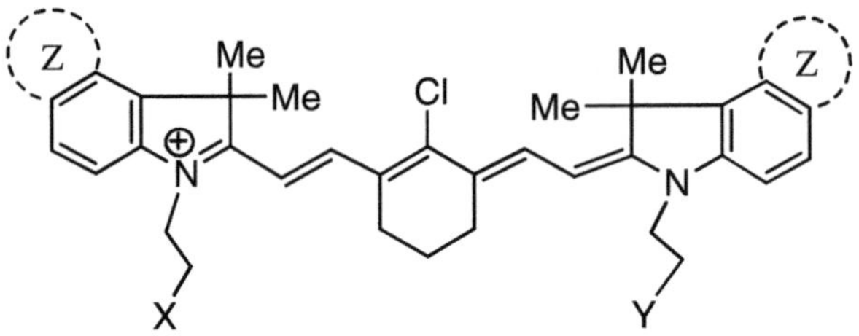

Z = Various aromatic or aliphatic groups; X,Y = Various functional groups

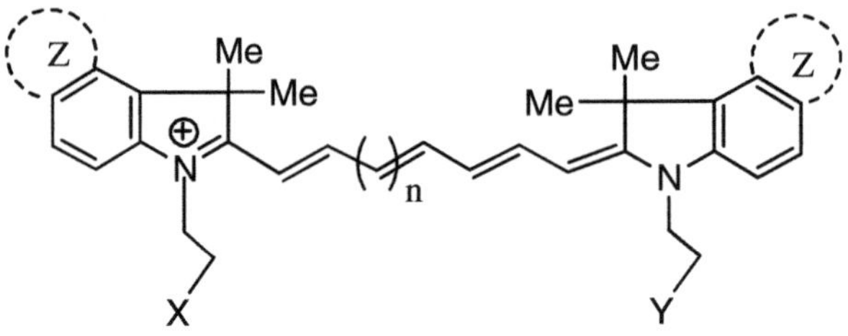

Fig. 16.8. Structures of NIR fluorophores belonging to a family of polymethine cyanine dyes.

widespread use as NIR probes and are currently being investigated in vitro and in vivo studies. General structural skeletons of these dyes are shown in **Fig. 16.8**.

Currently a variety of cyanine dyes are under investigation as the main class of NIR probes for in vivo fluorescence imaging because they usually possess large extinction coefficients, moderate-to-high fluorescence quantum yields, and broad wavelength tenability (52). However, most of these compounds are not tumor avid with poor pharmacokinetic properties. Thus conjugation of certain tumor-avid photosensitizers with near-infrared fluorochromes (NIRFs) ensures that these bifunctional agents exhibit a mutual symbiotic effect, in that, the enhanced tumor avidity of the NIR probes by the PS allows improved fluorescence imaging with photosensitizing ability.

2.5. Imaging and Therapeutic Potential of HPPH–Cyanine Dye Conjugates

It has been shown by Pandey and coworkers that tumor-avid photosensitizer, e.g., HPPH (a chlorophyll-*a* analog) on conjugating with a cyanine dye (modified IR-820) can be used as a bifunctional agent for tumor imaging and phototherapy (59). This conjugate was evaluated for tumor imaging and photosensitizing ability at variable doses and time intervals and shows promising tumor imaging capability at a dose of 0.3 μmol/kg in C_3H mice with RIF tumors or BALB/c mice bearing colon-26 tumors at 24, 48, and 72 h post-injection **(Figs. 16.9 and 16.10)**.

However, the therapeutic dose was much higher (10-fold) than the imaging dose to achieve the similar long-term tumor response as that of HPPH. Therefore for reducing the PDT drug dose, we structurally modified the conjugate by introducing one more HPPH moiety and the $(HPPH)_2$-CD conjugate thus obtained was evaluated for tumor imaging and photosensitizing efficacy. The tumor imaging, biodistribution, and in vivo photosensitizing data obtained from both conjugates are summarized in **Fig. 16.11a, b**, which indicate that introducing another HPPH moiety to HPPH-CD conjugate does not produce any significant enhancement in tumor imaging and PDT efficacy.

2.6. Spectroscopic Measurements

The in vitro electronic absorption spectra and the fluorescence spectra of HPPH-CD and $(HPPH)_2$-CD conjugates are shown in

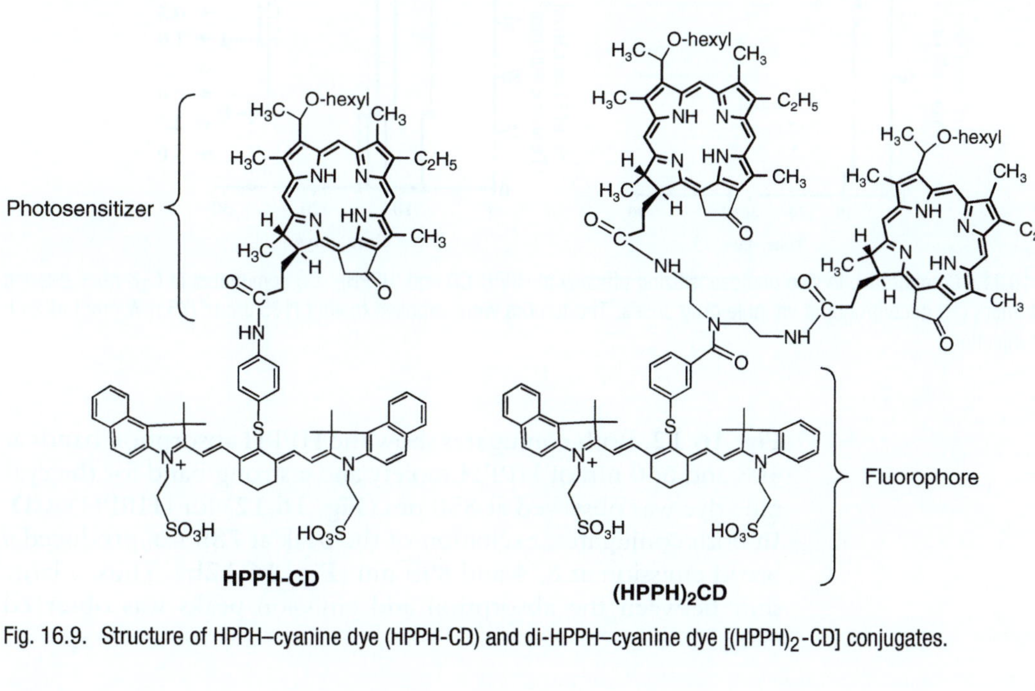

Fig. 16.9. Structure of HPPH–cyanine dye (HPPH-CD) and di-HPPH–cyanine dye [$(HPPH)_2$-CD] conjugates.

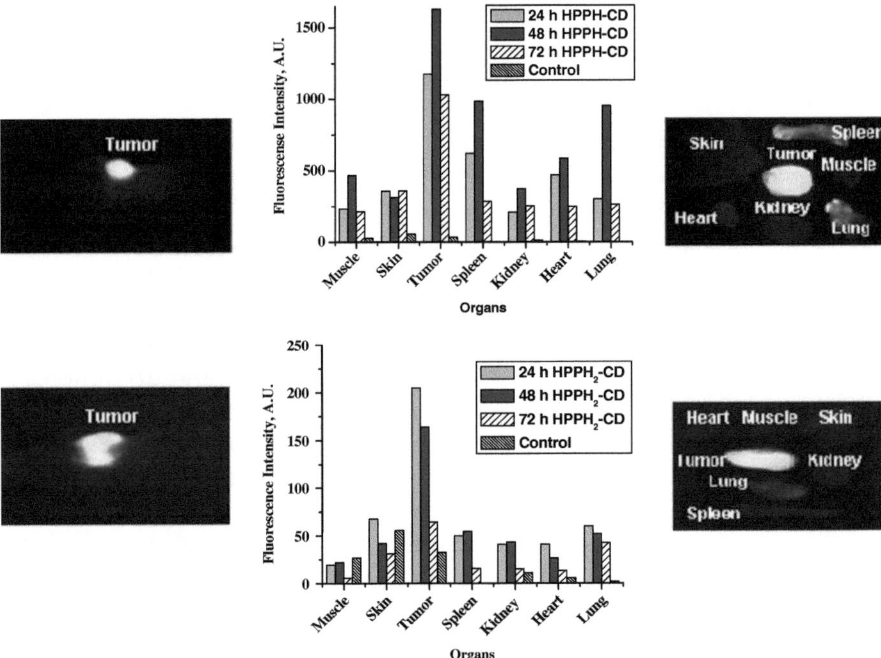

Fig. 16.10. Comparative tumor imaging, biodistribution, and organ specificity of HPPH-CD and $(HPPH)_2$-CD conjugates, respectively (dose: 0.3 μmol/kg), in BALB/c mice (three mice/group) bearing colon26 tumors at 48 h post-injection (λ_{ex}: 785 nm).

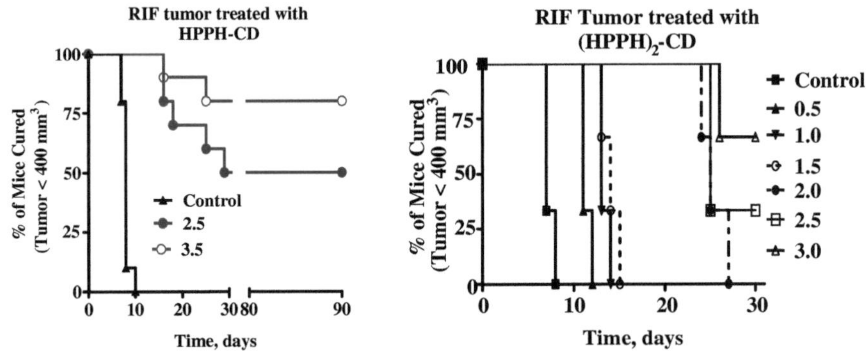

Fig. 16.11. Comparative in vivo photosensitizing efficacy of HPPH-CD and $(HPPH)_2$-CD conjugates in C_3H mice bearing RIF tumors (10 mice/group) at variable drug doses. The tumors were exposed to light (135 J/cm^2/75 mW/cm^2) at 24 h post-injection.

Fig. 16.12. Both conjugates show the HPPH absorption bands at 408 and 660 nm of HPPH moiety and a strong band for the cyanine dye was observed at 850 nm (**Fig. 16.12**) for $(HPPH)_2$CD. In both conjugates, excitation of the peak at 785 nm produced a broad emission at 874 and 890 nm (**Fig. 16.12b**). Thus, a large shift between the absorption and emission peaks was observed (90).

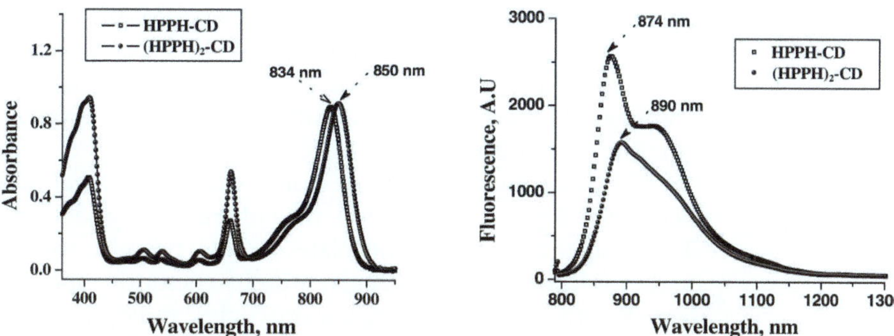

Fig. 16.12. (**a**) Absorbance spectrum and (**b**) fluorescence spectrum of HPPH-CD and $(HPPH)_2CD$ (Stokes shift of 40 nm).

2.7. Tumor-Targeted Bifunctional Agents

Folate receptors (FRs) are known to display limited distribution on normal cells but are significantly expressed on malignant cells and activated macrophages (91–93). The isoforms that are highly up-regulated on cancer cells and activated macrophages are FR-α and FR-β, respectively. FRs are usually overexpressed on epithelial cancers of the ovary, lung, endometrium, uterus, brain, kidney, colon, breast, prostate, head and neck, mesothelium, and hematopoietic cells of the myelogenous origin, including chronic and acute myelogenous leukemia (91–95). The up-regulation of FRs in various malignant tissues is significant because it aids in patient diagnosis, that is, FR expression helps to determine the histological stage and grade of the tumor. Highly undifferentiated metastatic tumors express more FRs and this leads to poor prognosis (92–94).

Overexpression of FRs is also prominent on activated macrophages because these are associated with a variety of inflammatory and autoimmune diseases such as rheumatoid arthritis, atherosclerosis, psoriasis, systemic lupus erythematosus, Crohn's disease, diabetes, ulcerative colitis, osteoarthritis, glomerulonephritis, and sarcoidosis (91).

FR expression was found on the apical or luminal surface of normal polarized epithelial cells, chiefly, choroid plexus, placenta, lung, intestine, and kidney (91, 95). These cells are mainly involved in retention and uptake of folate. Some concerns were raised that the development of folate-linked therapeutics could potentially be toxic to both malignant and normal cells, given that FRs are also present on the above-mentioned normal cells. However, these concerns were alleviated as ongoing research showed FRs that are apically distributed are mostly inaccessible to blood-borne folate conjugates and as a consequence have not been found to cause adverse toxicity in normal cells (91).

2.8. Folate as a Targeting Moiety

Having the knowledge that folic acid has a high affinity for FR, targeting folate-conjugated chemotherapeutic and imaging agents to specific pathological sites became feasible. This application is essential because drugs that would have otherwise been toxic toward both malignant and normal cells in their non-conjugated form could now be administered and delivered to specific sites when conjoined to folic acid.

To date, numerous folate-conjugated pharmaceuticals have been developed and applied to enhance drug delivery (96). These agents include antifolate drugs, protein toxins, cytotoxic molecules, low molecular weight chemotherapeutics, liposomes with enclosed drug, nanoparticles, radiopharmaceuticals, immunotherapeutic agents, near-infrared (NIR) fluorochromes, and photosensitizers used for photodynamic therapy (97). It is noteworthy that only a few articles exist on delivering PDT agents via FR. In order to circumvent some of the issues highlighted above in terms of selective and specific delivery of PS to tumor, Schneider (98) conjugated certain PSs with folic acid in order to compare the uptake of the drug in folate expressing (FR+, KB) cells versus non-folate expressing cancer cells (FR–, HT1080) in vitro and in vivo, respectively (71, 98). Schneider approached the PS-folate synthesis by tethering tetraphenylporphyrin (TPP) to folic acid via two linkers. In the first synthetic strategy, hexane-1,6-diamine was used a linker, which was later replaced with a small PEG, 2′2-(ethylenedioxy)-*bis*-ethylamine to increase water solubility and biocompatibility of the conjugate, **Fig. 16.13** (98).

A series of experiments was conducted in order to observe the accumulation, antiproliferation, and phototoxicity of the 4-carboxyphenylporphyrin–folic acid conjugates versus TPP in KB tumor cells. After 6 h incubation, it became evident that the conjugates significantly accumulated within KB cells compared to the non-conjugate analog.

Additionally, the cellular uptake of the conjugates was sevenfold higher after a 24 h exposure (98). In the phototoxicity experiments KB cells were incubated with TPP and the conjugates. The photosensitivity of the folate conjugates was significantly improved in comparison to TPP photosensitization (98). Based on the studies conducted, Schneider showed that folate-mediated targeting of the PS modified the photobiological activity of the reference molecule TPP because a higher and more selective intracellular folate-conjugated PS concentration was obtained which enhanced their cytotoxic effect after photoactivation (98). Another essential component of this work was that the nature of the linker also influenced drug efficacy.

Zheng and coworkers extended the foregoing approach in pyropheophorbide system and the pyropeptide–folic acid conjugate (**Fig. 16.14**) was synthesized to improve the delivery of the PDT agent with fluorescence-imaging capability (71). The construct was composed of three components: (i) a fluorescent

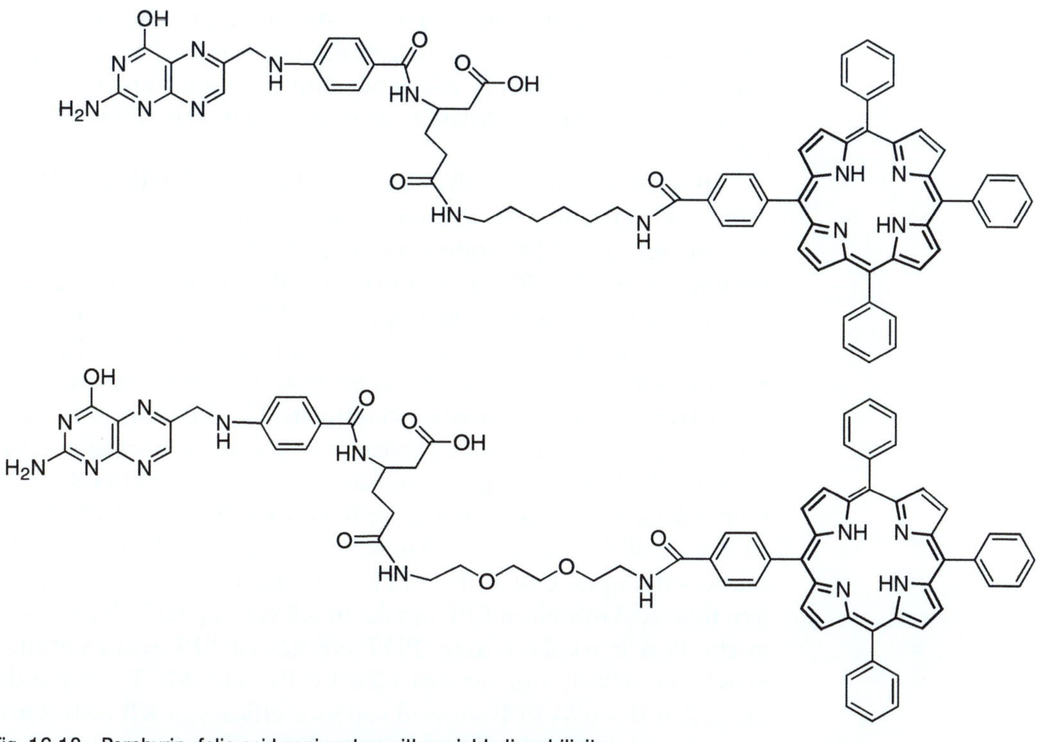

Fig. 16.13. Porphyrin–folic acid conjugates with variable lipophilicity.

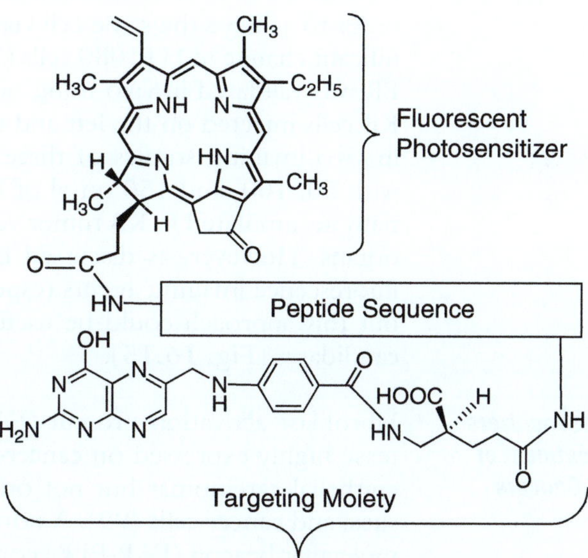

Fig. 16.14. Folate receptor targeting agent for imaging and PDT.

photosensitizer pyropheophorbide – a (Pyro) for NIR imaging (665 nm) and PDT (>50% singlet O_2 yield), (ii) a short peptide sequence that serves multiple functions such as (a) stable hydrophobic linker that enhances water solubility and (b) avoiding steric hindrance of FR targeting, and (iii) a pharmacomodulator for better delivery efficiency and decreased normal tissue toxicity (71), and (c) a folate moiety that guides the PS into FR + cells.

Its accumulation in FR+ (KB) and FR– (HT1080 and CHO) cells was monitored by confocal microscopy and flow cytometry. The selective PDT-induced cell killing and in vivo discrimination between KB (FR+) and HT1080 (FR–) tumors (71) was also investigated. The preferential uptake of PPF in KB and HT1080 cells was confirmed after incubating them with 50 μM PPF for 5 h and monitoring by confocal microscopy. These results indicated that PPF preferentially accumulated in KB cells (71). The FR delivery pathway was established as the main uptake mechanism for PPF by a competition assay, that is, KB, HT1080, and CHO (Chinese hamster oyster) cells were incubated with PPF and an excess of free folic acid. There was minimal influence of folic acid on the uptake of PPF in HT1080 and CHO cells, however, free folic acid inhibited PPF uptake in KB cells up to 70% as shown in the flow cytometry data. PDT efficacy of PPF was examined in KB, HT1080, and normal CHO cells. The MTT assay indicated that 0.5 μM PPF showed superior efficacy in KB cells when treated with a 5 J/cm^2 light dose. KB cell viability decreased to <10% at this treatment dose. The CHO cells required a 10-fold increase in PPF concentration and twice as much light dose in order to achieve the same cell viability, whereas there was no significant change in HT1080 cells (71). PPF targeting specificity for FR was validated in vivo using nude mice bearing HT 1080 and KB cells injected on the left and the right flank, respectively. The in vivo imaging studies of three double-tumored mice injected with 50, 100, and 150 nmol of PPF showed that PPF preferentially accumulated in KB tumor versus HT1080 and other normal organs. However, as discussed before, chlorins are not "ideal" fluorescence imaging agents (especially for deeply seated tumors) but this approach could be useful for developing more suitable candidates (**Fig. 16.15**).

2.9. Photosensitizers for the Treatment of Epithelial Cancers

Fibroblast activation protein (FAP) is a cell-surface serine protease highly expressed on cancer-associated fibroblasts of human epithelial carcinomas but not on normal fibroblasts, normal tissues, and cancer cells (99). A novel FAP-triggered photodynamic molecular beacon (FAP-PPB) comprising a fluorescent photosensitizer and a black hole quencher linked by a peptide sequence (TSGPNQEQK) specific to FAP was reported (100). FAP-PPB was effectively cleaved by both human FAP and murine FAP. By use of the HEK293 transfected cells (HEK-mFAP, FAP^+; HEK-vector, FAP^-), systematic in vitro and in vivo experiments validated the FAP-specific activation of FAP-PPB in cancer cells and

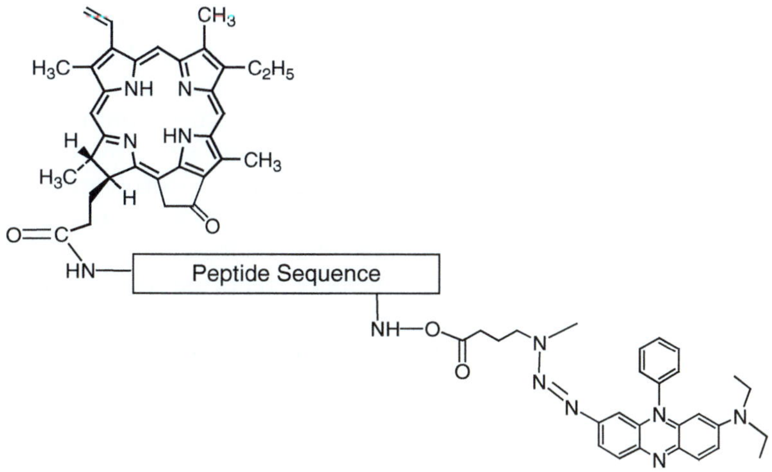

Fig. 16.15. Structure of fibroblast activation protein photosensitizer.

mouse xenografts, respectively. FAP-PPB was cleaved by FAP, allowing fluorescence restoration in FAP-expressing cells while leaving non-expressing FAP cells undetectable. Moreover, FAP-PPB showed FAP-specific photocytotoxicity toward HEK-mFAP cells whereas it was non-cytotoxic toward HEK-vector cells. This study suggested that the FAP-PPB is a potentially useful tool for epithelial cancer detection and treatment.

2.10. Bifunctional Agents for PET Imaging and PDT

Positron emission tomography (PET), a non-invasive imaging technique that exploits the unique decay physics of positron-emitting isotopes, has created enormous interest in tumor imaging in order to provide a functional or metabolic assessment of normal tissues or disease conditions (101). PET with 18F-FDG is approved by the Center for Medicare and Medicaid Services for diagnosing, staging, and restaging lung cancer, colorectal cancer, lymphoma, melanoma, head and neck cancer, and esophageal cancer (102). Although, ^{18}F-FDG is an exquisite tumor-localizing tracer; it is not tumor specific. The uptake of ^{18}F-FDG reflects glucose use in essentially any tissue; its increased uptake in tumors is a result of increased and inefficient use of glucose. Other benign processes associated with cells that have increased glucose use, such as inflammatory cells or hyperplastic bone marrow or thymic cells, also have enhanced ^{18}F-FDG uptake. Thus, increased ^{18}F-FDG uptake is usually observed in infectious and inflammatory processes, inflammatory changes after surgery or irradiation and thymic or bone marrow hyperplasia after treatment. Additionally, the short half-life of ^{18}F-isotope (110 min) limits its use in studies involving antibodies and in photodynamic therapy (PDT), where the photosensitizers take a considerably long time to both accumulate in tumors and clear from the non-targeted organs (66). In this respect, ^{124}I is a better choice due to its half-life of 4.2 days and because it enables longitudinal imaging studies using animal PET. The labeling technique for ^{124}I-isotope is now well established and this approach is continuously being used in labeling a variety of biologically active molecules (103). Speizer explored the utility of glucose by incorporating it to a fluorescent molecule into human erythrocytes and this approach was then extended in developing other analogs.

It has been reported by various investigators that introduction of glucose and β-galactose moieties in photosensitizers (104) leads to increased efficiency in tumor uptake. It is believed that ^{18}F-FDG, an analog of glucose, enters cells via glucose transporters (GLUT). In a recent similar approach, a pyropheophorbide-2-deoxyglucosamide has been reported as a new photosensitizer targeting the glucose transporters (105) and it is proposed to be trapped in tumor cells via the GLUT/hexokinase pathway. To investigate the utility of the carbohydrate moieties in developing target-specific photosensitizers, Pandey and coworkers conjugated an highly effective photosensitizer (HPPH, a chlorophyll derivative) with a series of carbohydrates and among all the compounds, the HPPH–β-galactose conjugate produced higher photosensitizing efficacy than HPPH in mice bearing RIF and colon 26 tumors (106). Based on these findings, a highly effective ^{124}I-labeled PET imaging agent [3-(1′-hexyloxyethyl)-3-devinyl pyropheophorbide-a or P-531] with significant PDT efficacy (non-labeled analog) was converted into the corresponding glucose (P-531-Glu) and galactose (P-531-Gal) derivatives (66); *see* **Fig. 16.16**.

With ^{124}I-labeled (half-life: 4.2 days) agent *P-531,* Pandey and coworkers were able to detect the tumors by PET imaging in two different models (RIF and colon-26). The long residence

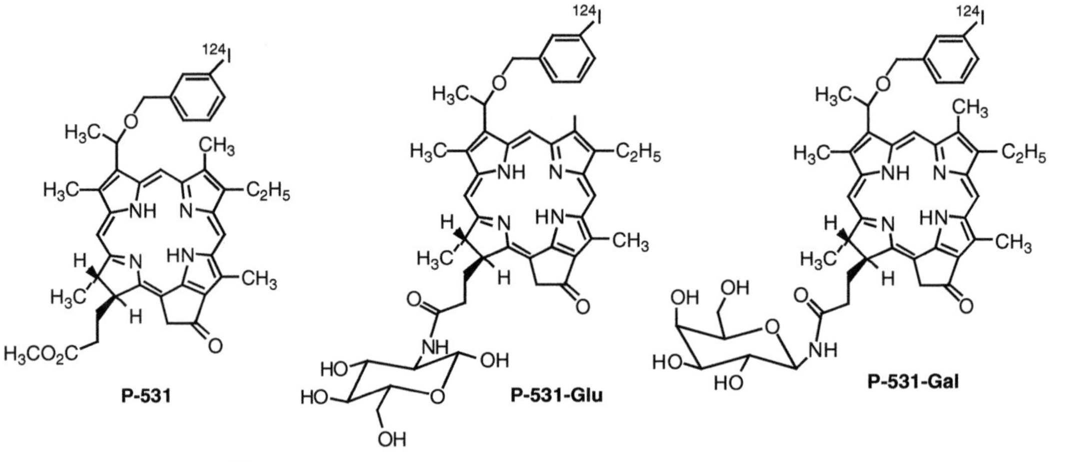

Fig. 16.16. Structure of ^{124}I-labeled chlorophyll-*a* analogs and its glucose (P531-Glu) and galactose (P-531-Gal) analogs.

time of the photosensitizer in tumor, as confirmed by the RUV and relative tumor activity values, also indicated great therapeutic potential. Compared to the compound *P-531* the corresponding glucose *P-531-Glu* and galactose *P-531-Gal* analogs showed higher uptake in both colon-26 and RIF cells. However, the in vivo biodistribution results obtained from the C3H mice bearing RIF tumors revealed that between the glucose and galactose conjugates, the galactose conjugate *P-531-Gal* had higher tumor uptake. Interestingly, due to a high uptake of the carbohydrate derivatives in liver and spleen, the parent molecule *P-531* produced the best tumor contrast in both RIF and colon-26 tumor models. The tumor images of mice bearing colon 26 tumors are shown in **Fig. 16.17** at variable time points. These photosensitizers also produced significant in vivo PDT efficacy and therefore, this approach provides a great opportunity to develop potential bifunctional agents for "see and treat" approach (**Fig. 16.17**).

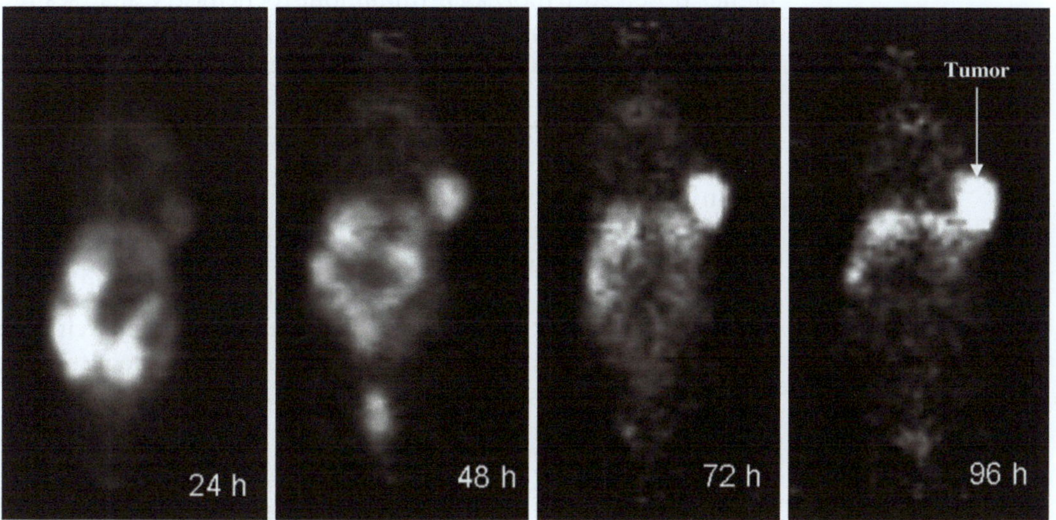

Fig. 16.17. The coronal view PET images of BALB/c mice bearing colon26 tumors on the right shoulder injected with 150 mCi ^{124}I-labeled photosensitizer P-531 (*see* **Fig. 16.16**). The studies were acquired for 30 min at 24, 48, 72, and 96 h post-injection.

2.11. Bifunctional Agents for MR Imaging and PDT

Among the MR agents developed so far, the Gd(III) chelates are the logical choice because they posses the highest relaxivity and a strong magnetic moment (107). Moreover, a key biological factor that influences the selection of Gd(III)-containing compounds for human use is that its ligands, like DTPA, circulate and are excreted intact. The metal ion buried in the chelation cage does not bind to donor groups of proteins and enzymes. This in vivo stability markedly reduces the potential for toxicity from Gd(III). Over the last decade magnetic resonance imaging has become the method of choice. As the contrast agent clears from the circulation, tumor enhancement may appear to increase, due to the rising of tumor-to-background ratio, but thereafter the tumor signal rapidly declines, as non-bound contrast medium leaches from the lesion (108). Slower clearance from the tumor would enable MR scanning of larger body volumes. Most of the Gd(III)-based MR agents which are not tumor specific do not retain in tumor for more than 10–15 min. Therefore for developing bifunctional agents for MR imaging and phototherapy, Pandey and coworkers conjugated the highly tumor-avid photosensitizer HPPH with the variable numbers of modified magnavist (a Gd(III) complex of DTPA). Among these analogs, the HPPH linked with three molecules of Gd(III)magnavist (containing a benzylamine functionality) produced enhanced tumor contrast (drug dose: 10 μmol/kg) than magnavist (100 μmol/kg) with significant in vivo PDT efficacy (**Fig. 16.18**). The normal organ toxicity of HPPH–3-Gd(III)DTPA chelate was investigated at the imaging dose (10 μmol/kg), a dose lower (5 μmol/kg), and at a higher dose (25 μmol/kg). Immunohistochemistry analyses did not show any normal organ (liver, spleen, kidney, lung, skin) toxicity. These results are of a particular interest, because the same molecule represents functions as both the contrast medium and a therapeutic agent; the lesion(s) can be continuously imaged during the PDT.

In another innovative development, Huber et al. (109) synthesized bifunctional contrast agents containing a metal chelator for binding of a paramagnetic ion such as gadolinium and a conjugated fluorescent dye such as tetramethylrhodamine to combine optical and MR imaging of experimental animals. Excitation of the rhodamine moiety at 547 nm produced the emission at 572 nm, and it was used for imaging *Xenopus laevis* embryos.

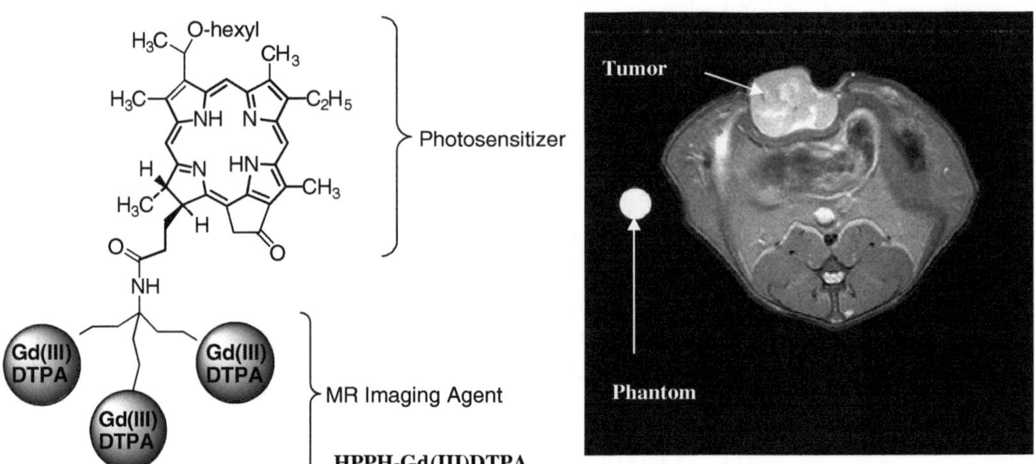

Fig. 16.18. MR images of a rat (Fischer) bearing Ward colon tumors with HPPH–3-Gd(III) conjugate (dose: 10.0 μmol/kg) at 24 h post-injection.

Although, this wavelength is not useful for treating deeply seated tumors, replacing rhodamine with dyes >800 nm may develop bifunctional contrast agents for MR and optical imaging.

3. Methods

3.1. Evaluation of In Vivo PDT Efficacy (Kaplan Meier Plot)

The female C3H/HeJ mice were intradermally injected with 2×10^5 RIF cells in 30 (l HBSS without Ca^{2+} and Mg^{2+} on the flank and tumors were grown until they reached 4–5 mm in diameter. The day before laser light treatment, all hair was removed from the inoculation site and the mice were injected intravenously with varying photosensitizers' doses. At 24 h post-injection, the mice were restrained without anesthesia in plastic holders and then treated with laser light from a dye laser tuned to emit drug-activating wavelengths. The treatment parameters consisted of an irradiated area of 1 cm^2, at a fluence rate of 75 mW/cm^2 for a dose of 135 J/cm^2. The mice were observed daily for signs of weight loss, necrotic scabbing, or tumor re-growth. If tumor growth appeared, the tumors were measured using two orthogonal measurements L and W (perpendicular to L) and the volumes were calculated using the formula $V = (L \times W^2)/2$ and recorded. Mice were considered cured if there was no sign of tumor re-growth by day 60 post-PDT treatment.

3.2. Fluorescence Imaging

The imaging potential of the conjugate was investigated at a dose of 0.3 μmol/kg in BALB/c mice (three mice/group) bearing colon 26 tumors on the right shoulder. The mice were naired near the tumor area prior to i.v. injections of the dye and the conjugate.

A frequency tripled pulsed Nd:YAG (neodymium:yttrium–aluminum–garnet) laser beam was used to pump an optical parametric oscillator (OPO) (Opotek Inc. Carlsbad, CA) and with the use of the proper IR filter (Omega optics, model # P7 0-700-S-LP, Brattleboro, VT) the signal beam was separated from the unwanted idler beam. Excitation light directly from the laser source through a beam expander, custom built in our laboratory with high-quality lenses from American Optical, Buffalo NY, projects a uniform beam on to the field of view (FOV). This area includes the tumor area plus a surrounding diameter of approximately 1″, in the peritumoral FOV.

The detection system was designed with the sensitivity necessary for recording the low levels of fluorescent photons emitted by the dye-photosensitizer conjugate and dye alone that are present in vivo. An intensified charge coupled device (ICCD) was used as the photon detector. This is comprised of Gen IV

18 mm multichannel plate (MCP) image intensifier coupled to a two-dimensional charge coupled device (CCD) 512 × 512 pixels, (IMAX, obtained from Princeton Instruments, Trenton, NJ). The ICCD camera system synchronization is controlled by an electronic interface (Princeton Instruments ST133) and pulse generator (PG535, Stanford Research) that is compatible with a standard computer. The ICCD camera is coupled to an Acton 150 spectrograph, Trenton NJ, equipped with a rotating turret. On one face of the turret is a 500 nm blaze, 300 lines/mm grating the other side is equipped with a first surface silver mirror. Either the grating or the mirror can be rotated into the beam path.

With the grating in place, the system was set up for spectroscopy analysis. Alternatively with the mirror in place the two-dimensional capability of the camera can be utilized to image drug distribution in the FOV. By placing the appropriate fluorescence emission filter in the filter wheel located behind the camera lens, a two-dimensional distribution of the drug concentration can be identified. Light is collected through a conventional zoom camera lens (Nikon model # AFNIKKOR) and projected through the spectrograph and grating onto the CCD for recording. Measurements were taken at 24, 48, and 72 h time points and experimental spectra were transferred to a PC for recording and processing.

The anesthetized mouse was taped upon a glass plate and mounted for imaging. Identical illumination settings (voltage, filters, focus (f/stop)) were used for image acquisitions. The tumor area was excited with laser light at 785 nm (total field of view is about 1″), rotating turret was set for mirror position, focus (f) set at 22, slit was properly positioned over tumor, and ROI (which typically ranged from 25 to 40 pixels upon progression of tumor volumes from time 24 to 72 h post-injection) was determined by visual inspection. Total 30 accumulations were acquired at the rate 0.1 s per accumulation, which provided a reasonably good image. Then, ROI was set and fluorescence spectrum was acquired after setting the rotating turret for grating position. Totally 30 accumulations were acquired at the rate 0.1 s per accumulation, which provided a spectrum with reasonably good intensity. A whole-body mouse image was acquired by setting the rotating turret for mirror position, f at 22, and a total of 30 accumulations were recorded. Acquired images were analyzed using WinSpec software, while the spectrum obtained was analyzed and plotted using MS Excel software. Data are presented as means and standard error of the mean.

3.3. PET Imaging

Mice were imaged in the microPET FOCUS 120®, a dedicated three-dimensional small-animal PET scanner (Concorde Microsystems Incorporated) at State University of New York at Buffalo under the Institutional Animal Care and Use Committee (IACUC) guidelines. The C3H mice were subcutaneously injected with 3×10^5 RIF cells in 30 μl complete α-MEM (into the axilla) and tumors were grown until they reached 4–5 mm in diameter (approximately 5 days). All tumored C3H mice were injected via intravenously with 72–200 μCi of 1–3 h and after 24, 48, 72, and 96 h post-injection the mice were anesthetized by inhalation of isoflurane/oxygen, placed head first prone for imaging and the acquisition time was set for 30 min. Radioiodine uptake by thyroid or stomach was not blocked. All mice going through imaging were marked with a cross-line on the back to provide a reference landmark for consistently positioning them in a series of imaging studies. The acquired data were re-binned with FORE algorithm (20) and reconstructed with two-dimensional OSEM algorithm. The dead-time and singles-based random coincidence corrections were applied to all the PET studies. The RUV results were calculated from PET images with attenuation and scatter corrections, in addition to the dead-time and random-coincidence corrections. The transmission scan for attenuation correction was carried out with a rotating ^{57}Co point source.

3.4. MR Imaging

MRI data sets were acquired for each animal to serve as baseline controls, and then animals were re-scanned 24 h after injection. For comparison to clinically administered MRI contrast agents, a separate group of rats ($n = 3$) were imaged immediately before and after the administration of Gd-DTPA (Magnevist®) via a tail-vein catheter at the clinically recommended dose of 100 μmol/kg.

Two SE imaging protocols were used with identical slice prescription parameters (5–6 axial slices, 1.5 mm slice thickness, 6 × 6 cm FOV). First, a moderately T1-weighted scan was acquired with a TE/TR of 10/1200 ms, and second, a heavily T1-weighted scan was acquired with chemical shift selective (CHESS) fat suppression with a TE/TR of 10/356.

Additionally, T1 relaxation rates for tissues were determined by acquiring a series of 6 RARE-encoded scans with TR's ranging from 360 to 6000 ms. Calculation of T1 relaxation rates were determined using non-linear regression fitting.

3.4.1. Image Processing

In vivo MR data sets were processed with Analyze by defining a region of interest (ROI) for tumor, muscle surrounding the backbone, and the 150 μM Gd-DTPA calibration standards. Following segmentation, the mean signal intensities for each ROI were sampled. To normalize signal intensity values acquired at different time points, all signal intensity values were divided by the average intensity value of the two Gd-DTPA phantoms. Normalized contrast between tumor and muscle was then determined by subtraction of the mean signal intensity of the two regions. T1 relaxation rates of tumor and back muscle were determined.

4. Notes

4.1. Drug Formulation and PDT

One of the major problems in the area of drug development (including the PDT agents) has been the biological evaluation of the compounds due to their poor solubility in water. Therefore, suitable in vivo injectable formulations are required and the concentration of the "drug" in resulting formulation(s) should be carefully determined. Fortunately, most of the photosensitizers/optical imaging agents show strong absorption in the UV–vis region and this characteristic can be used in calculating the extinction coefficient value(s) and the concentration of the desired agent(s) in the resulting formulation(s) by following the Beer–Lambert equation. Prior to biological evaluation, the purity/stability of the compound(s) in a particular formulation(s) should be ascertained by HPLC analysis. It is of utmost importance to make sure that treated area is under light exposure, and the wavelengths of light (in vitro versus in vivo) and light dose (treatment parameters) are carefully calculated. In animal model the size of the tumors to be treated should be in the same range (diameter 4.5–5.00 mm). The nature of the substituents in photosensitizer(s) makes a significant impact in their overall lipophilicity, which may alter their tumor uptake and pharmacokinetic profiles. Therefore, it becomes extremely important to determine the tumor uptake of the photosensitizer at variable time points and the tumors should be treated with light at a time of its maximum uptake.

4.2. Precautions in MR Imaging

Much of what is critical during a magnetic resonance imaging experiment lies not in the imaging, but in the proper planning of the experiment prior to execution and consistent data analysis. Issues such as the amount of samples used in the study, choice of animal species, and the position of the tumor are critical decisions which will affect the outcome of the study. Furthermore there are technical aspects of the scanning procedure which weigh heavily on the quality of images rendered.

Imaging live animals introduces multiple biological sources of variability into imaging data sets, and therefore careful choice of the number of animals per group needs to be given consideration. Tumors, for instance, can have dramatically different vascular, biochemical, and structural differences even when grown out of identical cell lines, which therefore will introduce a biologic variability that must be accounted for with inclusion of multiple animals from each type of group being studied. Cohorts no smaller than three must be used to apply tests for statistical relevance; more often five or greater animals are preferred to compensate for potential errors in the administration of contrast agent and scanner variability. Tumor size differences between animals should be minimized as the global vascular architecture of the tumor will vary with tumor size. Imaging should be carried out before the onset of necrosis within tumors, which may confound results.

Positioning of both the tumor on the animal and within the bore should be considered before the experiment. In our work, it has been found that tumors located on the posterior of the dorsal side of the subject (slightly above the tail) are optimal to minimize motion artifacts from the respiration of the animal. Respiratory artifacts can be "averaged out" by increasing the amount of scans acquired and averaged; however, this results in a corresponding increase in time required per animal. Although scans may be gated so as to acquire data between breaths, variations in breathing rates between animals will alter the repetition time (TR) of the scans, and therefore alter the contrast between tissues. This is especially apparent in T1-weighted imaging, where the TR is kept relatively short. It is also important to localize tumors at or near the same location of the bore of the MR scanner (isocenter is generally preferred), as spatial variability in the sensitivity of the radiofrequency coils is often present and may introduce added inter-animal variability in the signal intensities of tissues and tumors.

T1-weighted contrast will often be the type of contrast desired when using Gd(III)-based contrast agents. When acquiring multi-slice T1-weighted images using short repetition times, there is the possibility of introducing "cross-talk" between slices, which is the inadvertent excitations of hydrogen spins in adjacent slices to the slice the scanner is trying to excite. Interleaving the acquisition of the slice (e.g., first acquiring all odd-numbered slices, then acquiring all even-numbered slices) will help to reduce the effect of cross-talk, as will introducing a slight gap (10–20% of slice thickness) between slices. Even with these precautions, cross-talk may not be completely eliminated with very short TR's. Therefore, a phantom should be included (an NMR tube filled with 100 μM Gd-DTPA or similar Gd-based contrast agent) to determine the degree of inter-slice variability. Due to the geometry of the acquisition, outer slices will experience less cross-talk, and will often have increased signal intensity as compared to inner slices. Use of a phantom will allow the investigator to decide if this signal difference is significant; if so, data from outer slices should be excluded from analysis.

MR signal intensity is a relative measurement, as differences in receiver gain and RF coil intensity in the images. To account for this, sealed phantoms should be included within the imaging field of view to serve as normalization factors. Each data set should be normalized to signal intensity of the phantom. Multiple phantoms located at multiple locations around the animal offer greater stability of signal, though phantom location between scans should be consistent to account for RF coil sensitivity variability (see above). Choice of contrast agents used within phantoms is critical to the type of studies to be carried out within the animals. As a rule of thumb, the signal intensity of phantoms should be near the mean signal intensity of the tissues being imaged to serve as a suitable normalization factor. Distilled water (or low concentration of Gd(III)-based contrast agents) may be appropriate for T1-weighted imaging, but will dominate the signal in an image in T2-weighted image. A mixture of water and deuterium oxide (D_2O) will reduce the signal intensity arising from the phantom, as the deuterium isotope of hydrogen will not produce any signal in the MR image.

Lastly, anesthesia must be used for carrying out imaging using small animal models of disease. Unless addressed, anesthesia will cause core body temperature to drop, which will have an effect on signal intensity. First, T1 relaxation rates of tissues may increase at lower temperatures and the net population of spins in the lower energy state will also increase. Both of these factors will increase the signal to noise in acquired images, which will in turn increase contrast to noise measurements between tissues, which is often used as a metric for tissue conspicuity. To maintain body temperature of the animals for the dual purpose of (a) the health of the animal and (b) the quality of imaging data, either a flowing warm water bath or warm air blowing around the animal may be used. Flowing water may introduce phase artifacts within the image, therefore heating by warm air is generally preferred. Core body temperature of the animals should be monitored during imaging and should remain consistent between imaging sessions.

4.3. Precautions in PET Imaging

As the established PET protocol results from a combination of cellular, molecular biological, physiological, chemical, and imaging approaches, strong collaboration between the various groups is essential for its successful performance.

4.3.1. Image Reconstruction and Data Analysis

(a) Determine the framing sequence for the list mode data (i.e., 6–30 s, 2–1 min, 5–5 min, and 4–7.5 min) and reconstruct with filtered back projection (FBP) using ASIPro software.

(b) Reconstruct a single time frame using the three-dimensional iterative maximum a posteriori (MAP) algorithm to improve organ identification and the accuracy of positioning regions of interest (ROI).

(c) Determine the 2–3 slices in which the kidney or liver is best visualized and draw circular ROIs (same size ROI in all the slices) on the kidney or liver areas of the MAP image.

(d) Reposition the ROIs on the corresponding slices of the kinetically reconstructed data and generate time activity curves (TACs) for each region.

(e) Convert the counts/pixel/min obtained from the ROI to counts/ml/min by using the calibration constant obtained from scanning a cylinder phantom filled with a known concentration of activity in the microPET scanner.

(f) Convert the ROI counts/ml/min to counts/g/min.

4.3.2. Troubleshooting

(a) Problem: chromatogram aberrant, failure to collect the peak of right compound.
Reason: the column had contact with a wrong eluent.
Solution: flush the column for at least 30 min with the right eluent, inject second half of the reaction mixture.

(b) Problem: mouse moved during scanning.
Reason: the level of anesthesia is insufficient.
Solution: carefully control the levels of component gases to maintain a proper state of anesthesia. The quality of imaging critically depends on the condition of the experimental animal. Therefore, continuously monitor the vital parameters during the scanning. If animal moves during scanning, reliable time activity curves (TACs) cannot be obtained unless sophisticated movement correction algorithms are applied, which are currently not adequately validated for mice full-body imaging.

(c) Problem: tumors are not detected by PET imaging or poor signal-to-background ratio was observed.
Reason: several possibilities.
Solution:
(i) It is critical to have high quality of tumors. PET signals will be reduced with low quality of tumors.
(ii) High background signals from the gut may be detectable due to endogenous kinases. In our experience, this background signal varies between individual animals.
(iii) Critical steps:
(a) Radioactive compound should be smoothly injected to the tail of the mice.
(b) When tumoring mice, restrict spread of the cells to a limited area; if the needle is inserted too far, the tumor could spread to many organs by capillary traveling.
(c) Use mice bearing clean and intact tumors.
(d) Animals should have free access to water and are fully hydrated prior to scanning so that renal function is good.

(f) The quality of imaging critically depends on the condition of the experimental animal. Therefore, it is advisable to monitor vital parameters during anesthesia: respiratory and pulse rate, pO_2/pCO_2, and maintain body temperature with a lamp placed above the animal or a water-heated pad. There should be no animal movement during scanning since reliable time activity curves (TACs) cannot be obtained.

4.4. Precautions in Fluorescence Imaging

The imaging methodology described in this chapter is basically a planar illumination technique. This technique is also known as fluorescence reflectance imaging, whereby the illumination source, laser light, and the detection device, EMCCD, are placed on the same side of the sample being imaged. The laser diode used to excite the sample should be set at an oblique angle in order to minimize any back-reflected laser light. Precaution should be taken to spread the light uniformly in the sample area or field of view (FOV) via a beam expander to a plate of diffusing glass. Field homogeneity should be tested using a white sample (imaged with the EMCCD camera through a neutral density filter), and an ideal imaging area should be identified. All subsequent measurements should be conducted within this area.

A proper filter should be used to remove any back-reflected laser light before being recorded by the EMCCD. The exposure time and EM gain should be adjusted to maximize the dynamic range of the strongest expected signal.

Acknowledgments

We are highly thankful to our collaborators over the years for their contributions. There name can be found in various citations. We also thank the NIH (CA55791, CA109914, CA114053, CA127639), Roswell Park Alliance, the Oncologic Foundation of Buffalo, and the shared resources of the RPCI (support Grant P30CA16056) for the financial support.

References

1. Dougherty, T. J., Gomer, C. J., Henderson, B. W., Jori, G., Kessel, D., Korbelik, M., Moan, J., and Peng, Q. (1998) Photodynamic therapy. *J Natl Cancer Inst*, **90**, 889–905.
2. Jori, G. (2004) Photodynamic therapy: basic and preclinical aspects. In: Horspool, W. and Francesco, L. (eds.) CRC Handbook of Organic Photochemistry and Photobiology. Boca Raton: CRC Press, Chapter 146.
3. Kessel, D. (2004) Delivery of photosensitizing agents. *Adv. Drug Delivery Rev*, **56**(**1**), 7–8.
4. Dolmans, D. E. J. G., Fukumura, D., and Jain, R. K. (2003) Photodynamic therapy for cancer. *Nat Rev Cancer*, **3**(**5**), 380.

5. Pandey, R. K. and Zheng, G. (2000) Porphyrins as photosensitizers in photodynamic therapy. *Porphyrin Handb,* **6**, 157–230. and the references therein.
6. Pandey, R. K., James, N., Chen, Y., and Dobhal, M. P. (2008) *Topics in Heterocyclic Chemistry*. Berlin/Heidelberg: Springer, Vol. 14/2008, 41–74.
7. Henderson, B. W. and Dougherty, T. J. (1992) How does photodynamic therapy work? *Photochem Photobiol,* **55**, 145–157.
8. Sternberg, E. D., Dolphin, D., and Bruckner, C. (1998) Porphyrin-based photosensitizers for the use in photodynamic therapy. *Tetrahedron,* **54**(**17**), 4151–4202.
9 Sherman, W. M., Allen, C. M., and van Lier, J. E. (2000) Role of activated oxygen species in photodynamic therapy. *Methods Enzymol,* **319**, 376–386.
10. MacDonald, I. and Dougherty, T. J. (2001) Basic principles of photodynamic therapy. *J Porphyrins Phthalocyanines,* **5**(**105**), 2001–2011.
11. Weishaupt, K. R., Gomer, C. J., and Dougherty, T. J. (1976) Identification of singlet oxygen as the cytotoxic agent in photoinactivation of murine tumor. *Cancer Res,* **90**, 889–899.
12. Ali, H. and Van Lier, J. E. (1999) Metal complexes as photo- and radiosensitizers. *Chem Rev (Washington, DC),* **99**, 2379–2450.
13. Bonnett, R. (1995) Photosensitizers of the porphyrin and phthalocyanine series for photodynamic therapy. *Chem Soc Rev,* **24**, 19–33.
14. Chen, Y., Sumlin, A., Morgan, J., Gryshuk, A., Oseroff, A., Henderson, B. W., Dougherty, T. J., and Pandey, R. K. (2004) Synthesis and photosensitizing efficacy of isomerically pure bacteriopurpurinimides. *J Med Chem,* **47**, 4814–4817.
15. Ethirajan, M., Saenz, C., Gupta, A., Dobhal Mahabeer, P., and Pandey Ravindra, K. (2008) In: Hamblin, M. R. and Mroz, P. (eds.), *Photosynsitizers for Photodynamic Therapy and Imaging: Advances in Photodynamic Therapy.* Boston: Artech House Series.
16. Kessel, D. (2004) Delivery of photosensitizing agents. *Adv Drug Delivery Rev,* **56**, 7–8.
17. Oleinick, N. L., Morris, R. L., and Belichenko, I. (2002) The role of apoptosis in response to photodynamic therapy: what, where, why, and how. *Photochem Photobiol Sci,* **1**, 1–21.
18. Pandey, R. K., Goswami, L. N., Chen, Y., Gryshuk, A., Missert, J. R., Oseroff, A., and Dougherty, T. J. (2006) Nature: a rich source for developing multifunctional agents. Tumor-imaging and photodynamic therapy. *Lasers Surg Med,* **38**, 445–467.
19. Pandey, R. K. and Herman, C. K. (1998) Shedding some light on tumors. *Chem Ind (London),* 739–743.
20. Brown, S. B., Brown, E. A., and Walker, I. (2004) The present and future role of photodynamic therapy in cancer treatment. *Lancet Oncol,* **5**, 497–508.
21. Fingar, V. H., Wieman, J., Wiehle, S. A., and Cerrito, P. B. (1992) The role of microvasulature damage in photodynamic therapy: the effect of treatment on vessel constriction, permeability and leukocyte adhesion. *Cancer Res,* **53**, 4914–4924.
22. Fingar, V. H., Wieman, T. J., Karavolos, P. S., Doak, K. W., Ouellet, R., and van Lier, J. E. (1993) The effects of photodynamic therapy using different substituted phthalocyanines on vessel constriction, vessel leakage and tumor response. *Photochem Photobiol,* **58**, 251.
23. Pandey, R. K., Sumlin, A. B., Constantine, S., Aoudia, M., Potter, W. R., Bellnier, D. A., Henderson, B. W., Rodgers, M. A., Smith, K. M., and Dougherty, T. J. (1996) Alkyl ether analogs of chlorophyll-*a* derivatives, Part 1: synthesis, photophysical properties and photodynamic efficacy. *Photochem Photobiol,* **64**, 194–204.
24. Tarantola, R. M., Law, J. C., Recchia, F. M., Sternberg, P., Jr., and Agarwal, A. (2008) Photodynamic therapy as treatment of chronic idiopathic central serous chorioretinopathy. *Lasers Surg Med,* **40**, 671–675.
25. Betz, C. S., Rauschning, W., Stranadko, E. P., Riabov, M. V., Albrecht, V., Nifantiev, N. E., and Hopper, C. (2008) Optimization of treatment parameters for Foscan-PDT of basal cell carcinomas. *Lasers Surg Med,* **40**, 300–311.
26. Berkovitch, G., Doron, D., Nudelman, A., Malik, Z., and Rephaeli, A. (2008) Novel multifunctional acyloxyalkyl ester prodrugs of 5-aminolevulinic acid display improved anticancer activity independent and dependent on photoactivation. *J Med Chem,* **51**, 7356–7369.
27. Ohshiro, T., Nakajima, T., Sasaki, K., Fujii, S., and Taniguchi, Y. (2008) Photodynamic therapy with Talaporfin sodium for capillary hemangioma in a chicken comb model. *Laser Surg Med, Suppl 20, Meeting Abstract,* **339**, 102.
28. Woodhams Josephine, H., MacRobert Alexander, J., Novelli, M., and Bown Stephen, G. (2006) Photodynamic therapy with WST09 (Tookad): quantitative studies in normal colon and transplanted tumours. *Int J Can (Journal international du cancer),* **118**, 477–482.

29. Pandey, R. K. et al. Unpublished results.
30. Ke, M. S., Xue, L. -y, Feyes, D. K., Azizuddin, K., Baron, E. D., McCormick, T. S., Mukhtar, H., Panneerselvam, A., Schluchter, M. D., Cooper, K. D. et al. (2008) Apoptosis mechanisms related to the increased sensitivity of Jurkat T-cells vs A431 epidermoid cells to photodynamic therapy with the phthalocyanine Pc 4. *Photochem Photobiol,* **84**, 407–414.
31. Taquet, J. -p., Frochot, C., Manneville, V. and Barberi-Heyob, M. (2007) Phthalocyanines covalently bound to biomolecules for a targeted photodynamic therapy. *Curr Med Chem,* **14**, 1673–1687.
32. Milgrom, L. R. (2008) Towards recombinant antibody-fragment targeted photodynamic therapy. *Sci Prog,* **91**, 241–263.
33. Chen, B., Pogue, B. W., Hoopes, P. J., and Hasan, T. (2006) Vascular and cellular targeting for photodynamic therapy. *Crit Rev Eukaryot Gene Expr,* **16**, 279–305.
34. Henry, J. M. and Isaacs, J. T. (1989) Synergistic enhancement of the efficacy of the bioreductively activated alkylating agent RSU-1164 in the treatment of prostatic cancer by photodynamic therapy. *J Urol,* **142**, 165–170.
35. Urizzi, P., Allen, C. M., Langlois, R., Ouellet, R., La Madeleine, C., and Van Lier, J. E. (2001) Low-density lipoprotein-bound aluminum sulfophthalocyanine: targeting tumor cells for photodynamic therapy. *J Porphyr Phthalocyanines,* **5**, 154–160.
36. Henderson, B. W., Bellnier, D. A., Greco, W. R., Sharma, A., Pandey, R. K., Vaughan, L. A., Weishaupt, K. R., and Dougherty, T. J. (1997) An in vivo quantitative structure-activity relationship for a congeneric series of pyropheophorbide derivatives as photosensitizers for photodynamic therapy. *Cancer Res,* **57**, 4000–4007.
37. Raab, O. (1900) Action of fluorescent materials on infusorial substances. *Zeitschrift fuer Biologie (Munich),* **39**, 524–546.
38. Winkelman, J. and Rasmussen-Taxdal, D. S. (1960) Quantitative determination of porphyrin uptake by tumor tissue following parenteral administration. *Bull Johns Hopkins Hosp,* **107**, 228–233.
39. Lipson, R. L. and Baldes, E. J. (1960) The photodynamic properties of a particular hematoporphyrin derivative. *Arch Dermatol,* **82**, 508–516.
40. Dougherty, T. J., Grindey, G. B., Fiel, R., Weishaupt, K. R., and Boyle, D. G. (1975) Photoradiation therapy. II. Cure of animal tumors with hematoporphyrin and light. *J Natl Cancer Inst,* **55**, 115–121.
41. Dougherty, T. J., Grindley, G. B., and Weishaupt, K. R. (1975) Photoradiation therapy of animal tumors. *Proc Am Assoc Cancer Res,* **16**, 29–29.
42. Yumita, N., Han, Q. -S., Kitazumi, I., and Umemura, S.-i. (2008) Sonodynamically-induced apoptosis, necrosis, and active oxygen generation by mono-l-aspartyl chlorin e6. *Cancer Sci,* **99**, 166–172.
43. Gurfinkel, M., Thompson, A. B., Ralston, W., Troy, T. L., Moore, A. L., Moore, T. A., Gust, J. D., Tatman, D., Reynolds, J. S., Muggenburg, B. et al. (2000) Pharmacokinetics of ICG and HPPH-car for the detection of normal and tumor tissue using fluorescence, near-infrared reflectance imaging: a case study. *Photochem Photobiol,* **72**, 94–102.
44. Foster, A. E., Kwon, S., Ke, S., Lu, A., Eldin, K., Sevick-Muraca, E., and Rooney, C. M. (2008) In vivo fluorescent optical imaging of cytotoxic T lymphocyte migration using IRDye800CW near-infrared dye. *Appl Opt,* **47**, 5944–5952.
45. Poellinger, A., Martin Jan, C., Ponder Steven, L., Freund, T., Hamm, B., Bick, U., and Diekmann, F. (2008) Near-infrared laser computed tomography of the breast first clinical experience. *Acad Radiol,* **15**, 1545–1553.
46. Hawrysz, D. J. and Sevick-Muraca, E. M. (2000) Developments toward diagnostic breast cancer imaging using near-infrared optical measurements and fluorescent contrast agents. *Neoplasia (New York, NY),* **2**, 388–417.
47. Mahmood, U., Tung, C. -H., Tang, Y., and Weissleder, R. (2002) Feasibility of in vivo multichannel optical imaging of gene expression: experimental study in mice. *Radiology,* **224**, 446–451.
48. Dougherty, T. J. and Levy, J. G. (2003) Photodynamic therapy (PDT) and clinical applications. *Biomed Photonics Handb,* 38/31–38/16.
49 Henderson, B. W. and Miller, A. C. (1986) Effects of the scavengers of reactive oxygen and radical species on cell survival following photodynamic treatment in vitro: comparison to ionizing radiation. *Radiat Res,* **108**, 196.
50. Chin, W. W. L., Heng, P. W. S., and Olivo, M. (2007) Chlorin e6 – polyvinylpyrrolidone mediated photosensitization is effective against human non-small cell lung carcinoma compared to small cell lung carcinoma xenografts. *BMC Pharmacol,* 7, 15.
51. Chin, W. W. L., Heng, P. W. S., Thong, P. S. P., Bhuvaneswari, R., Hirt, W., Kuenzel, S., Soo, K. C., and Olivo, M. (2008) Improved

formulation of photosensitizer chlorin e6 polyvinylpyrrolidone for fluorescence diagnostic imaging and photodynamic therapy of human cancer. *Euro J Pharm Biopharma,* **69**, 1083–1093.

52. Pandey, R. K. et al. Unpublished results.
53. Chin, W. W. L., Lau, W. K. O., Heng, P. W. S., Bhuvaneswari, R., and Olivo, M. (2006) Fluorescence imaging and phototoxicity effects of new formulation of chlorin e6-polyvinylpyrrolidone. *J Photochem Photobio B, Biol,* **84**, 103–110.
54. Jiang, F. -L., Wong, W. -K., Zhu, X. -J., Zhou, G. -J., Wong, W. -Y., Wu, P. -L., Tam, H. -L., Cheah, K. -W., Ye, C., and Liu, Y. (2007) Synthesis, characterization, and photophysical properties of some heterodimetallic bisporphyrins of ytterbium and transition metals – enhancement and lifetime extension of Yb3+ emission by transition-metal porphyrin sensitization. *Euro J Inorg Chem,* 3365–3374.
55. Gravier, J., Schneider, R., Frochot, C., Bastogne, T., Schmitt, F., Didelon, J., Guillemin, F., and Barberi-Heyob, M. (2008) Improvement of meta-tetra(hydroxyphenyl)chlorin-like photosensitizer selectivity with folate-based targeted delivery. Synthesis and in vivo delivery studies. *J Med Chem,* **51**(**13**), 3867–3877.
56. Li, G., Slansky, A., Dobhal, M. P., Goswami, L. N., Graham, A., Chen, Y., Kanter, P., Alberico, R. A., Spernyak, J., Morgan, J. et al. (2005) Chlorophyll-a analogues conjugated with aminobenzyl-DTPA as potential bifunctional agents for magnetic resonance imaging and photodynamic therapy. *Bioconjug Chem,* **16**, 32–42.
57. Liu, J., Ohta, S. -I., Sonoda, A., Yamada, M., Yamamoto, M., Nitta, N., Murata, K., and Tabata, Y. (2007) Preparation of PEG-conjugated fullerene containing Gd3+ ions for photodynamic therapy. *J Control Release,* **117**, 104–110.
58. Chang, T. C., Chang, C. -C., Kang, C. -C., Chen, C. -T., and Lin, Y. -C. (2007) A new BMVC-porphyrin binary photosensitizer for PDT selectivity. *Mol Cancer Ther,* **6**, 3526S.
59. Chen, Y., Gryshuk, A., Achilefu, S., Ohulchansky, T., Potter, W., Zhong, T., Morgan, J., Chance, B., Prasad, P. N., Henderson, B. W. et al. (2005) A novel approach to a bifunctional photosensitizer for tumor imaging and phototherapy. *Bioconjug Chem,* **16**, 1264–1274.
60. Chen, Y., Ohkubo, K., Zhang, M., Wenbo, E., Liu, W., Pandey, S. K., Ciesielski, M., Baumann, H., Erin, T., Fukuzumi, S. et al. (2007) Photophysical, electrochemical characteristics and cross-linking of STAT-3 protein by an efficient bifunctional agent for fluorescence image-guided photodynamic therapy. *Photochem Photobiol Sci,* **6**, 1257–1267.
61. Isakau, H. A., Parkhats, M. V., Knyukshto, V. N., Dzhagarov, B. M., Petrov, E. P., and Petrov, P. T. (2008) Toward understanding the high PDT efficacy of chlorin e6-polyvinylpyrrolidone formulations: photophysical and molecular aspects of photosensitizer-polymer interaction in vitro. *J Photochem Photobiol B, Biol,* **92**, 165–174.
62. Boisbrun, M., Vanderesse, R., Engrand, P., Olie, A., Hupont, S., Regnouf-de-Vains, J. -B., and Frochot, C. (2008) Design and photophysical properties of new RGD targeted tetraphenylchlorins and porphyrins. *Tetrahedron,* **64**, 3494–3504.
63. Thomas, N., Tirand, L., Chatelut, E., Plenat, F., Frochot, C., Dodeller, M., Guillemin, F., and Barberi-Heyob, M. (2008) Tissue distribution and pharmacokinetics of an ATWLPPR-conjugated chlorin-type photosensitizer targeting neuropilin-1 in glioma bearing nude mice. *Photochem Photobiol Sci,* **7**(**4**), 433–441.
64. Li, Y., Jang, W. -D., Nishiyama, N., Kishimura, A., Kawauchi, S., Morimoto, Y., Miake, S., Yamashita, T., Kikuchi, M., Aida, T. et al. (2007) Dendrimer generation effects on photodynamic efficacy of dendrimer porphyrins and dendrimer-loaded supramolecular nanocarriers. *Chem Mater,* **19**, 5557–5562.
65. Pandey, S. K., Gryshuk, A. L., Sajjad, M., Zheng, X., Chen, Y., Abouzeid, M. M., Morgan, J., Charamisinau, I., Nabi, H. A., Oseroff, A. et al. (2005) Multimodality agents for tumor imaging (PET, fluorescence) and photodynamic therapy. A possible "see and treat" approach. *J Med Chem,* **48**, 6286–6295.
66. Pandey, S. K., Sajjad, M., Chen, Y., Zheng, X., Yao, R., Missert, J. R., Batt, C., Nabi, H. A., Oseroff, A. R., and Pandey, R. K. (2009) Comparative positron-emission tomography (PET) imaging and phototherapeutic potential of 124I-labeled methyl-3-(1′-iodobenzyloxyethyl)pyropheophorbide-a vs the corresponding glucose and galactose conjugates. *J Med Chem,* **52**, 445–455.
67. Pandey, S. K., Sajjad, M., Chen, Y., Pandey, A., Missert, J. R., Batt, C., Yao, R., Oseroff, A. R., and Pandey, R. K. (2009) Compared to purpurinimides, the pyropheophorbide containing an iodobenzyl group showed enhanced PDT efficacy and tumor imaging ability. *Bioconjug Chem,* **20**(**2**), 274–282.

68. Kang, C. -C., Chen, C. -T., Cho, C. -C., Lin, Y. -C., Chang, C. -C., and Chang, T. -C. (2008) A dual selective antitumor agent and fluorescence probe: the binary BMVC-porphyrin photosensitizer. *ChemMedChem,* **3**, 725–728.
69. Zheng, G., Graham, A., Shibata, M., Missert, J. R., Oseroff, A. R., Dougherty, T. J., and Pandey, R. K. (2001) Synthesis of beta -galactose-conjugated chlorins derived by enyne metathesis as galectin-specific photosensitizers for photodynamic therapy. *J Org Chem,* **66**, 8709–8716.
70. Li, G., Pandey, S. K., Graham, A., Dobhal, M. P., Mehta, R., Chen, Y., Gryshuk, A., Rittenhouse-Olson, K., Oseroff, A., and Pandey, R. K. (2004) Functionalization of OEP-based benzochlorins to develop carbohydrate-conjugated photosensitizers. Attempt to target beta -galactoside-recognized proteins. *J Org Chem,* **69**, 158–172.
71. Stefflova, K., Chen, J., and Zheng, G. (2007) Killer beacons for combined cancer imaging and therapy. *Curr Med Chem,* **14**, 2110–2125.
72. Stefflova, K., Li, H., Chen, J., and Zheng, G. (2007) Peptide-based pharmacomodulation of a cancer-targeted optical imaging and photodynamic therapy agent. *Bioconjug Chem,* **18**, 379–388.
73. Massoud, T. F. and Gambhir, S. S. (2003) Molecular imaging in living subjects: seeing fundamental biological processes in a new light. *Genes Dev,* **17**, 545–580.
74. Chance, B. (1998) Near-infrared images using continuous, phase-modulated, and pulsed light with quantitation of blood and blood oxygenation. *Ann N Y Acad Sci,* **838**, 29–45.
75. Chance, B., Cope, M., Gratton, E., Ramanujam, N., and Tromberg, B. (1998) Phase measurement of light absorption and scatter in human tissue. *Rev Sci Instrum,* **69**, 3457–3481.
76. Choy, G., Choyke, P., and Libutti, S. K. (2003) Current advances in molecular imaging: noninvasive in vivo bioluminescent and fluorescent optical imaging in cancer research. *Mol Imaging,* **2**, 303–312.
77. Achilefu, S., Dorshow, R. B., Bugaj, J. E., and Rajagopalan, R. (2000) Novel receptor-targeted fluorescent contrast agents for in vivo tumor imaging. *Invest Radiol,* **35**, 479–485.
78. Choi, H., Choi Seok, R., Zhou, R., Kung Hank, F., and Chen, I. W. (2004) Iron oxide nanoparticles as magnetic resonance contrast agent for tumor imaging via folate receptor-targeted delivery. *Acad Radiol,* **11**, 996–1004.
79. Gao, X., Cui, Y., Levenson Richard, M., Chung Leland, W. K., and Nie, S. (2004) In vivo cancer targeting and imaging with semiconductor quantum dots. *Nat Biotechnol,* **22**, 969–976.
80. Kelly, K., Alencar, H., Funovics, M., Mahmood, U., and Weissleder, R. (2004) Detection of invasive colon cancer using a novel, targeted, library-derived fluorescent peptide. *Cancer Res,* **64**, 6247–6251.
81. Sevick-Muraca, E. M., Godavarty, A., Houston, J. P., Thompson, A. B., and Roy, R. (2003) Near-infrared imaging with fluorescent contrast agents. *Handb Biomed Fluoresc,* 445–527.
82. Bouteiller, C., Clave, G., Bernardin, A., Chipon, B., Massonneau, M., Renard, P. -Y., and Romieu, A. (2007) Novel water-soluble near-infrared cyanine dyes: synthesis, spectral properties, and use in the preparation of internally quenched fluorescent probes. *Bioconjug Chem,* **18**, 1303–1317.
83. Weissleder, R. and Ntziachristos, V. (2003) Shedding light onto live molecular targets. *Nat Med (New York, NY, US),* **9**, 123–128.
84. Frangioni, J. V. (2003) In vivo near-infrared fluorescence imaging. *Curr Opin Chem Biol,* **7**, 626–634.
85. Klohs, J., Wunder, A., and Licha, K. (2008) Near-infrared fluorescent probes for imaging vascular pathophysiology. *Basic Res Cardiol,* **103**, 144–151.
86. Ntziachristos, V. (2006) Fluorescence molecular imaging. *Ann Rev Biomed Eng,* **8**, 1–33.
87. Sevick-Muraca, E. M., Kuwana, E., Godavatry, A., Houston, J. P., Thompson, J. P., and Roy, R. (2000) Near infra-red fluorescence imaging and spectroscopy in random media and tissues. In: Vo-Dinh, T. (ed.) Biomedical Photonics. Boca Raton: CRC Press.
88. Stranc, M. F., Sowa, M. G., Abdulrauf, B., and Mantsch, H. H. (1998) Assessment of tissue viability using near-infrared spectroscopy. *Br J Plast Surg,* **51**, 210–217.
89. Klohs, J., Graefe, M., Graf, K., Steinbrink, J., Dietrich, T., Stibenz, D., Bahmani, P., Kronenberg, G., Harms, C., Endres, M. et al. (2008) In vivo imaging of the inflammatory receptor CD40 after cerebral ischemia using a fluorescent antibody. *Stroke,* **39**, 2845–2852.
90. James, N. S., Goswami, L. N., Chen, Y., Sunar, U., Ohulchansky, T., and Pandey, R. K. Versatile Cyanine Dye Based Compounds for Tumor Imaging and Photodynamic Therapy. International Conference of Porphyrins and Phthalocyanines (ICPP-5), Moscow, July 2008.

91. Hilgenbrink, A. R. and Low, P. S. (2005) Folate receptor-mediated drug targeting: from therapeutics to diagnostics. *J Pharm Sci,* **94**, 2135–2146.
92. Low, P. S., Henne, W. A., and Doorneweerd, D. D. (2008) Discovery and development of folic-acid-based receptor targeting for imaging and therapy of cancer and inflammatory diseases. *Acc Chem Res,* **41**, 120–129.
93. Lu, Y. and Low, P. S. (2002) Folate-mediated delivery of macromolecular anticancer therapeutic agents. *Adv Drug Delivery Rev,* **54**, 675–693.
94. Leamon, C. P. and Low, P. S. (2001) Folate-mediated targeting: from diagnostics to drug and gene delivery. *Drug Discov Today,* **6**, 44–51.
95. Salazar, M. D. A. and Ratnam, M. (2007) The folate receptor: what does it promise in tissue-targeted therapeutics? *Cancer Metastasis Rev,* **26**, 141–152.
96. Mueller, C., Schibli, R., Krenning, E. P., and de Jong, M. (2008) Pemetrexed improves tumor selectivity of 111In-DTPA-folate in mice with folate receptor-positive ovarian cancer. *J Nucl Med,* **49**, 623–629.
97. Sega, E. I. and Low, P. S. (2008) Tumor detection using folate receptor-targeted imaging agents. *Cancer Metastasis Rev,* **27**, 655–664.
98. Schneider, R., Schmitt, F., Frochot, C., Fort, Y., Lourette, N., Guillemin, F., Mueller, J. -F., and Barberi-Heyob, M. (2005) Design, synthesis, and biological evaluation of folic acid targeted tetraphenylporphyrin as novel photosensitizers for selective photodynamic therapy. *Bioorg Med Chem,* **13**, 2799–2808.
99. Hofmeister, V., Schrama, D., and Becker, J. C. (2007) Anti-cancer therapies targeting the tumor stroma. *Cancer Immunol Immunother,* **57**, 1–17.
100. Lo, P. -C., Chen, J., Stefflova, K., Warren, M. S., Navab, R., Bandarchi, B., Mullins, S., Tsao, M., Cheng, J. D., and Zheng, G. (2009) Photodynamic molecular beacon triggered by fibroblast activation protein on cancer-associated fibroblasts for diagnosis and treatment of epithelial cancers. *J Med Chem,* **52**, 358–368.
101. Nestle, U., Weber, W., Hentschel, M., and Grosu, A. -L. (2009) Biological imaging in radiation therapy: role of positron emission tomography. *Phys Med Biol,* **54**, R1–R25.
102. Magne, N., Chargari, C., Vicenzi, L., Gillion, N., Messai, T., Magne, J., Bonardel, G., and Haie-Meder, C. (2008) New trends in the evaluation and treatment of cervix cancer: the role of FDG-PET. *Cancer Treat Rev,* **34**, 671–681.
103. Verel, I., Visser Gerard, W. M., and van Dongen Guus, A. (2005) The promise of immuno-PET in radioimmunotherapy. *J Nucl Med: official publication, Society of Nuclear Medicine,* **46(Suppl 1)**, 164S–171S.
104. Laville, I., Pigaglio, S., Blais, J. -C., Doz, F., Loock, B., Maillard, P., Grierson David, S., and Blais, J. (2006) Photodynamic efficiency of diethylene glycol-linked glycoconjugated porphyrins in human retinoblastoma cells. *J Med Chem,* **49**, 2558–2567.
105. Zhang, M., Zhang, Z., Blessington, D., Li, H., Busch, T. M., Madrak, V., Miles, J., Chance, B., Glickson, J. D., and Zheng, G. (2003) Pyropheophorbide 2-deoxyglucosamide: a new photosensitizer targeting glucose transporters. *Bioconjug Chem,* **14**, 709–714.
106. Zhang, X., Morgan, J., Pandey, S. K., Chen, Y., Tracy, E., Baumann, H., Missert, J. R., Batt, C., Jackson, J., Bellnier, D. A., Henderson, B. W., and Pandey, R. K. (2009) Conjugation of HPPH to carbohydrates changes its subcellular distribution and enhances photodynamic activity in vivo. *J Med Chem,* **52**, 4306–4318.
107. Munoz, A. and Castillo, M. (2008) Indications for adult and pediatric magnetic resonance imaging gadolinium-enhanced cisternography and myelography: experience and review of the literature. *Curr Med Imaging Rev,* **4**, 170–180.
108. Caravan, P., Ellison, J. J., McMurry, T. J., and Lauffer, R. B. (1999) Gadolinium (III) chelates as MRI contrast agents: structure, dynamics and applications. *Chem Rev,* **99**, 2293–2352.
109. Hueber, M. M., Staubli, A. B., Kustedjo, K., Gray, M. H. B., Shih, J., Fraser, S. E., Jacobs, R. E., and Meade, T. J. (1998) Fluorescently detectable magnetic resonance imaging agents. *Bioconjug Chem,* **9**, 242–249.

Chapter 17

Photodynamic Diagnosis and Therapy and the Brain

Herwig Kostron

Abstract

Photodynamic techniques such as photodynamic diagnosis (PDD), fluorescence-guided tumour resection (FGR) and photodynamic therapy (PDT) are currently undergoing intensive clinical investigations as adjuvant treatment for malignant brain tumours. The following chapter provides an overview on the current clinical data and trials of PDT as well as photosensitizers, technical developments and indications for photodynamic application in neurosurgery. Besides many clinical phase I/II trials for PDT for malignant brain tumours, there are only few controlled clinical trials following tumour resection. Variations in treatment protocols, variation of photosensitizers and light dose make the evaluation scientifically difficult; however there is a clear trend towards prolonging median survival after one single photodynamic treatment as compared to standard therapeutic regimens. According to the meta analysis the median survival after PDT for primary glioblastoma multiforme (WHO grade IV) was 22 months and for recurrent GBM was 9 months as compared to standard conventional treatment, in which it is 15 and 3 months, respectively. Fluorescence-guided resection of the tumour demonstrated significant greater reduction of tumour burden. The combination of PDD/ FGR and intraoperative PDT ("to see and to treat") offers an exciting approach to the treatment of malignant brain tumours. PDT was generally well tolerated and side effects consisted of occasionally increased intracranial pressure and prolonged skin sensitivity against direct sunlight.

Key words: Photodynamic therapy, Fluorescence-guided resection, Neurosurgery, Malignant brain tumour, Photofrin®, 5-ALA, Foscan®.

1. Introduction

Malignant brain tumours such as anaplastic gliomas WHO grade III and glioblastoma multiforme WHO grade IV carry a lethal prognosis. Current treatment regimes, such as surgery, chemotherapy and radiotherapy, prolong the lifespan to a median survival of 15 months and recurrent glioblastoma demonstrate

C.J. Gomer (ed.), *Photodynamic Therapy*, Methods in Molecular Biology 635,
DOI 10.1007/978-1-60761-697-9_17,

a median survival of 3 months (1, 2) (**Table 17.1**). The natural lifespan of patients after diagnosis suffering from glioblastoma multiforme WHO grade IV is around 3 months. The 5-year survival is under 1%. The incidence of malignant brain tumours varies from 4/100.000 in the United States to 14/100.000 in the Scandinavian countries with an increase of up to 70/100.000 in the elderly population above 65 years (3).

Table 17.1
Outcome of malignant gliomas WHO gradings and therapeutic strategies (1)

Histology WHO	Therapy	Recurrence time	Median survival
Glioblastoma multiforme WHO grade IV (GBM)	Surg, CHT, XRT	6 months	15 months
Anaplastic astrocytoma WHO grade III (AA)	Surg, CHT, XRT	18 months	3 years
Astrocytoma II	Surg, XRT	3 years	6 years
Astrocytoma I	Surg	8 years	10 years

Surg, surgery; XRT, radiotherapy; CHT, chemotherapy

Surgery is the first and most important step in the treatment of malignant gliomas and remains the mainstay of therapy. However, radical resection is hardly possible due to infiltrating growth into normal brain parenchyma. Recurrences occur 95% locally within 2 cm from the initial site and arise from tumour cells (guerrilla or satellite cells) embedded in the area of oedematous or normal brain adjacent to tumour brain adjacent to tumour (BAT) region) (4).

Photodynamic therapy (PDT) is currently undergoing intensive clinical investigations as adjunctive treatment for malignant brain tumours (5–7). Photosensitizers are accumulated in pathological brain tissue to a higher extent than in normal brain parenchyma (8, 9). Subsequent light activation produces a variety of cytotoxic oxidative reactions which induce selective tumour destruction via vascular or direct cellular mechanisms (10, 11).

Therefore PDT offers a more selective treatment of such malignancies as compared to other currently available treatment modalities and seems to be a logical concept for brain tumours infiltrating into normal brain (12). Clinical studies demonstrated a benefit for the patients treated with PS-mediated PDT in terms of prolongation of median survival time as well as quality of life (8).

In the past, intraoperative fluorescence-guided delineation had been under investigation with fluorescine and tetracyclines or autofluorescence (13, 14); however, the sensitivity and specificity were too low to be of clinical significance, especially for neurosurgery. Modern intraoperative imaging techniques now include techniques such as MRT and CT, neuronavigation and ultrasound, which are very expensive tools, except for the last one. The fluorescence properties of photosensitizers such as HPD, 5-aminolevulinic acid (5-ALA) and chlorine compounds such as *meta*-tetrahydroxyphenylchlorin (*m*THPC) are used for photodynamic diagnosis (PDD) and FGR has already gained wide attention of neurosurgeons (14–16). This intraoperative photodynamic diagnosis allows a "real-time" optical delineation of normal and malignant tissues, which facilitates intraoperative orientation and allows fluorescence-guided resection, which results in a more radical resection. This translates directly in a significant longer survival (4, 17).

Intraoperative mTHPC-mediated photodynamic diagnosis (PDD) followed by intraoperative PDT has been reported for the first time for patients suffering from recurrent glioblastoma with promising results (17–19). A just completed randomized phase III trial with 5-ALA-mediated FGR has proven high selectivity and specificity and demonstrated a significant advantage over conventional resection and provides evidence level II according to Oxford standards. FGR has now been introduced into clinical practice (4).

In cases where brain regions of functional areas are infiltrated by tumour, tumour tissue has to be left behind in order not to impair neurological function and quality of life (20). Therefore, simultaneous intraoperative PDT offers a logical supplement to PDD according to the slogan "to see and to treat" (15, 17).

The intention of this review is to critically analyse the available data and draw the future potential of PDD and PDT for its application in neurosurgery.

2. Photosensitizers

The photosensitizers for brain tumours must have a different profile than for any other indication. The tumour burden is much larger and radical resection is hardly possible because of infiltration of tumour into normal brain tissue of 3 cm and deeper.

The ideal neurosurgical sensitizer should (1) have a high selectivity for tumour and tumour cells sensitizing only tumour tissue and tumour island (guerrilla cells) embedded in normal brain tissue; (2) not cross the blood–brain barrier (BBB); (3) have photoactivation in the near-infrared range of 700 nm and beyond;

(4) have strong fluorescence properties; (5) have no systemic toxicity .The photosensitizer of first-generation haematoporphyrin derivative (HPD) is a complex mixture of various porphyrins (21), which was used for most of the basic experimental work and almost exclusively in the clinical brain tumour studies. HPD has its optimum absorption between 628 and 635 nm and allows a penetration depths of up to 5 mm depending on the tissue. The dose in clinical use is 2 mg/kg injected intravenously. Energies required range from 60 to 260 J/cm^2. The ratio of the concentration in tumour to normal brain ranges from 2.5 to 4:1 and in animal experiments it ranges up to 12:1. In human GBM the concentrations vary significantly from 1.46 to 4.00 μg/g wet weight. The concentration in the BAT region ranged from 0.6 to 1.2 μg/g. In this series the amount of PS correlated positively with the survival of the patients (8).

meta-tetrahydroxyphenylchlorin (mTHPC; Tempoforin, Foscan®) has been used as a second-generation sensitizer with a higher tumour to brain ratio in humans of 10:1 at a dose of 0.15 mg/kg and light doses of up to 20 J/cm^2 (17, 22, 23). The ratio in the BAT region is around 1:20. Clinical results of FGR mediated by mTHPC followed by intraoperative PDT have demonstrated a significant benefit for survival in recurrent malignant gliomas (17). Light hypersensitization of the skin was observed for 4 weeks.

5-Aminolevulinic acid (ALA)-induced protoporphyrin IX produces excellent fluorescence for diagnostic purposes and is activated at 635 nm. Sufficient cell kill of superficial tumours such as bladder and skin tumour is achieved at energies of up to 100 J/cm^2 (5, 16). The ratio of ALA concentration in tumour to normal brain is around 4:1. Currently there is a phase I/II trial for PDT mediated by ALA under investigation (24). A randomized phase III trial investigating the effect of ALA (Gliolan®)-mediated FGR demonstrated a higher incidence of almost radical tumour removal, which also translated in a significant greater survival (4). Skin phototoxicity of ALA is only for few hours after instillation.

A promising approach is the use of infrared sensitizers or sensitizers which are activated by ultrasound or by two-photon activation. Chloraluminium phthalocyanine (AlClPc), benzoporphyrin (BPD), tin ethyl purpurin (SnET2), texaphyrin, methylene blue, bacteriochlorin and boronated porphyrins are further sensitizers with great potential for its use in brain tumour (25, 26). Bacteriochlorin A has been reported to be more effective at wavelengths of 765 nm; however, there are no clinical data (27). The search for new sensitizer is intensive in order to increase tumour selectivity, fluorescence detection, phototoxicity, penetration depths and reduced skin toxicity.

3. PDT Mechanisms

The mechanisms of PDT are based on photo-oxidative reactions and the primary target depends on the pathology, the absorbance and chemistry of the sensitizer and the incubation time (6, 9, 10, 28).

Three different main mechanisms at the cellular level are involved in PDT-mediated cytotoxicity. The regular performed parenteral injection, whether intravenously or (in animals) intraperitoneally, results in primary vascular damage (8), whereas the direct intratumoural injection results in a more pronounced direct cellular effect (8). The third mechanisms are mediated by cytokine modulation. Transforming growth factor, fibroblastic growth factor, interleukin-1 and interleukin-6 but also PDGF and TNF play a role in mediating the photooxidative cytotoxic process (28, 29). IL-6, an auto-endocrine stimulator for glial tumours, is significantly reduced in cell cultures after PDT (22). Oxidative stress activates early response genes and further modulates apoptosis depending on the cell lines employed. Since porphyrins are incorporated into lipoproteins, the low-density lipoprotein receptor pathway is an important factor for the selective accumulation of porphyrins by tumour cells and by subcellular structures such as liposomes and mitochondria. This mechanism is particularly important for brain tumours as malignant and reactive glial cells express significant amounts of low-density lipoprotein (LDL) receptor-related protein.

These mechanisms outlined above could well explain that the PDT effect exceeds by far the penetration depths of the activating light. However, all these mechanisms depend strongly on the type of photosensitizers, light dose regime and investigated tumour cells.

4. Effect of PDT on Normal Brain

Despite a high selectivity of PS towards tumour cells, injury to normal glial and neurones had been observed in the normal brain (8, 23, 28, 29). This damage depends on the type of sensitizer used, the concentration of the sensitizer, the time interval of sensitization to light exposure and the light density. The blood–brain barrier, which protects the normal brain from toxic substances, plays an important part. Since the blood–brain barrier does not exist within the tumour, and the surrounding oedema, this barrier is well intact in the brain embedding tumour island (29). However, the evidence is mostly derived from experimental work. HPD is taken up by normal brain in a dose-dependent fashion, varying between 0.2 and 1.2 μg/g wet weight of brain tissue at a dose of 10 and 20 mg HPD/kg body weight. Twenty milligrams of HPD per kilogram body weight and 100 J cause death of the animals due to severe swelling. Fluorescence diagnosis demonstrated the presence of the sensitizer mostly along the fibre bundles of the white matter. Upon light activation, first break down of blood–brain barrier, swelling of astrocytes and neurones are observed and after 2 days, coagulation necrosis occurs in a dose-dependent fashion at concentrations higher than 5 mg HPD (8, 12). Intratumoural or intraparenchymal instillation of the sensitizer does not exhibit selectivity. Whereas in experimental studies, high doses of HPD had been used, in clinical relevant doses of 2.0–5 mg/kg, only few reports described morphological changes in the normal human brain (29).

Focal necrosis around the vessels 24 h after intra-arterial injection was found in only one series (8), whereas oedema post-PDT was described by almost all authors. Muller reported a significant increase in intracranial pressure despite avoiding hyperthermia effects (30). After stereotactic PDT, cerebral oedema was observed in most of the cases. The amount of postoperative swelling correlates with the residual tumour volume, so the tumour resection has to be performed to the utmost possible extent (8).

5. Interaction of PDT with Various Drugs

Since the introduction of temozolomide in the therapy of malignant brain tumours, chemotherapy is the third mainstay of adjuvant therapy after surgery and ionizing radiation (31, 32). Steroids (like dexamethasone) are widely used in neurosurgery for the treatment of tumour-associated oedema. The mechanism in closing loose junctions in the endothelium and tightening the blood–brain barrier might jeopardize the uptake of sensitizers into the tumour tissue. Patients on higher doses than 12 mg dexamethasone daily demonstrated a lower uptake of radiolabelled 111-In-Photofrin®. Furthermore an ameliorating effect of methylprednisolone on PDT was observed when given after light irradiation but not when given prior (8).

There are experimental data which show a synergistic or a potentiating effect of chemotherapeutic agents on PDT. However, this varies strongly within the various cell lines and tumour. Doxorubicin, e.g., potentiates therapeutic efficacy of mTHPC-mediated PDT significantly when given after light irradiation, but to a lesser extent when given prior (33). There are no reported clinical data on the interaction of PDT and chemotherapy.

PDT might be of advantage in the treatment of tumours not responding to chemotherapy because cells which express multidrug resistance features are less likely to be cross-resistant to PDT (34). The combination of PDT and drugs acting at the molecular level of cancerogenicity, such as VGF, PDGF, EPGF as well as factors enhancing apoptosis and phagocytoses, enhances or potentiates the efficacy of PDT (35–38).

6. Interaction of PDT and Ionizing Radiation

Ionizing radiation is a standard therapy in the postoperative course after surgery of malignant brain tumours (1, 2, 31).

To investigate the interaction of HPD-mediated PDT and ionizing radiation, a rat gliosarcoma model 9L was subcutaneously implanted. In low doses of HPD after intraperitoneal injection an additive effect of both treatment modalities could be observed, whereas direct injection with high intratumoural concentration and high light doses of 120 J/cm^2 and 4 Gy resulted in significant greater response, indicating a potentiating mechanism. The effect was more pronounced when PDT was followed by XRT within 30 min (8). The underlying mechanism is thought to be the inhibition of the potential lethal damage induced by PDT. In a more recent study employing human glioma, spheroids study, it was shown that gamma radiation and PDT interact in a synergistic manner only if both light fluence and gamma radiation dose exceed approximately 25 J/cm^2 and 8 Gy, respectively (39).

In an early series at our own institution, patients with de novo glioblastomas were treated with one single dose of 4 Gy of electrons within 30 min after PDT (8). The results remained unchanged to those without immediate X-radiation treatment; therefore this treatment protocol was not continued. Radiotherapy was commenced in addition in all de novo patients within 10 days after surgery and PDT. We did not see any side effect from this radiotherapy. There were also no side effects reported in the 5-ALA-mediated PDD/FGR trial where ionizing radiation of 60 Gy was commenced within 4 weeks after sensitization (4).

Gamma knife irradiation has not been used in combination with PDT.

7. Instrumentation

Initial work was performed with argon-dye laser systems or xenon arc lamps with adequate filtering. LEDs and diode lasers are available in almost all desired wavelengths and are much reliable and cost effective than, for example, neodymium YAG/ KTP lasers. Laser light delivery in neurosurgery has become the state of the art and interstitial PDT has become possible. Light delivery and dosimetry are critical points in PDT, especially in neurosurgery with no ideally geometrically shaped or superficial lesions, and irregular and large volumes must be treated (30, 40, 42).

An inflatable balloon is employed to facilitate dosimetry. In general the cavity or the balloon is filled with a 0.1% concentration of intralipid solution or plane water to achieve a homogeneous light distribution (8, 30). The superficial light delivery is performed mostly by bare fibres. Interstitial light application is either performed by bare or cylindrical fibres, the latter allowing higher power density (350 mW/cm^2) without producing carbonization at the fibre tip. The placements of up to four fibres are done by 3D planning and stereotactic methods (41–43). Repetitive PDT treatments were given using 100 J/cm^2 of a diode laser at 630 nm (44, 45). Important parameters such as fluence rate, sensitizer fluorescence intensity, and changes in local blood oxygen saturation can be measured with the same fibres that deliver the therapeutic light (46).

8. Photodynamic Diagnosis and Fluorescence-Guided Resection

Next to the phototoxic properties, the fluorescence abilities of the photosensitizer can also be used for optical discrimination of normal and malignant tissue allowing intraoperative photodynamic diagnosis and fluorescence-guided resection, thus minimizing residual tumour.

Intraoperative fluorescence is induced by a UV light source at 370–440 nm, which spectrally matches the main absorption peak of the sensitizer for fluorescence excitation which is delivered via a liquid light guide to the surgical microscope. The induced fluorescence light is collected by the same optical fibre, separated from the blue excitation light by passing through a dichroic beam splitter and focused to the entrance slit of a modified CCD camera and a spectrograph in connection with an electric tuneable optical filter. In regions of faint fluorescence intensities (especially in the region of the tumour border), spatially resolved spectra can be taken with a very sensitive spectrometer to delineate tumour borders. The pictures are converted digitally by a standard frame grabber and processed in real time. Standard neurosurgical microscopes (Zeiss, Leica) modified for fluorescence detection have become commercially available. Normal white light illumination of the surgical microscope can be switched to blue light excitation with simultaneous observation by the naked eye. The induced fluorescence could be seen directly through the observer light path (**Figs. 17.1a,b** and **17.2a,b**) (14, 15, 18).

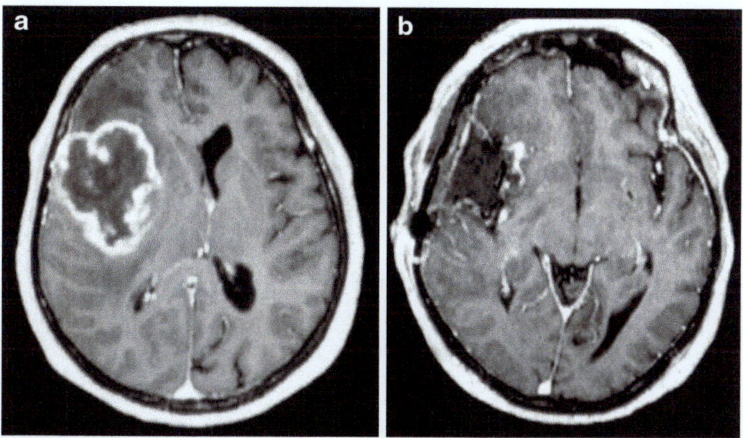

Fig. 17.1. (**a**) Typical appearance of a glioblastoma multiforme WHO IV right temporal. (**b**) Tumor after fluorescence-guided resection.

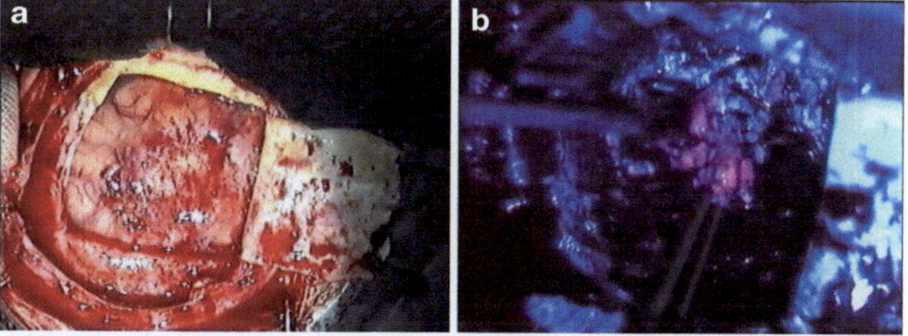

Fig. 17.2. (**a**) White light appearance of the glioblastoma of **Fig. 17.1a**, the differentiation of normal to tumor tissue is hardly visible. (**b**) Fluorescence-guided resection; note the strong fluorescence of mTHPC.

9. Methods and Patients

The indication for PDT are primary and recurrent malignant brain tumours. Slow-growing tumours such as low-grade astrocytomas or other benign lesions are currently no indication for PDT or PDD because of the lack of uptake of photosensitizers. Scull base tumours are a good indication for PDD/PDT because there is no BBB. Most recent case reports are including now metastasis, malignant meningiomas and recurrent pituitary tumours also.

Patients presenting with primary or recurrent brain tumours were enrolled in various clinical trials, which are detailed in **Table 17.2**.

Table 17.2
Clinical studies of PDT (+) in braintumors and results

Author	Number of patients	Histology	Median survival
Eljamel (19)	**103**	Various[a] brain tumours	13 months for GBM
Muller (30)	**112**	HGG	10.5 months
Kaneko (48)	**60**	GBM	20.5 months
		AA	36.2 months
Kostron (8, 17)	**116**	GBM	19 months
		Recurrent GBM	7–9 months
Stylli (49)	**350**	GBM	14.3 months
		AA	76.7 months
Pichlmeier + (4)	**243**	GBM	GBM cr 16.7 months
			GBM ir 11.8 months

[a]Various brain tumours: GBM, metastasis, meningioma, pituitary tumour + fluorescence guided resection only followed by radiotherapy
GBM, glioblastoma multiforme WHO grade IV; AA, anaplastic astrocytoma WHO grade III; HGG, high-grade glioma WHO grade IV and WHO grade III; GBM cr, GBM with complete resection > 95%; GBM ic, GBM with incomplete resection

The patients received either various formulations of haematoporphyrin derivative (HPD, Photofrin I, DHE, Photofrin II, Photosan 3,) or mTHPC. In order to utilize also intraoperative diagnostics, the combination of Photofrin and 5-ALA is used (19, 47).

At our institution the following protocol is used: After fulfilling the criteria for informed consent the patients are sensitized with HPD (Photofrin) 2.5 mg/kg or with Foscan® 0.15 mg/kg BW 24–48 h prior to a standard craniotomy (8, 17). Steroids were withdrawn 2–3 days prior to sensitization, so far tolerated. A standard craniotomy and maximal tumour resection were performed. Patients sensitized by mTHPC underwent additionally intraoperative photodynamic diagnosis and fluorescence-guided resection.

PDT was performed by a KTP-pumped dye laser (Laser Sonics) or a diode laser emitting at 652 nm (Diamed 2 W). The light was delivered by bare fibres coupled into a modified balloon system by a spherical distributor or by a 20-mm-long cylinder for interstitial treatment. The power density varied from 2500 mW/s

(KTP dye) to 870 mW/s (diode laser) for surface illumination. For interstitial treatment the power density was 350 mW. For treatments of HPD-mediated PDT, the light dose was increasing from 20 J/cm^2 for the first patients to the majority receiving 240 J/cm^2. Treatment times ranged from 9 to 75 min.

In cases of significant amount of residual tumour in critical areas, an interstitial PDT was performed at a power density of 250–350 mW/s to a total dose of 150 J. The dose for the mTHPC-sensitized patients was 20 J/cm^2 and the interstitial therapy was performed at a power density of 350 J/cm^2 to a dose of 20 J/cm^3. The fibres were placed according to preoperative 3D planning by means of neuronavigation or stereotactically. Anaesthesia was induced by neuroleptanalgesia without barbiturates. During light irradiation 100% oxygen was used and after light treatment was terminated a bolus of 40 mg dexamethasone was given, followed by the generally used dose regimen for postoperative steroid treatment. Postoperative, the patients were kept in ambient room light. After mobilization the patients were slowly exposed to normal sunlight to allow pigmentation of the skin. A light meter was provided for the patients to control light exposure. The patients were followed by clinical exams and CT scans every 3 months.

10. Clinical Trials and Results

Since 1980, over 984 patients had been treated meanwhile worldwide (8, 30, 48–50) (**Table 17.2**). This number is relatively low as compared to the amount of patients treated with lung, bladder or skin cancers. The reason might be that the incidence of brain tumours is lower and their treatment more complicated since it requires highly sophisticated surgery and instrumentation. In general the patients were sensitized with HPD–Photofrin in various formulations and only one study used mTHPC as sensitizer (17). The majority of the patients were sensitized parenterally and few patients received intratumoural or intra-arterial sensitization (8).

Light irradiation was performed with photoradiation lamps, dye laser, gold vapour KTP dye laser and diode lasers. Patients presenting with primary glioblastomas underwent 45 Gy of irradiation within 4 weeks after PDT. The light dose was initially low at 70–180 J/cm^2, which was finally increased to 240 J/cm^2 in the majority of the patients. Most of the patients underwent standard craniotomies and open tumour resection (8). Stereotactic approach was chosen by several authors (24, 43). Muller observed complete response with excellent survival in cases where a cystic geometric tumour cavity allowed a very homogeneous light distribution (30).

The results of the reported cases are difficult to evaluate because the histology are in general not detailed and high-grade gliomas consisting of WHO grade IV and grade III gliomas are often pooled.

10.1. Primary Glioblastoma

Primary glioblastomas were initially treated with various formulations of HPD (Photofrin I, HPD-Adelaide, Photosan 3) 24–72 h prior to treatment.

Photofrin® is now easily commercially available. The activation sources ranged from various lamps, by argon-dye laser (Aurora M), KTP dye laser and gold vapour lasers, whereas now diode lasers and LEDs are the current standard. The light dose ranged from 15 to 260 J/cm^2 delivered with a power density of up to 1600 mW/s (for details, *see* **Section** 7). These patients received in addition a conventional radiotherapy of total 55–60 Gy as well as conventional chemotherapy (nitrosourea and cytosine arabinoside). The median time to progression was 13 months. Patients with recurrent glioblastomas underwent retreatment with PDT without any other treatment. Their median survival was 10 months. There was no adverse effect from a second photosensitization and photoradiation (8).

The total median survival of primary glioblastomas in the compiled series was 14.3 months (range 9, 0–27 months).

In the Canadian study 112 patients were treated with PDT and adjuvant radiotherapy of 45 Gy. The median survival was 9 months. Furthermore at this institution a randomized phase III was conducted enrolling 77 primary GBM patients who underwent either surgery plus PDT and XRT or surgery and XRT. The results were not significant with a median survival of 11 months versus 8 months, respectively (30). A similar result was reported enrolling 31 patients who had a median survival of 13 months after FGR and PDT as compared to 6 months in the controls (19).The largest series enrolling more than 350 high-grade gliomas was reported by Stilly 2006 in an uncontrolled trial (49). Primary gliomas received 45 Gy in addition and reached a median survival of 27 months.

10.2. Recurrent Glioblastomas

Thirty-nine patients with recurrent glioblastomas were treated photodynamically because of treatment failures. The median time to first recurrence without any other treatment was 7 months and the median survival time after PDT was 9 months (range 3–18 months). Fourteen patients were reoperated after 12 months having presented with a first recurrence. No further treatment was commenced. These patients suffered another recurrence within 3 months. After a third surgical procedure and PDT the median time to recurrence was 6 months (3–8 months).

Stylli reported a median survival of 18 months for patients with recurrent high-grade gliomas and PDT (49). Muller reported on 64 recurrent glioblastomas which underwent a dose escalation study. Patients receiving more than 1700 J had a median survival of 9.2 months, whereas those receiving less than that had a survival of 6.6 months (30).

Kaneko had treated 60 patients mostly bearing glioblastomas with a median survival of 18 months (48). Fifteen recurrent glioblastomas were treated by multiple interstitial fibres which were based on a computed 3D image. The light dose was 100 J/ cm^2 with median survival of 6 months. Stereotactically placed interstitial fibres with light dose of up to 400 J/cm^2 were also used (17, 24, 47).

10.3. High-Grade Gliomas WHO Grade III

Over 120 recurrent anaplastic astrocytomas were treated photodynamically with energies varying from 45 to 175 J/cm^2 and with a median survival of 56 months (range 36.0 to 76.7 months). Malignant mixed oligoastrocytomas and ependymomas had a 2-year survival of 37% and 75%, respectively (13, 30, 48, 49).

10.4. Brain Tumours of Other Origin

Malignant meningiomas were treated with light dose up to 260 J/cm^2 and the median survival was 6.15 and 23 months, respectively.

10.5. Pituitary Tumours

These are benign tumours; however, when they recur they produce anatomical malignancy. Thirty patients suffering from recurrent pituitary tumours were treated in combination with fluorescence-guided localization and resection because of repeated recurrence and treatment failures. All cases responded favourable, all showing no progression or recurrence of tumours for 2.5 years (50, 51).

10.6. Metastasis

There are 46 reported cases of metastasis of various origins. All except for melanoma metastasis showed complete or partial response and patients usually died of systemic progress with local control.

10.7. mTHPC-Mediated PDT

Twenty-four patients with primary or recurrent GBM were enrolled in this trial. Two patients with primary glioblastoma multiforme WHO grade IV (GBM) were treated in addition with 60 Gy of XRT and died 9 and 15 months afterwards. The patients with recurrent GBM ($n = 22$) demonstrated a median time to progression of 4 months and a median survival time of 9 months (17).The patients with metastasis demonstrated complete tumour control in two cases for up to 28 months, two were progressing 6 months after treatment and were lost to follow-up. One scull base tumour demonstrated a complete response with a follow-up of 24 months; the other relapsed within 7 months. All patients tolerated mTHPC-mediated treatment well; one patient suffered swelling of the treated area. Two patients experienced severe toxic reaction to sunlight due to unintentional exposure to direct sunlight requiring conventional treatment.

10.8. Photodynamic Diagnosis (PDD) and Fluorescence-Guided Resection (FGR)

An outmost surgical resection with maximal cytoreduction is directly correlated with a longer survival (1, 2, 4, 31), which can be accomplished by intraoperative PDD and FGR. 5-ALA (Gliolan®) will be given orally at 20 mg/kg BW 3–4 h prior to surgery or also Foscan® at 0.15 mg/ kg BW 12 or 96 h prior to surgery. A randomized phase III trial proved that FGR mediated by 5-ALA results in a significantly higher amount of almost complete resection than without, which translated in greater survival of 16.7 versus 11.8, respectively (4, 52). Foscan-mediated PDD and FGR were investigated in recurrent GBM and compared to a cohort of paired patients. The histological specimens of fluorescent tissue correlated to a sensitivity and specificity of 89% and 96%, respectively. Complete resection was achieved in 68% as compared to 35% in the control group, which was demonstrated by MRI within 48 h after surgery. These latter patients underwent immediate PDT after FGR tumour resection was accomplished. The results were significantly longer in the treatment group with 9 months as compared to the matched pair group, which lived 3 months in the median (17). Since tumour grows invasively in also functional areas such as speech, motor function or psychic function, complete resection cannot be performed in order not to harm the patient. In such cases, interstitial PDT can be performed in those functional areas (17, 20). Care has to be taken not to harm the patients since an impaired neurological status (KPI < 60%) correlates with a shorter overall survival (1).

11. Discussion

The purpose of this review is to summarize the current available data on brain tumours which underwent photodynamic-mediated therapies, which include FGR/PDD and PDT. This poses some difficulties since the data are hardly comparable among various investigators differing in photosensitizer, time interval from sensitization to surgery, instrumentation and light dose. There are two randomized phase III trials: one trial with paired controls and 15 uncontrolled trials in comparison with historical controls. Therefore scientific evaluation with standard statistics cannot be applied.

The largest series currently comes from Melbourne, which recruited more than 350 patients presenting with high-grade gliomas, the majority being recurrent tumours (49). The median survival for primary glioblastomas undergoing Photofrin-mediated PDT (180–240 J/cm^2) and 45 Gy of radiation was 24 months; anaplastic gliomas WHO grade III had a median survival of 76.7 months. Recurrent gliomas demonstrated a 10-month median survival after PDT as compared to historical controls which lived in the median 12 months.

Muller reported on 112 patients with recurrent high-grade gliomas which were sensitized with 2 mg Photofrin 12–36 h prior to operation (30). This randomized phase III study enrolling 43 patients in the treatment arm and 33 patients in the control did not show a trend towards prolonged survival; however, statistical significance was not reached. A larger number would have been needed to show a difference. Also the comparison of high-dose to low-dose light radiation did not show a difference in survival, whereas a prior study reported significant better results. Patients undergoing PDT greater than 1700 J had a survival of 9.2 months as compared to 6.6 months in those who were treated with a lower dose than 1700 J. A high light dose was always associated with a longer survival.

The results of primary glioblastomas at our own institution showed a median survival of 19 months and for patients suffering from recurrent tumours, the range was 6–9 months. Direct intratumoural and intra-arterial injection performed in few patients yielded high intratumoural sensitizer concentration; however the results were not improved as compared to intravenous sensitization. The concentration of the sensitizer varied significantly among the tumours, even in tumours of the same histology (8, 29). Photosensitizer kinetics depends on the tumour blood flow and oxygenation of the tumour and is highly inconsistent within tumour entities and varies significantly in in vivo and in vitro models. After PDT the relapses always recur locally and there is no difference in the patterns as after conventional treatment modalities. The reasons are multiple for the only temporary response of gliomas to PDT. In comparison to tumours localized elsewhere in the body, brain tumours exceed 100 cm^3 and more. Even after most radical resection the tumour cells remain infiltrating normal brain.

BAT area is often the site of tumour recurrence. At the critical area a low light dose and a low sensitizer dose coincide. To overcome this problem and to circumvent the blood–brain barrier, the sensitizers were injected directly into the tumour cavity, resulting in significant higher intratumoural concentration; however, the clinical results were not improved. Muller irradiated patients within 12 h after sensitization to prevent the rapid washout of sensitizer at the BAT region (14). Therefore, most likely a low penetration of activating light seems to be the most realistic reason for recurrences on that site. On the contrary, interstitial radiation improved depth penetration to about 2 cm and dosimetry at this critical area, but this also did not improve the results (17).The best results were actually achieved by Kaye using high dose of superficial irradiation. A different approach for light delivery and inducing phototoxicity has to be aimed for (40–42). Different approaches in varying light delivery, timing of light delivery, varying photosensitizer concentrations and also drugs changing the microenvironment of the tumour had been investigated which will induce and prolong different photochemical and phototoxic reactions (10, 11, 14, 38, 53, 54). Metronomic or multiple treatment sessions after one time sensitization with Photofrin have been reported with favourable effects. Multiple investigations are currently performed to elucidate metronomic PDT (14, 19, 44, 45).

Ionizing radiation was applied to the patients either almost simultaneously or consecutively within 4 weeks after PDT. There was no observed advantage or disadvantage for the patients despite an additive or synergistic effect was reported experimentally (8, 39).

A synergistic response of hyperthermia to PDT was observed when delivered simultaneously or within 30 min after PDT (5, 6, 11); however, there is no clinical relevance of hyperthermia in neurooncology. Of greater importance in neurooncology might be the fact that PDT does not induce resistance to chemotherapy and might be effective in tumours expressing multidrug resistance features (33, 34). PDT in combination with targeted therapies changing the molecular signature of the tumour cells could further improve the treatment response (35–37). However, the interactions of PDT with current standard treatment modalities such as ionizing radiation and chemotherapy are by far not yet fully elucidated and investigated. The use of carrier systems such as liposomal encapsulated photosensitizers or photochemical internalization (PCI) enhances selectivity and PDT-mediated cytotoxic effects significantly (26, 55–57).

PDT-specific side effects were temporarily increased intracranial pressure and prolonged skin sensitivity, reported from various centres (17, 30, 49). In five cases a reversible diencephalic syndrome and neuropathy were reported during PDT of the middle cerebral fossa, most probably due to hyperthermic effect on the midline structures (18, 30); however this did not impair the patient's outcome. The sensitizers in clinical practice such as Photofrin, 5-ALA and Foscan show efficacy in regard to cytotoxicity and gave proof of principle of the effect of PDT in neurooncology. Foscan-mediated PDD/FGR has the advantage that PDT can also be very efficiently performed (17), whereas the combination of Photofrin and ALA allows "to see and to treat" (19, 47). Currently a pilot study investigates PDT mediated by 5-ALA following FGR (24). The development of instrumentation has to be, however, as intensive as for sensitizers. Light dosimetry is critical for PDT response and underdosing might often be the cause for therapeutic failures. Online dosimetry could prevent such failures (46). Computer-aided planning with 3D reconstruction of the remaining tumour and an exact planning of dosimetry, which can be archived by multiple stereotactic interstitial fibres placed by neuronavigation systems, should be considered mandatory for treating brain lesions (41, 42).

The prime indication for PDT in neurosurgery are infiltrating high-grade gliomas. Pituitary tumours, spinal tumours, cystic lesion at the scull base and scull base tumours and metastatic lesions are also good indications in second-line therapy. Low-grade gliomas demonstrate a significant longer survival and may be not good candidates for PDT. Also tumours in delicate areas such as brain stem must be excluded from PDT, whereas it can be used, for example, in the motor strip or other functional areas without impairing function (17, 20). Novel indications are scull base tumours and tumour in the field of ENT (57) as well as osseous tumour such as metastasis of the vertebrae or bone at the scull base (58).

PDT is currently offered in only a few selected centres, although it is slowly gaining acceptance in addition to conventional cancer therapies. The clinical potential and the implementation of PDD and FGR have brought general PDT to a wider acknowledgment to the neurosurgical community and might increase the awareness in neurosurgery and have significant impact for its clinical application. Here, we show the developmental steps of PDT and summarize the current clinical applications. The data show that PDT especially in combination with PDD/FGR is a safe and an effective treatment for a second-line therapy in neurooncology.

References

1. Lacroix, M., Abi-Said, D., Fourney, D. R., Gokaslan, Z. L., Shi, W., DeMonte, F., Lang, F. F., McCutcheon, I. E., Hassenbusch, S. J., Holland, E., Hess, K., Michael, C., Miller, D., and Sawaya, R. (2001) A multivariate analysis of 416 patients with glioblastoma multiforme: prognosis, extent of resection, and survival. *J Neurosurg*, **95**, 190–198.
2. Obwegeser, A., Ortler, M., Seiwald, M., Ulmer, H., and Kostron, H. (1995) Therapy of glioblastoma multiforme: a cumulative experience of 10 years. *Acta Neurochir*, **137**, 29–33.
3. Radhakrishnan, K., Bohnen, N. I., and Kurland, L. T. (1994) Epidemiology of brain tumors. In: Morantz R. A. and Wals J. W. (eds.) Brain Tumors. New York: Marcel Dekker Inc, pp. 1–18.
4. Pichlmeier, U., Bink, A., Schackert, G., and Stummer, W. (2008) Resection and survival in glioblastoma multiforme: an RTOG recursive partitioning analysis of ALA study patients. *Neuro Oncol*, **10**, 1025–1034.
5. Dougherty, T. J., Gomer, C. J., Henderson, B. W., Jori, G., Kessel, D., Korbelik, M., Moan, J., and Peng, Q. (1998) Photodynamic therapy. *J Natl Cancer Inst*, **17**, 889–905.
6. Triesscheijn, M., Baas, P., Schellens, J. H. M., and Stewart, F. A. (2006) Photodynamic therapy in oncology. *Oncologist*, **11**, 1034–1044.

7. Mitton, D. and Ackroyd, R. (2008) A brief overview of photodynamic therapy in Europe. *Photodiagnosis Photodyn Ther*, **5**, 103–111.
8. Kostron, H., Obwegeser, A., and Seiwald, M. (1996) PDT in neurosurgery; a review. *J Photochem Photobiol B*, **36**, 157–168.
9. Castano, A. P., Demidova, T. N., and Hamblin, M. R. (2004) Mechanisms in photodynamic therapy: part one—photosensitizers, photochemistry and cellular localization. *Photodiagnosis Photodyn Ther*, **1**, 279–293.
10. Seshadri, M., Bellnier, D. A., Vaughan, L. A., Spernyak, J. A., Mazurchuk, R., Foster, T. H., and Henderson, B. W. (2008) Light delivery over extended time periods enhances the effectiveness of photodynamic therapy. *Clin Cancer Res*, **1**, 2796–2805.
11. Angell-Petersen, E., Spetalen, S., Madsen, S. J., Sun, C. H., Peng, Q., Carper, S. W., Sioud, M., and Hirschberg, H. (2006) Influence of light fluence rate on the effects of photodynamic therapy in an orthotopic rat glioma model. *J Neurosurg*, **104**, 109–117.
12. Stylli, S. S. and Kaye, A. H. (2006) Photodynamic therapy of cerebral glioma – a review part I – a biological basis. *J Clin Neurosci*, **13**, 615–625.
13. Eljamel, S. M. (2008) Brain photodiagnosis (PD), fluorescence guided resection (FGR) and photodynamic therapy (PDT): past, present and future. *Photodiagnosis Photodyn Ther*, **5**, 29–35.
14. Bogaards, A., Varma, A., Zhang, K., Zach, D., Bisland, S. K., Moriyama, E. H., Lilge, L., Muller, P. J., and Wilson, B. C. (2005) Fluorescence image-guided brain tumour resection with adjuvant metronomic photodynamic therapy: pre-clinical model and technology development. *Photochem Photobiol Sci*, **4**, 438–442.
15. Kostron, H., Zimmermann, A., and Obwegeser, A. (1998) MTHPC-mediated photodynamic detection for fluorescence guided resection of brain tumors. In: Bogner S.M., Charles S.T., Grundfest W.S., Harrington J.A., Katzir A., Lome L.S., Vannier M.W., and von-Hanwehr R., (eds.) Surgical-Assist Systems. SPIE proceedings-series, Bellingham, WA, US: International-Biomedical-Optics-Society, SPIE, 3262, pp. 259–264.
16. Kennedy, J. C., Marcus, S. L., and Potier, R. H. (1996) Photodynamic therapy and photodiagnosis using endogenous photosensitisation induced by 5-aminolevulinic acid (ALA): mechanism and clinical results. *J Clin Laser Med Surg*, **15**, 289–304.
17. Kostron, H., Fiegele, Th., and Akatuna, E. (2006) Combination of FOSCAN® mediated fluorescence guided resection and photodynamic treatment as new therapeutic concept for malignant brain tumors. *Laser Med*, **24**, 285–290.
18. Zimmermann, A., Ritsch-Marte, M., and Kostron, H. (2001) mTHPC-mediated photodynamic diagnosis of malignant brain tumors. *Photochem Photobiol*, **74**, 611–616.
19. Eljamel, M. S., Goodman, C., and Moseley, H. (2008) ALA and Photofrin® fluorescence-guided resection and repetitive PDT in glioblastoma multiforme: a single centre phase III randomised controlled trial. *Lasers Med Sci*, **23**, 361–367.
20. Schmidt, M. H., Meyer, G. A., Reichert, K. W., Cheng, J., Krouwer, H. G., Ozkerand, K., and Whelan, H. T. (2004) Evaluation of photodynamic therapy near functional brain tissue in patients with recurrent brain tumors. *J Neurooncol*, **67**, 201–207.
21. Kessel, D. (2004) Photodynamic therapy: from the beginning. *Photodiagnosis Photodyn Ther*, **1**, 3–7.
22. Kostron, H., Obwegeser, A., Jakober, R., Zimmermann, A., and Rueck, A. (1998) Experimental and clinical results of mTHPC (Foscan®)– mediated photodynamic therapy for malignant brain tumors. In: Dougherty T.J. (ed.) Optical Methods for Tumor Treatment and Detections: Mechanisms and Techniques in Photodynamics Therapy VII. Bellingham, WA, US: International-Society-for-Optical-Engineering, SPIE, 3247, pp. 40–45.
23. Obwegeser, A., Jakober, R., and Kostron, H. (1998) Uptake and kinetics of C-14 labelled m-THPC and 5-ALA in C-6 rat glioma model. *Br J Cancer*, **78**, 733–738.
24. Beck, T. J., Kreth, F. W., Beyer, W., Mehrkens, J. H., Obermeier, A., Stepp, H., Stummer, W., and Baumgartner, R. (2007) Interstitial photodynamic therapy of nonresectable malignant glioma recurrences using 5-aminolevulinic acid induced protoporphyrin IX. *Lasers Surg Med*, **39**, 386–393.
25. Allison, R. R., Downie, G. H., Cuenca, R., Hu, X. H., Carter, J. H., and Sibata, C. H. (2004) Photosensitizers in clinical PDT. *Photodiagnosis Photodyn Ther*, **1**, 27–42.
26. Jori, G. (1996) Tumour photosensitizers: approaches to enhance the selectivity and efficiency of photodynamic therapy. *J Photochem Photobiol B*, **36**, 87–93.
27. Rovers, J. P., Schuitmaker, J. J., Vahrmeijer, A. L., Van-Dierendonck, J. H., and Terpstra, O. T. (1998) Interstitial photodynamic

therapy with the second-generation photosensitizer bacteriochlorin in a rat model for liver metastases. *Br J Cancer*, 77, 2098–2103.

28. Peng, Q., Moan, J., Wei-Ma, L., and Nesland, J. M. (1995) Uptake, localisation and photodynamic effect of meso-tetrahydroxyphenylporphyrine and its corresponding chlorin in normal and tumor tissue of mice bearing mammary carcinoma. *Cancer Res*, **55**, 2260–2266.
29. Kostron, H., Bellnier, D. A., Lin, C. W., Swarzt, M. R., and Martuza, R. L. (1986) Distribution and retention and phototoxicity of HPD in a rat glioma: intraneoplastic versus intraperitoneal injection. *J Neurosurg*, **64**, 768–774.
30. Muller, P. J. and Wilson, B. C. (2006) Photodynamic therapy of brain tumors – a work in progress. *Lasers Surg Med*, **38**, 384–389.
31. Stupp, R., Hegi, M. E., Gilbert, M. R., and Chakravarti, A. (2007) Chemoradiotherapy in malignant glioma: standard of care and future directions. *J Clin Oncol*, **25**, 4127.
32. Stupp, R., Mason, W. P., van den Bent, M. J., Weller, M., Fisher, B., Taphoorn, M. J. B., Belanger, K., Brandes, A. A., Marosi, C., Bogdahn, U. et al. for the European Organisation for Research and Treatment of Cancer Brain Tumor and Radiotherapy Groups and the National Cancer Institute of Canada Clinical Trials Group (2005) Radiotherapy plus concomitant and adjuvant Temozolomide for glioblastoma. *N Engl J Med*, **10**, 987–996.
33. Kirveliene, V., Grazeliene, G., Dabkeviciene, D., Micke, I., Kirvelis, D., Juodka, B., and Didziapetriene, J. (2006) Schedule-dependent interaction between Doxorubicin and mTHPC-mediated photodynamic therapy in murine hepatoma in vitro and in vivo. *Cancer Chemother Pharmacol*, **57**, 65–72.
34. Hornung, R., Walt, H., Crompton, N. E., Keefe, K. A., Jentsch, B., Perewusnyk, G., Haller, U., and Köchli, O. R. (1998) *m*-THPC-mediated photodynamic therapy (PDT) does not induce resistance to chemotherapy, radiotherapy or PDT on human breast cancer cells in vitro. *Photochem Photobiol*, **68**, 569–574.
35. Chen, B., Pogue, B. W., Hoopes, P. J., and Hasan, T. (2005) Combining vascular and cellular targeting regimens enhances the efficacy of photodynamic therapy. *Int J Radiat Oncol Biol Phys*, **61**, 1216–1226.
36. Ferrario, A., Rucker, N., Wong, S., Luna, M., and Gomer, C. J. (2007) Survivin, a member of the inhibitor of apoptosis family, is induced by photodynamic therapy and is a target for improving treatment response. *Cancer Res*, **67**, 4989–4995.
37. Fanuel-Barret, D., Patrice, T., Foultier, M. T., Vonarx-Coinsmann, V., Robillard, N., and Lajat, Y. (1997) Influence of epidermal growth factor on photodynamic therapy of glioblastoma cells in vitro. *Res Exp Med*, **197**, 219–233.
38. Kessel, D. and Oleinick, N. L. (2009) Chapter 1 initiation of autophagy by photodynamic therapy. *Methods Enzymol*, **453**, 1–16.
39. Madsen, S. J., Sun, C. H., Tromberg, B. J., Yeh, A. T., Sanchez, R., and Hirschberg, H. (2002) Effects of combined photodynamic therapy and ionizing radiation on human glioma spheroids. *Photochem Photobiol*, **76**, 411–416.
40. Mang, T. S. (2004) Lasers and light sources for PDT: past, present and future. *Photodiagnosis Photodyn Ther*, **1**, 43–48.
41. Mang, T. S. (2008) Dosimetric concepts for PDT. *Photodiagnosis Photodyn Ther*, **5**, 217–223.
42. Krishnamurthy, S., Powers, S. K., Witmer, P., and Brown, T. (2000) Optimal light dose for interstitial photodynamic therapy in treatment for malignant brain tumors. *Lasers Surg Med*, **27**, 224–234.
43. Kaneko, S., Kobayashi, H., and Kohama, Y. (1999) Stereotactic intratumoral photodynamic therapy on malignant brain tumors, *Abstract*, International Symposium on Photodynamic Therapy in Clinical Practice, Innsbruck
44. Bisland, S. K., Lilge, L., Lin, A., Rusnov, R., and Wilson, B. C. (2004) Metronomic photodynamic therapy as a new paradigm for photodynamic therapy: rationale and preclinical evaluation of technical feasibility for treating malignant brain tumors. *Photochem Photobiol*, **80**, 222–230.
45. Hirschberg, H., Sørensen, D. R., Angell-Petersen, E., Peng, Q., Tromberg, B., Sun, C. H., Spetalen, S., and Madsen, S. (2006) Repetitive photodynamic therapy of malignant brain tumors. *J Environ Pathol Toxicol Oncol*, **25**, 261–279.
46. Thompson, M. S., Johansson, A., Johansson, T., Andersson-Engels, S., Svanberg, S., Bendsoe, N., and Svanberg, K. (2005) Clinical system for interstitial photodynamic therapy with combined on-line dosimetry measurement. *Appl Opt*, **1**, 4023–4031.
47. Kaneko, S., Shírasaka, T., Yoshimuzi, T., Fujimoto, S., Yamouchi, T., Yoshimoto, T., Tokuda, K., Kashiwaba, T., and Kohama, Y.

(2002) Fluorescence diagnosis and PDT using two types of photosensitizer. In: Recent progress on clinical and basic research of ALA, Proceedings of 2nd international ALA Symposium, Fukuoka, 17–24.

48. Kaneko, S. (2008) A current overview: photodynamic diagnosis and photodynamic therapy using 5-ALA in neurosurgery. *JJSLSM*, **29**, 135–146.
49. Stylli, S. S. and Kaye, A. H. (2006) Photodynamic therapy of cerebral glioma – a review part II – clinical studies. *J Clin Neurosci*, **13**, 709–717.
50. Marks, P. V., Belchetz, P. E., Saxena, A., Igbaseimokumo, U., Thomson, S., Nelson, M., Stringer, M. R., Holroyd, J. A., and Brown, S. B. (2000) Effect of photodynamic therapy on recurrent pituitary adenomas: clinical phase I/II trial – an early report. *Br J Neurosurg*, **14**, 317–325.
51. Stummer, W., Pichlmeier, U., Meinel, T., Wiestler, O. D., Zanella, F., and Reulen, H. J. (2006) Fluorescence-guided surgery with 5-aminolevulinic acid for resection of malignant glioma: a randomised controlled multicentre phase III trial. *Lancet Oncol*, **7**, 392–401.
52. Henderson, B. W., Busch, T. M., and Snyder, J. W. (2006) Fluence rate as a modulator of PDT mechanisms. *Lasers Surg Med*, **38**, 489–493.
53. Peng, Q., Warloe, T., Moan, J., Godal, A., Apricena, F., Giercksky, K. E., and Nesland, J. M. (2001) Antitumor effect of 5-aminolevulinic acid-mediated photodynamic therapy can be enhanced by the use of a low dose of Photofrin in human tumor xenografts. *Cancer Res*, **61**, 5824–5832.
54. Norum, O. J., Gaustad, J. V., Angell-Petersen, E., Rofstad, E. K., Peng, Q., Giercksky, K. E., and Berg, K. (2009) Photochemical internalization of bleomycin is superior to photodynamic therapy due to the therapeutic effect in the tumor periphery. *Photochem Photobiol* Sci, **85**, 740–749.
55. Jain, K. K. (2007) Use of nanoparticles for drug delivery in glioblastoma multiforme. *Expert Rev Neurother*, **7**, 363–372.
56. Chen, Y., Gryshuk, A., Achilefu, S., Ohulchansky, T., Potter, W., Zhong, T., Morgan, J., Chance, B., Prasad, P. N., Henderson, B. W., Oseroff, A., and Pandey, R. K. (2005) A novel approach to a bifunctional photosensitizer for tumor imaging and phototherapy. *Bioconjug Chem*, **16**, 1264–1274.
57. Jerjes, W., Upile, T., Betz, C. S., El Maaytah, M., Abbas, S., Wright, A., and Hopper, C. (2007) The application of photodynamic therapy in the head and neck. *Dent Update*, **34**, 478–486.
58. Burch, S., London, C., Seguin, B., Rodriguez, C., Wilson, B. C., and Bisland, S. K. (2009) Treatment of canine osseous tumors with photodynamic therapy: a pilot study. *Clin Orthop Relat Res*, **22**, 44–47.

Chapter 18

Photodynamic Therapy of Head and Neck Cancers

Merrill A. Biel

Abstract

Over 1,500 patients have been treated with PDT using Photofrin, HPD, ALA, or Foscan for head and neck cancers. These patients include a mixture of presentations including primary, recurrent, and metastatic lesions. The predominant histology is squamous cell carcinoma, but other histologies treated include mucosal melanoma, Kaposi's sarcoma, adenocarcinoma, metastatic breast carcinoma, and adenoid cystic carcinoma. Several multi-institutional phase II clinical trials evaluating PDT treatment of head and neck cancers have demonstrated the efficacy of this minimally invasive therapy in the treatment of early oropharyngeal primary and recurrent cancers as well as the palliative treatment of refractory head and neck cancers. Patients with early stage cancers or early recurrences in the oral cavity and larynx (Cis, T1, T2) tend to have an excellent response to PDT. Of 518 patients treated with Cis, T1, or T2 cancers of the oral cavity, larynx, pharynx, and nasopharynx, 462 (89.1%) obtained a complete clinical response after one PDT treatment. Laryngeal cancers, comprising 171 patients in this group, obtained a durable complete response rate of 89% with up to a 16-year follow-up. Photodynamic therapy is as effective as conventional therapies for the treatment of early (Cis, T1, T2) squamous cell cancers of the head and neck. It is also a promising therapy to be used in association with surgery to increase tumor-free margins and therefore increase cure rates.

Key words: Photodynamic therapy, head and neck cancer, oral cancer, laryngeal cancer, intraoperative photodynamic therapy, interstitial photodynamic therapy.

1. Review

Photodynamic therapy (PDT) is an FDA–approved, minimally invasive medical treatment modality that utilizes light in the presence of oxygen to activate photosensitizing agents that are relatively selectively concentrated in abnormal or neoplastic cells, resulting in cell death. At the present time, PDT has been approved for clinical treatment in the United States, the European Union, Canada, Russia, and Japan. In the United

C.J. Gomer (ed.), *Photodynamic Therapy*, Methods in Molecular Biology 635,
DOI 10.1007/978-1-60761-697-9_18, © Springer Science+Business Media, LLC 2010

States, US Food and Drug administration approval has been given for the use of PDT in the treatment of Barrett's esophagus, obstructing esophageal carcinoma, and early and obstructing tracheobronchial carcinoma using the photosensitizer Photofrin; actinic keratosis using the photosensitizer Levulan (aminolevulinic acid); and macular degeneration using the photosensitizer BPD. In the EU, the above noted indications have also been approved in addition to the treatment of early head and neck cancers and palliative treatment of head and neck cancer using the photosensitizer Foscan and treatment of basal and squamous cell skin cancers using the photosensitizer Metvix.

The method of PDT involves the use of a photosensitizing agent that is relatively selectively concentrated in abnormal or neoplastic cells. Depending on the type of photosensitizer, it may be injected intravenously, ingested orally, or applied topically. After application of the photosensitizer, it is relatively selectively retained by tumor cells so that after several hours to days, determined by the kinetics of the compound's distribution, there is more sensitizer in the neoplastic tissue than in the normal tissue. The photosensitizer is then activated with a specific wavelength of light matching the absorption characteristics that are unique to that specific photosensitizer, usually using a laser. This results in tumor necrosis via several mechanisms including oxygen radical production as well as vascular shutdown to the tumor (1). Because there is less sensitizer in the adjacent normal tissue, only the neoplastic tissue necroses and the normal tissue are preserved. The advantage of PDT over the other conventional modalities of surgery, radiation, and chemotherapy is that it is a minimally invasive treatment technique that lacks systemic toxicity yet results in selective tumor destruction with normal tissue preservation. This advantage is of particular importance for cancers of the head and neck, where excessive tissue loss results in significant functional debilities. In addition, since this is an entirely different process, the use of chemotherapy, ionizing radiation, or surgery does not preclude the use of photodynamic therapy. Also, unlike ionizing radiation, repeated applications of the photosensitizer and activating light treatments can be performed indefinitely. The following is a retrospective review of the author's 410 patients treated with photodynamic therapy for head and neck neoplasia between 1990 and 2008.

2. Materials and Methods

The author 's clinical experience with PDT for the treatment of the head and neck spans 18 years. Four hundred and ten patients with various processes of the upper aerodigestive tract were treated with PDT from February 1990 to July 2008. Patients were divided into seven groups: those with advanced cancer where the intent of therapy was purely palliative; those with clinically focal early cancers (CIS, T1, and T2) with or without previous radiotherapy; those with T2 and T3 superficial oral cavity cancers; those with T2 and T3 invasive cancers that failed or refused conventional therapy; those with Kaposi's sarcoma; those with recurrent juvenile laryngotracheal papillomatosis that was uncontrolled with conventional therapies; and those with recurrent infiltrating carcinomas of the head and neck treated with adjuvant intraoperative PDT at the time of surgical resection. This present review will discuss only the treatment and outcome of 358 patients from the following three treatment groups: those with clinically focal early primary cancers with N0 necks (CIS, T1, and T2) with or without previous radiotherapy; those with T2 and T3 superficial oral cavity cancers; and those with recurrent infiltrating carcinomas of the head and neck treated with adjuvant intraoperative PDT at the time of surgical resection.

All patients were treated according to specific protocols in accordance with FDA and local IRB approvals. Pretreatment evaluation included a history and physical examination, an endoscopic examination with tumor mapping and biopsy, a routine laboratory evaluation, and a photographic documentation. All treatments were performed using the photosensitizer Photofrin (Axcan Pharma, Montreal, Canada) as an off-label use indication. The male-to-female ratio was 248:110, with an age range of 24–90 years.

Photofrin was injected intravenously at a dose of 2.0 mg/kg over a 5-min period as an outpatient procedure. Forty-eight hours after the injection, the patients underwent treatment with light from an Nd:YAG pumped dye laser (Laserscope) at 630 nm wavelength. Light was delivered to the tissue bed with a 400-μm fused silica optical fiber (Laserguide, Inc., Buellton, CA). A microlens treatment was used for all tumors with a depth of less than 3 mm. These treatments were performed at a dose rate of 50–75 J/cm^2 and 150 mW/cm^2 in the oral cavity, nasopharynx, and skin and 80 J/cm^2 and 150 mW/cm^2 in the larynx. For tumors greater than 3 mm in depth or T2 laryngeal tumors with paraglottic involvement, cylindrical diffusers 0.5–2.5 cm in length were placed in the tumor bed using an 18-gauge catheter under local or general anesthesia. These treatments were performed at a dose rate of 100 J/cm fiber length and 400 mW/cm fiber length. Adjuvant intraoperative PDT was performed following tumor resection, covering the entire surgical resection site with a microlens fiber at 50 J/cm^2 and 150 mW/cm^2. All treatments were performed on an outpatient basis under local or general anesthesia except for those patients with intraoperative adjuvant PDT. Those treatments were performed at the time of surgical resections under general anesthesia and the patients were hospitalized for their usual postoperative course.

On completion of treatment, each patient received 10 mg Decadron intravenously for one dose to reduce tissue edema and was discharged on oral pain medications. All patients were instructed to avoid daylight for 30 days. Tumor response was evaluated at 1 week, 1 month, and then monthly thereafter for 1 year and every 3 months thereafter. Multiple biopsy specimens of the treated area were obtained for most patients 1 month after treatment to evaluate a complete histopathologic response.

3. Results

One hundred and thirty-three patients with recurrent or primary CIS, T1N0, and T2N0 laryngeal tumors were treated with PDT for cure. Three patients had recurrent CIS, 115 patients had T1N0 carcinomas of the true vocal cord of which 25 were radiation failures, and 15 patients had T2N0 carcinomas of the true vocal cord of which 8 were radiation failures. All patients underwent a single microlens light treatment and most T2 tumors also underwent cylindrical diffuser implants into the paraglottic space. All treatments were performed under general anesthesia with standard laryngoscopy and all patients were discharged to home the same day of PDT treatment. All patients obtained a complete histopathologic response after a single light treatment. With follow-up of up to 211 months (mean 96 months), there were 11 recurrences for a 5-year cure rate of 90%. Importantly all the recurrences were salvaged using either PDT, surgery, or radiation for a total 5-year cure rate of 100%. In the entire treatment group there were no episodes of airway compromise and the degree of postoperative pain was minimal and easily controlled with oral analgesics. All patients after treatment developed an immediate breathy voice that persisted for 2–3 weeks. At 4–6 weeks after treatment, the quality of voice was universally much improved over the pretreatment state. In addition, videostroboscopy 6 weeks post-PDT treatment demonstrated a normal vocal cord mucosal fluid wave on the treated vocal cord.

One hundred and thirty-eight patients with recurrent or primary CIS and T1N0 squamous cell carcinomas of the oral cavity were treated. Three patients had recurrent CIS and 135 patients had T1N0 lesions. All patients were treated with a microlens and if the tumors were clinically invasive greater than 3 mm, they were also treated with cylindrical diffuser implantation to distribute the light deeper into the tissues. The diffusers were spaced 1 cm apart from each other. All patients obtained a complete pathologic and clinical response after a single PDT treatment. With follow up of up to 211 months (mean 99 months), there were seven local recurrences within 8 months of PDT treatment. These were all salvaged with either repeat PDT treatment or surgical resection. Two patients with T1 tongue tumors developed regional lymph nodes within 3 months of PDT treatment and went on to conventional neck dissection and have remained free of disease for at least 5 years. Five-year cure rate for these patients therefore remains at 100%. Unfortunately, there was one peri-PDT treatment death unrelated to PDT due to a drug overdose.

Fifty-two patients with superficial T2N0 and T3N0 squamous cell carcinomas of the oral cavity were treated. All of these patients had extensive areas of tumor involvement up to 7 cm in size. The maximal depth of the tumor, however, was clinically less than 1 cm. These patients were treated with a microlens and for those areas where there was clinical invasion greater than 3 mm, cylindrical diffusers of 0.5–1.0 cm were employed to distribute the 630 nm light deeper into the tissues. All patients obtained a complete clinical and pathologic response after a single PDT treatment. With follow-up of up to 137 months (mean 66 months), there were six recurrences at the edge of the PDT treatment field. These were all salvaged with either repeat PDT treatment or surgical resection. No patient developed regional lymph node involvement. Three-year cure rate for these patients is 100%. Importantly, the post-PDT healing of these patients demonstrated normal mobile oral mucosa without scar formation and preservation of the patency of the submandibular and parotid salivary ducts. Histologic evaluation of the post-PDT healing process demonstrated preservation of the cellular collagen matrix with repopulation of the normal mucosal cells into the preserved collagen matrix, resulting in normal mucosa and submucosa.

Intraoperative adjuvant PDT was performed in 35 patients. These patients were divided into two treatment groups: (1) PDT for curative intent following gross tumor debulking. The goal of this treatment is to achieve complete tumor eradication with preservation of normal vital structures such as the larynx and tongue. (2) PDT of the surgical resection bed following *complete* resection of T3 and T4 tumors. The goal of this treatment is to increase local regional disease control by increasing tumor-free resection margins and destroy microscopic skip lesion disease while preserving uninvolved normal structures.

In the first treatment group, PDT for curative intent following gross tumor debulking, 17 patients were treated, 11 laryngeal and 6 oral cavity. Of the 11 laryngeal, 8 were supraglottic and 3 were glottic. The oral cavity lesions were tongue and floor of mouth. The treatment consisted of the patient receiving 2 mg/kg Photofrin preoperatively and 2 days after the injection the patient underwent general anesthesia and gross but incomplete resection of the tumor mass. Residual microscopic disease was confirmed with frozen section biopsies intraoperatively. PDT was then performed to the resection site using a microlens fiber at 75–80 J/cm^2 and 150 mW/cm^2. Cylindrical diffuser implantation 0.5 cm in length was placed wherever the location was safe to do so and illumination performed at 100 J/cm fiber length and 400 mW/cm fiber length. Most of the treatments were performed on an outpatient basis. For the laryngeal tumors treated, with follow-up of up to 92 months, there have been no recurrences. For the six oral cavity tumors, with follow-up of up to 78 months there was one recurrence that went on to conventional surgical resection and remains free of disease.

In the second treatment group, intraoperative adjuvant PDT of the surgical resection bed following *complete* resection of T3 and T4 tumors, 18 patients with recurrent infiltrating squamous cell carcinoma of the head and neck were treated. Each patient had undergone previous treatment of the primary lesion of the head and neck with surgical resection, radiotherapy, and chemotherapy. The initial primary carcinomas were in the larynx; tongue and floor of mouth; branchial cleft cyst; medial canthal skin and ethmoid sinus; and tonsil. The sites of recurrence included the pharyngoesophagus and anterior neck skin; mandible and neck; medial orbit, ethmoid, and anterior skull base; neck skin, parotid, and lateral skull base; tongue and floor of mouth; and neck. In all cases, extensive skin involvement with tumor was present with deep infiltration into the soft tissues as determined by CT, MRI, and angiographic scanning. All lesions were determined to be surgically resectable.

Intraoperative adjuvant photodynamic therapy was performed as follows: Photofrin was injected intravenously at a dose of 2.0 mg/kg over a 5-min period as an outpatient procedure 2 days prior to surgery. Forty-eight hours after injection, the patient underwent planned surgical resection of the recurrent tumor. All uninvolved skin was covered during the surgical procedures, which lasted up to 10 h. Lighting during the surgical resection was with headlights. The resected tumor underwent frozen section pathologic evaluation of the margins in order to ensure a complete surgical resection. PDT was then performed of the entire tumor resection bed at a dose rate of 50 J/cm^2 and 150 mW/cm^2 using a microlens fiber tip (Laserguide, Inc., Buellton, CA). The areas involved in the PDT treatment were up to 8×10 cm and included the carotid artery and internal jugular veins. Following PDT treatment, the patients underwent surgical reconstruction of the defect using microvascular free flaps in 14 of 18 patients.

The postoperative course of all of the patients was uncomplicated and each patient healed without difficulty with only one self-limited fistula. The time of hospitalization and the time to total healing were not altered with the use of PDT. There was increased facial swelling postoperatively that lasted up to 1 week. As well, there was prolonged serous drainage from the neck drains that lasted an average of 2 days longer than an equivalent non-PDT-treated patient. There were no postoperative vascular complications.

All patients were followed postoperatively (minimum 157 months, maximum 189 months) with only six patients developing recurrent or metastatic disease, two inside the field of PDT treatment, and four outside the field of surgical and PDT therapy. Importantly, the first 10 patients admitted to the trial were randomized to surgery only or surgery and intraoperative adjuvant PDT. Of the first 10 patients, five patients in the surgery-only control group were all dead at 10 months post-surgery and three of five surgery and PDT patients were alive and free of disease for more than 5 years post-treatment.

Although this represents a small single institution trial, based on these results there is some indication that adjuvant intraoperative PDT may improve cure rates of recurrent head and neck malignancies by providing for larger tumor-free margins of resection while preserving normal structures. It may also be of benefit as an adjuvant intraoperative treatment at the time of primary resection of tongue base and hypopharyngeal carcinomas and skull base tumors, as well as at the time of neck dissection for lymph node involvement with extracapsular spread.

In the entire series, of 358 patients, only two patients sustained a significant sun-induced photosensitivity reaction with significant facial edema. This resolved with oral steroids in 5 days without sloughing of skin. In all patients the treated area demonstrated maximal necrosis by 7 days after light treatment, and there was complete healing by 4 weeks after treatment. The degree of treatment-related pain was quite variable with some patients having mild pain and others, usually those with extensive oral tumors, having severe pain. In all cases, however, the pain was adequately controlled with oral analgesics. The pain was uniformly resolved within 2–3 weeks of treatment.

4. Discussion

Data are available for over 1,500 patients treated with PDT using Photofrin, HPD, ALA, or Foscan for the treatment of head and neck cancers. These patients include a mixture of presentations including primary, recurrent, and metastatic lesions. The predominant histology is squamous cell carcinoma, but other histologies treated include mucosal melanoma, Kaposi's sarcoma, adenocarcinoma, metastatic breast carcinoma, and adenoid cystic carcinoma. Fortunately, the first multi-institutional phase II–III clinical trials evaluating PDT treatment of head and neck cancers have been completed. These trials have demonstrated the efficacy of this minimally invasive therapy in the treatment of early oropharyngeal primary and recurrent cancers as well as the palliative treatment of refractory head and neck cancers. Although this author has presented the results of Photofrin-based PDT for the treatment of head and neck cancers, it is important to recognize that other photosensitizers have been used and continue to be investigated for the treatment of head and neck cancers with very similar results.

4.1. Early Stage Head and Neck Cancer: Photofrin–HPD-Based PDT

Patients with early stage cancers or early recurrences in the oral cavity and the larynx (Cis, T1, T2) tend to have an excellent response to PDT. Of 518 patients treated with Cis, T1, or T2 cancers of the oral cavity, the larynx, the pharynx, and the nasopharynx, 462 (89.1%) obtained a complete clinical response after one PDT treatment. Laryngeal cancers, comprising 171 patients in this group, obtained a durable complete response rate of 89% with up to a 16-year follow-up (2–19).

4.2. Early Stage Head and Neck Cancer: Foscan (mTHPC)-Mediated PDT

Second-generation photosensitizers have the potential to improve the effectiveness of PDT by providing for greater tumor selectivity and deeper light penetration into tissue with the use of longer wavelengths of activating light. In addition, side effects such as the length of skin photosensitivity are reduced.

Foscan (mTHPC; Biolitec, Germany) is a potent second-generation photosensitizer that is activated at 652 nm light. To date, this is the only photosensitizer that has been evaluated in multi-institutional trials for the treatment of head and neck cancers. Numerous single investigator trials have demonstrated the efficacy of Foscan PDT in treating head and neck cancers (20–25).

Two large multi-institutional phase II trials have been completed evaluating the efficacy of Foscan PDT in the treatment of primary oropharyngeal cancers and recurrent and second primary oral carcinomas. The trial evaluating Foscan PDT for the treatment of primary oropharyngeal cancers involved 114 patients with Tis–T2 oropharyngeal cancers. These patients received 0.15 mg/kg Foscan intravenously and underwent light activation at 652 nm at 20 J/cm^2 at 100 mW/cm^2. Up to three light treatments were allowed under the protocol. A complete response rate of 85% (97/114) was achieved at completion of therapy. With 2-year follow-up, there was a 77% complete response rate at 2 years with disease-free survival of 89 and 75% at 1 and 2 years after PDT treatment, respectively. This trial demonstrated complete durable response rates that are equivalent to those obtained with conventional therapies (26, 27). The second trial evaluated Foscan PDT in 96 patients with recurrent or second primary carcinomas in the oral cavity. These patients demonstrated a 50% histologically confirmed complete response rate with a 79% survival rate at 1 year (28). Adverse events in these two trials consisted of pain at the treatment site, easily treated with oral analgesics and narcotics, and residual skin photosensitivity which lasted up to 2 weeks post-Foscan injection. Both of these events were expected and manageable. These two clinical trials, the first multi-institutional PDT trials to be performed in the treatment of head and neck cancers, demonstrated that Foscan PDT results in cure rates that are equivalent to conventional therapy with less treatment-associated morbidity, especially systemic toxicities (26–28).

4.3. Early Stage Head and Neck Cancer: ALA-Mediated PDT

Grant treated four patients with oral carcinoma following the oral administration of ALA (29). Six hundred and thirty-nanometer wavelength light of 50–100 J/cm^2 was delivered 6 h after oral ingestion of the ALA. All patients sustained tumor necrosis but normal surrounding tissue also necrosed, indicating no tumor selectivity. Fan treated 18 patients with dysplasia and malignant lesions of the oral cavity with ALA. Only two of six patients with carcinomas obtained a complete response (30). Sieron treated five patients with larynx and hypopharynx carcinomas using ALA-PDT. All five patients achieved only a partial response (31). Transient liver function abnormalities occurred in all patients. Due to the limited depth of accumulation of ALA and the limited penetration of 635-nm light, tumors greater than 2 mm depth are not consistently cured (29–31).

Kubler treated 12 patients with oral leukoplakia with 20% ALA cream and 630-nm light. Five patients demonstrated a complete response, four patients a partial response, and three patients no response. One patient with a partial response was retreated, resulting in a complete response (32). Chen treated 24 patients with oral leukoplakia with ALA topically twice a week. Eight patients had a complete response and 16 patients had a partial response. Significant pain during light treatment was noted (33).

4.4. Intraoperative Adjuvant Photodynamic Therapy for Massive Recurrent Head and Neck Cancers

Biel reported the first human clinical trial with long-term follow-up using PDT as an intraoperative adjuvant treatment for recurrent head and neck cancer (15, 34). Eighteen patients with recurrent infiltrating squamous cell carcinoma of the head and neck were treated. Each patient had undergone previous treatment of the primary lesion of the head and neck with surgical resection, radiotherapy, and chemotherapy. All patients were followed postoperatively (minimum 133 months, maximum 164 months) with only six patients developing recurrent or metastatic disease, two inside the field of PDT treatment, and four outside the field of surgical and PDT therapy. In another treatment group, PDT was performed for curative intent following gross tumor debulking in 17 patients, 11 laryngeal and 6 oral cavity. Of the 11 laryngeal, 8 were supraglottic and 3 were glottic. The oral cavity lesions were of tongue and floor of mouth. For the laryngeal tumors treated, with follow-of up to 69 months, there have been no recurrences. For the six oral cavity tumors, with follow-up of up to 58 months, there was one recurrence that went on to conventional surgical resection and remains free of disease.

This investigator determined that adjuvant intraoperative PDT may improve cure rates of recurrent head and neck malignancies by providing for larger tumor-free margins of resection while preserving normal structures. It may also be of benefit as an adjuvant intraoperative treatment at the time of resection of tongue base and hypopharyngeal carcinomas and skull base tumors, as well as at the time of neck dissection for lymph node involvement with extracapsular spread.

Dilkes treated 14 patients with intraoperative Foscan-mediated PDT. Two patients remain free of disease with up to 5-month follow-up. Two patients suffered carotid blowouts (21).

Lou described the method of interstitial PDT using Foscan to treat 39 patients with recurrent unresectable head and neck cancers. The overall median survival was 14 months with 72% overall palliative benefit achieved. Importantly, the local control rate at 12 months was 41% (35).

The present studies indicate the effectiveness of PDT in the treatment of specific anatomic areas in the head and neck. In particular, Tis and T1 carcinomas of the larynx appear to be particularly effectively treated with PDT. This clinical series demonstrates the efficacy of Photofrin-mediated photodynamic therapy as a curative treatment for Tis, T1 (85–91%), and T2 (72%) squamous cell carcinomas of the larynx. PDT for laryngeal carcinomas results in no glottic scarring as compared to conventional laser or surgical excision or vocal cord stripping. For recurrent carcinomas of the larynx that have failed conventional radiation therapy, PDT allows excellent voice preservation and may eliminate the need for partial or total laryngectomy. Also, PDT can be repeated without additional functional laryngeal compromise that can occur from repeated conventional laser surgery or cordectomy. Importantly, PDT treatment of primary T1 and T2 laryngeal carcinomas reserves radiation therapy for treatment of recurrences or of second head and neck primaries that may occur in these high-risk patients.

The side effects of PDT treatment of laryngeal carcinomas are quite minimal as compared to conventional radiotherapy or surgery. PDT treatment is performed as a single outpatient procedure as compared to 6–7 weeks of radiotherapy or the hospitalization associated with a partial or total laryngectomy.

The photosensitivity of Photofrin is a temporary inconvenience not associated with systemic toxicity and is minimized by patient education and temporary changes in daily outdoor activities.

Photodynamic therapy for treatment of T1 and T2 laryngeal carcinomas in the present series has cure rates that are comparable to, if not better than, those of conventional therapies with less morbidity of treatment. PDT should be considered as a reasonable option for the treatment of primary and recurrent Tis, T1, and T2 squamous cell carcinomas of the larynx.

PDT is also effective in the treatment of Tis and T1 primary and recurrent carcinomas of the oral cavity including the palate, the floor of mouth, the nasopharynx, and posterior pharyngeal walls. These results have been demonstrated in the multi-institutional phase II Foscan PDT clinical trials and in single investigator Photofrin trials in which cure rates were comparable to those of conventional therapy with less morbidity.

The adjuvant intraoperative use of PDT to treat recurrent infiltrating carcinomas of the head and neck has been impressive to date. In this group of patients with a very high incidence of recurrence, adjuvant intraoperative PDT may improve cure rates by providing for larger tumor-free margins of resection while preserving normal structures. In addition, the use of interstitial PDT for the treatment of large recurrent head and neck cancers appears to provide good local control and palliation for this difficult patient population.

5. Conclusion

Photodynamic therapy is an excellent modality for the treatment of carcinomas of the head and neck. Great advances have been achieved in the past few years in defining the role of PDT in the treatment of head and neck cancers. The future for the use of PDT in the treatment of head and neck cancers lies in its ability to treat early carcinomas of the head and neck with minimal morbidity and its potential use as an adjuvant therapy intraoperatively to treat surgical margins following resection for T3 and T4 head and neck and skull base tumors via superficial or interstitial light applications. In order to further assess the effectiveness of this treatment on various areas within the head and neck, further standardized controlled studies are necessary. In addition, the development of new, more tumor-specific photosensitizing agents and user-friendly light delivery systems will improve the effectiveness of this therapy. The present studies indicate that photodynamic therapy is an effective primary or alternative treatment modality for carcinomas in specific areas of the head and neck.

References

1. Henderson, B. W. and Dougherty, T. J. (1992) How does photodynamic therapy work? *Photochem Photobiol*, **55**, 145–157.
2. Keller, G. S., Doiron, D. R., and Fisher, C. U. (1985) Photodynamic therapy in otolaryngologyhead and neck surgery. *Arch Otolaryngol*, **111**, 758–761.
3. Feyh, J., Goetz, A., Muller, W., Konigsberger, R., and Kastenbauer, E. (1990) Photodynamic therapy in head and neck surgery. *J Photochem Photobiol B: Biol*, 7, 353–358.
4. Feyh, J., Gutmann, A., and Leunig, A. (1993) A photodynamic therapy in head and neck surgery. *Laryngo Rhino Otol*, **72**, 273–278.
5. Wenig, B. L., Kurtzman, D. M., Grossweiner, L., Mafee, J. F., Harris, D. M., Lobraico, R. V., Prycz, R. A., and Appelbaum, E. L. (1990) Photodynamic therapy in the treatment of squamous cell carcinoma of the head and neck. *Arch Otolaryngol Head Neck Surg*, **116**, 1267–1270.
6. Grossweiner, L. I., Hill, J. H., and Lobraico, R. V. (1987) Photodynamic therapy of head and neck squamous cell carcinoma: optical dosimetry and clinical trial. *Photochem. Photobiol*, **46**, 911–917.
7. Freche, C. and DeCorbiere, S. (1990) Use of photodynamic therapy in the treatment of vocal cord carcinoma. *J Photochem Photobiol*, **6**, 291–296.
8. Schweitzer, V. G. (1990) Photodynamic therapy for treatment of head and neck cancer. *Otolaryngol Head Neck Surg*, **102**, 225–232.
9. Schweitzer, V. G. (1990) Photofrin-mediated photodynamic therapy for treatment of early stage oral and laryngeal malignancies. *Lasers Surg Med*, **29**, 305–313.
10. Gluckman, J. L. (1991) Hematoporphyrin photodynamic therapy: is there truly a future in head and neck oncology? Reflections on a 5-year experience. *Laryngoscope*, **101**, 36–42.
11. Grant, W. E., Hopper, C., Speight, P. M., Macrobert, A. D., and Bown, S. C. (1993) Photodynamic therapy of malignant and premalignant lesions in patients with "field cancerization": of the oral cavity. *J Laryngol Otol*, **107**, 1140–1145.
12. Biel, M. A. (1994) Photodynamic therapy and the treatment of neoplastic diseases of the larynx. *Laryngoscope*, **104**, 399–403.
13. Biel, M. A. (1995) Photodynamic therapy of head and neck cancers. *Semin Surg Oncol*, **11**, 355–359.
14. Biel, M. A. (1998) Photodynamic therapy and the treatment of head and neck neoplasia. *Laryngoscope*, **108**, 1259–1268.
15. Biel, M. A. (2002) Photodynamic therapy in head and neck cancer. *Curr Oncol Rep*, **4**, 87–96.
16. Zhao, F. Y., Zhang, K. H., Ma, D. Q., He, Z. Q., Chen, S., Ni, X. M., and Yu, G. Y. (1989) Treatment of 510 cases of oral squamous cell carcinoma. *Ann Acad Med Singapore*, **18**, 533–536.
17. Zhao, F. Y., Zhang, K. H., Huang, H. N., Sun, K. H., Ling, Q. B., and Xu, B. (1986) Use of hematoporphyrin derivative as a sensitizer for radiotherapy of oral and maxillofacial tumors: a preliminary report. *Lasers Med Sci*, **1**, 253–256.
18. Kulapaditharom, B. and Boonkitticharoen, V. (2000) Photodynamic therapy in management of head and neck cancers and precancerous lesions. *J Med Assoc Thai*, **83**, 249–258.
19. Kulapaditharom, B. and Boonkitticharoen, V. (1999) Photodynamic therapy for residual or recurrent cancer of the nasopharynx. *J Med Assoc Thai*, **82**, 1111–1117.
20. Dilkes, M. G. and DeJode, M. L. (1996) m-THPC photodynamic therapy for head and neck cancer. *Lasers Med Sci*, **11**, 23–29.
21. Dilkes, M. G., Alusi, G., and Djaezeri, B. J. (1999) The treatment of head and neck cancer with photodynamic therapy: clinical experience. *Rev Contemp Pharmacother*, **10**, 47–57.
22. Dilkes, M. G., Benjamin, E., Ovaisi, S., and Banerjee, A. S. (2003) Treatment of primary mucosal head and neck squamous cell carcinoma using photodynamic therapy: results after 25 treated cases. *J Laryngol Otol*, **117**, 713–717.
23. Savary, J. F., Monnier, P. H., and Fontolliet, C. (1997) Photodynamic therapy for early squamous cell carcinomas of the esophagus, bronchi, and mouth with *m*-tetra(hydroxyphenyl) chlorin. *Arch Otolaryngol Head Neck Surg*, **123**, 162–168.
24. Fan, K. F., Hopper, C., and Speight, P. M. (1997) Photodynamic therapy using mTHPC for malignant disease in the oral cavity. *Int J Cancer*, **73**, 25–32.
25. Kubler, A. D., de Carpentier, J., Hopper, C., Leonard, A. G., and Putnam, G. (2001) Treatment of squamous cell carcinoma of the lip using Foscan-mediated photodynamic therapy. *Int J Oral Maxillofac Surg*, **30**, 504–509.
26. Hopper, C., Kubler, A., Lewis, H., Tan, I. B., and Putnam, G. mTHPC-mediated photodynamic therapy for early oral squamous cell carcinoma. *Int J Cancer*, **111**, 138–146.

27. Copper, M. P., Tan, B. I., Oppelaar, H., Ruevekamp, M. C., and Stewart, F. A. Meta-tetra(hydroxyphenyl)chlorine photodynamic therapy in early-stage squamous cell carcinoma of the head and neck. *Arch Otolaryngol Head Neck Surg*, **129**, 709–711.
28. Biel, M. (2000) Foscan-mediated photodynamic therapy in recurrent and second primary oral cavity cancers. Oral presentation 5th International Conference on Head and Neck Cancer, San Francisco, CA.
29. Grant, W. E., Hopper, C., MacRobert, A. J., Speight, P. M., and Bown, S. C. (1993) Photodynamic therapy of oral cancer: photosensitisation with systemic amino levulinic acid. *Lancet*, **342**, 147–149.
30. Fan, K. F. M., Hopper, C., Speight, P. M., Buonaccorsi, G., MacRobert, A. J., and Bown, S. G. (1996) Photodynamic therapy using 5-aminolevulinic acid for premalignant and malignant lesions of the oral cavity. *Cancer*, **78**, 1374–1383.
31. Sieron, A., Namyslowski, G., Misiolek, M., Adamek, M., and Dawczyk, K. (2001) Photodynamic therapy of premalignant lesion and local recurrence of laryngeal and hypopharyngeal cancers. *Eur Arch Otorhinoloarygol*, **258**, 349–352.
32. Kubler, A., Haase, T., Rheinwald, M., Barth, T., and Muhling, J. (1998) Treatment of oral leukoplakia by topical application of 5-aminolevulinic acid. *Int J Oral Maxillofac Surg*, **27**, 466–469.
33. Chen, H., Yu, C., Tu, P., Yeh, C., Tsai, T., and Chiang, C. (2005) Successful treatment of oral verrucous hyperplasia and oral leukoplakia with topical 5-aminolevulinic acid-mediated photodynamic therapy. *Lasers Surg Med*, **37**, 114–122.
34. Biel, M. A. (1996) Photodynamic therapy as an adjuvant intraoperative treatment of recurrent head and neck carcinomas. *Arch Otolaryngol Head Neck Surg*, **122**, 1261–1265.
35. Lou, P. J., Jager, H. R., Jones, L., Theodossy, T., Bown, S. G., and Hopper, C. (2004) Interstitial photodynamic therapy as salvage treatment for recurrent head and neck cancer. *Br J Cancer*, **91**, 441–446.

Subject Index

C.J. Gomer (ed.), *Photodynamic Therapy*, Methods in Molecular Biology 635,
DOI 10.1007/978-1-60761-697-9, © Springer Science+Business Media, LLC 2010

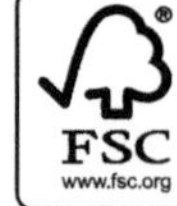

MIX
Papier aus verantwortungsvollen Quellen
Paper from responsible sources
FSC® C105338

If you have any concerns about our products,
you can contact us on
ProductSafety@springernature.com

In case Publisher is established outside the EU,
the EU authorized representative is:
Springer Nature Customer Service Center GmbH
Europaplatz 3, 69115 Heidelberg, Germany

Printed by Libri Plureos GmbH
in Hamburg, Germany